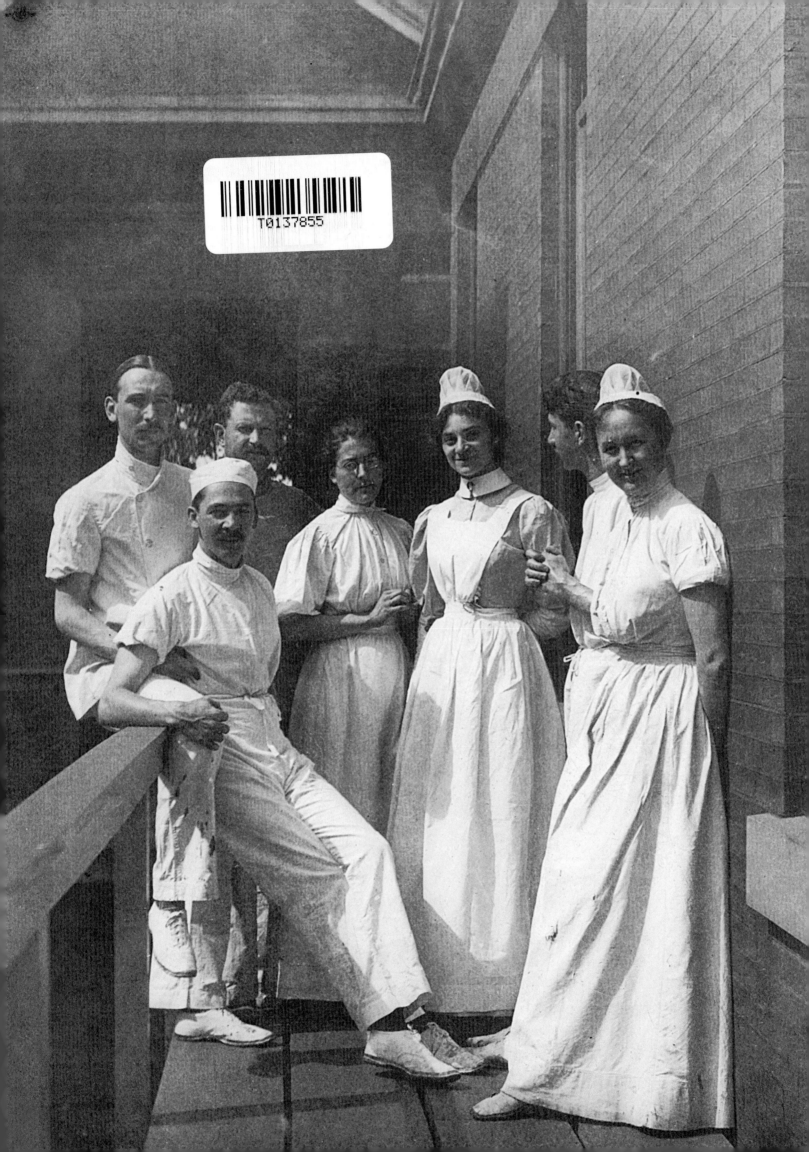

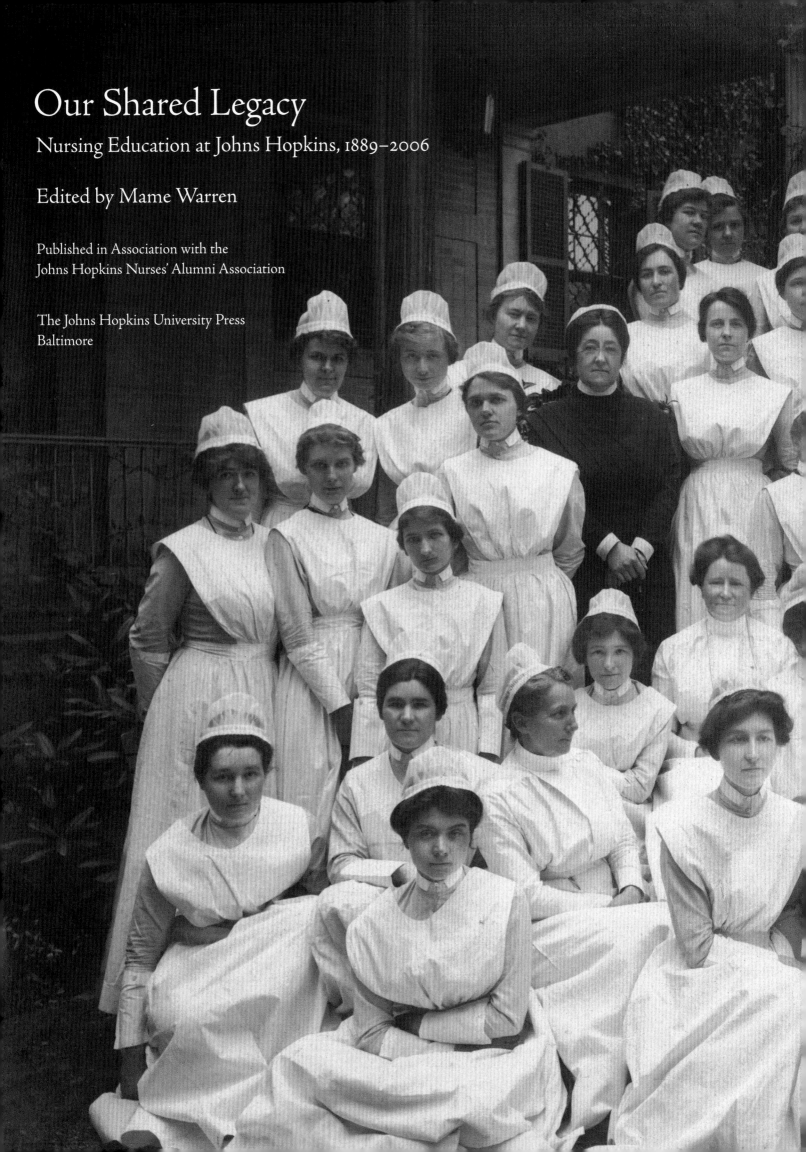

Our Shared Legacy

Nursing Education at Johns Hopkins, 1889–2006

Edited by Mame Warren

Published in Association with the
Johns Hopkins Nurses' Alumni Association

The Johns Hopkins University Press
Baltimore

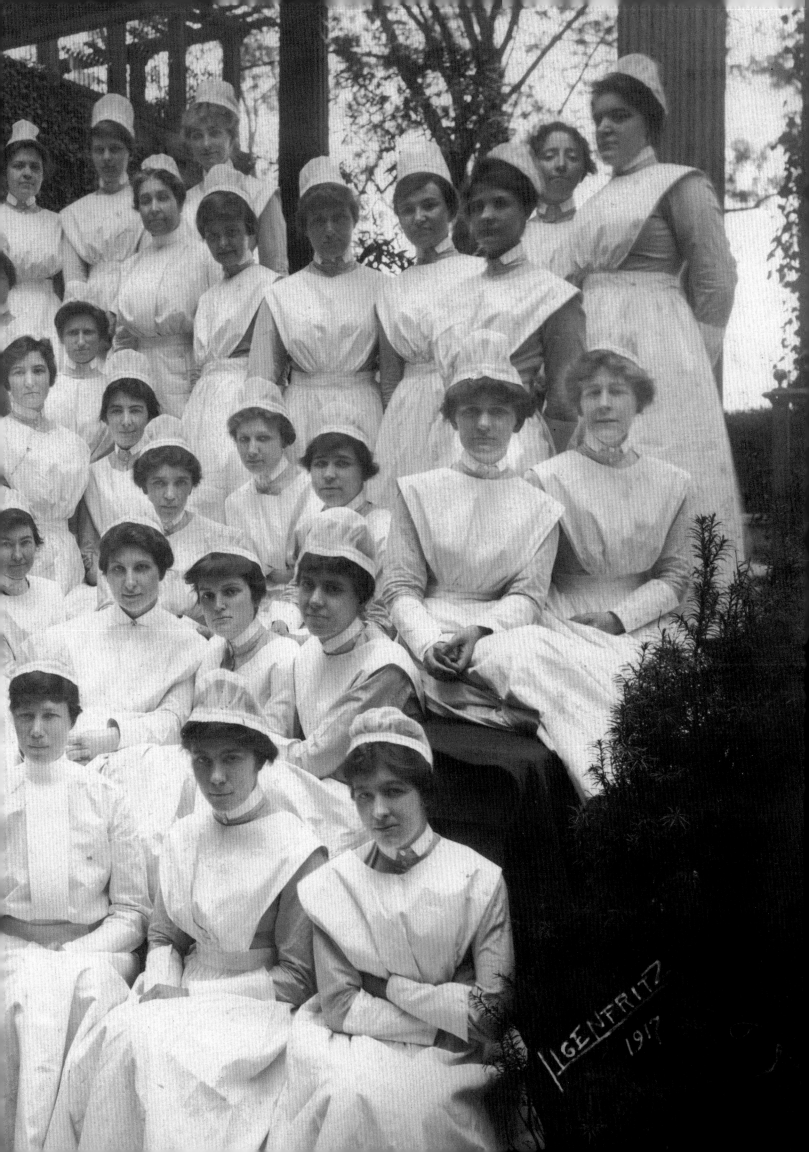

ILGENFRITZ
1917

Printed in Italy on acid-free paper

9   8   7   6   5   4   3   2   1

The Johns Hopkins University Press
2715 North Charles Street
Baltimore, Maryland 21218-4363

www.press.jhu.edu

Library of Congress Cataloging-in-Publication Data

Our shared legacy : nursing education at Johns Hopkins,
1889–2006 / edited by Mame Warren.
      p. ;   cm.
   Includes bibliographical references and index.
   ISBN 0-8018-8473-x (hardcover : alk. paper)
   1. Johns Hopkins Hospital. School of Nursing—History.
2. Johns Hopkins University. School of Nursing—History.
3. Nursing schools—Maryland—Baltimore—History.
I. Warren, Mame, 1950– . II. Johns Hopkins Nurses'
Alumni Association. III. Title: Nursing education at Johns
Hopkins, 1889–2006.
   [DNLM: 1. Johns Hopkins Hospital. School of Nursing.
2. Johns Hopkins University. School of Nursing.
3. Schools, Nursing—history—Maryland. 4. History,
19th Century—Maryland. 5. History, 20th Century—
Maryland. 6. History, 21st Century—Maryland.   WY 19
093 2006]
   RT80.M32B346 2006
   610.73071'17526—dc22   2005036843

Composed in Adobe Jenson (designed by Robert Slimbach),
Legacy Sans (designed by Ronald Arnholm), and Durer
Titling (designed by Robert L. Wiser)

Book design by Robert L. Wiser, Silver Spring, Maryland

Front endsheet: When members of the class of 1987, who were
about to receive baccalaureate degrees, posed with Dean Carol
Gray in the garden of the Phipps Building, they personified the
dreams of determined alumni.

Page i: Sporting their distinctive organdy caps, two graduates of
the Johns Hopkins Hospital Training School for Nurses stepped
outside with colleagues for a breath of fresh air in 1899.

Pages ii–iii: Apron-clad nursing students of 1917 gathered
around Elsie Lawler, an 1899 graduate, who led the school for
thirty years, from 1910 to 1940.

Pages iv–v: Members of the nursing choir in 1950, many with
bulging pockets, may have been singing the school's anthem,
"Within the Gates."

Pages vi–vii: As students of the new Johns Hopkins University
School of Nursing left the Billings Administration Building in
1985, they were following in the footsteps of generations of
Johns Hopkins nursing students.

Page 1: Christine Wright, Rebecca Hanson, Colleen Frei, Janet
Schnider, Karen Rodgers, Mary Flynn George, Pam Baretto, and
Margaret Porter Jones won the top graduation prizes in 1987.

Back endsheet: The enclosed courtyard behind the Anne M.
Pinkard Building provided students with a sunny oasis in 2004.

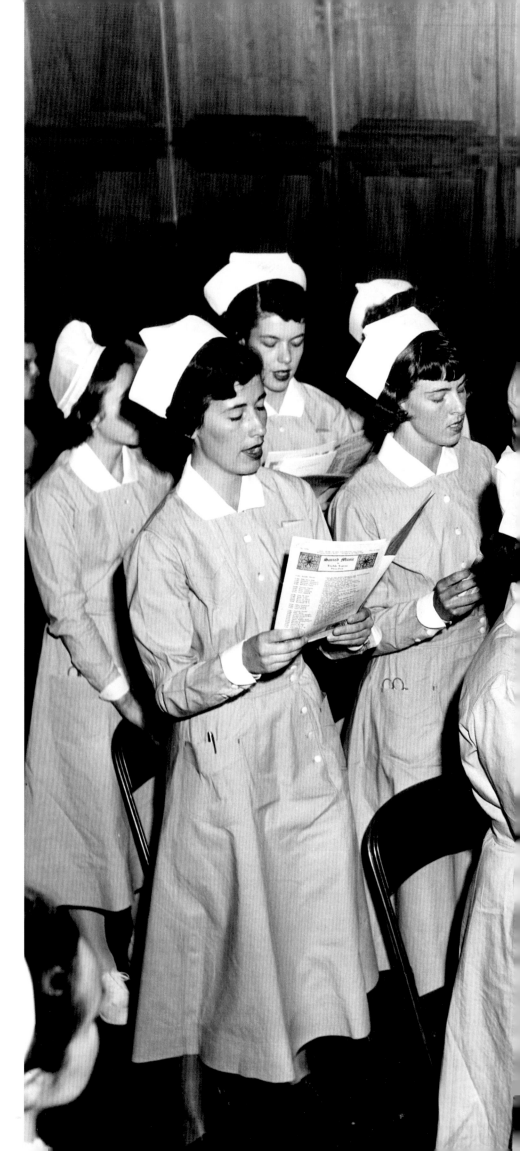

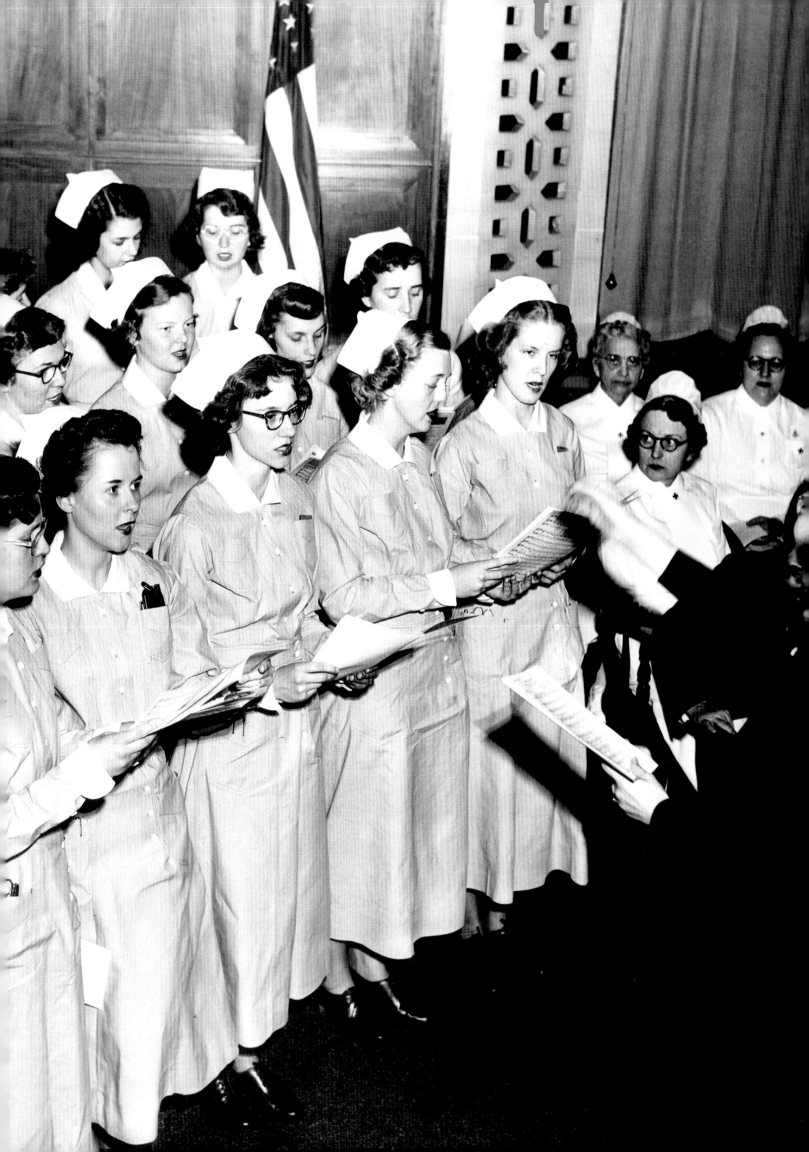

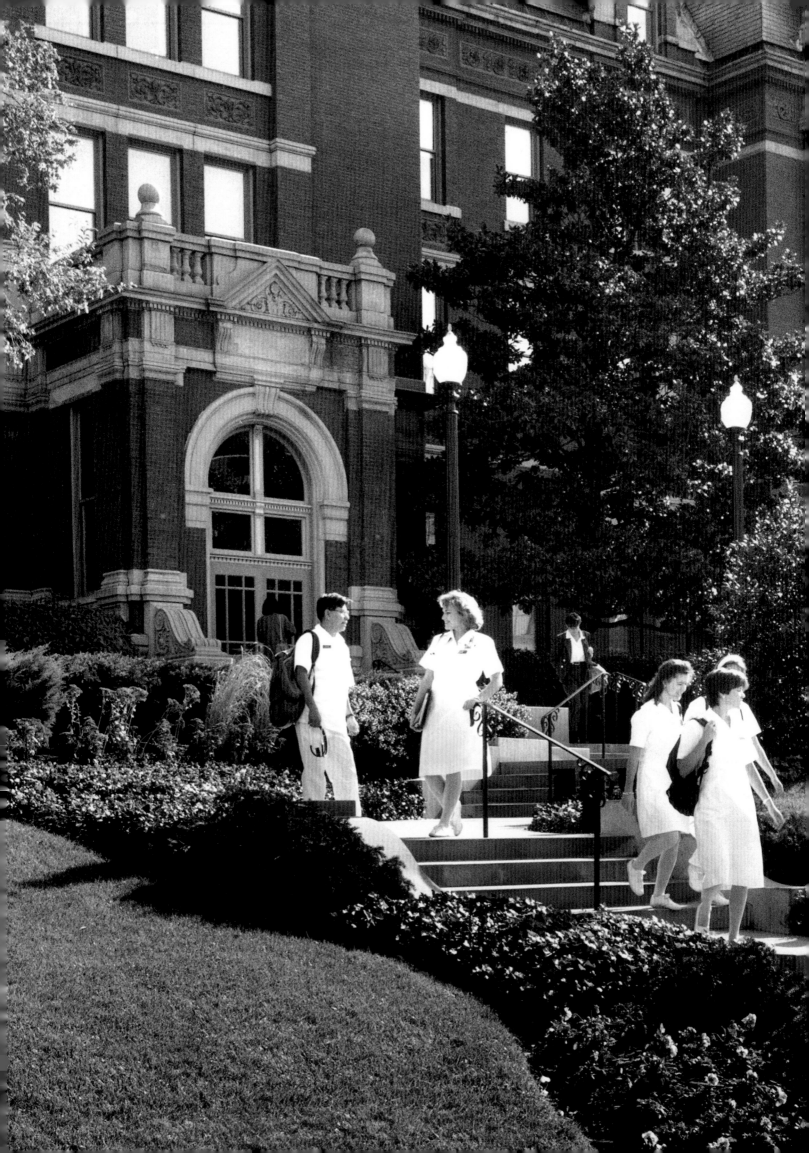

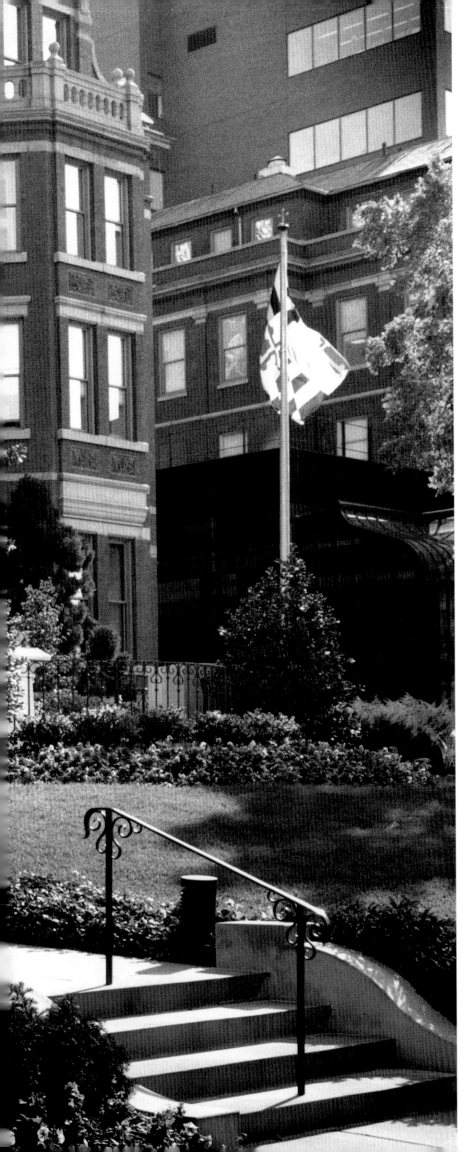

Contents

Foreword · ix
DEBORAH BAKER

Introduction · xi
GERT BRIEGER

"Proud of Our Heritage" · xvi

One · An Auspicious Beginning, 1889–1940 · *3*
LINDA SABIN

Two · Rapid Change, 1940–1950 · *47*
LINDA SABIN

Three · Nursing at the Crossroads, 1950–1960 · *83*
LINDA SABIN

"The Dreaded Uniforms" · 116

Four · The Handwriting on the Wall, 1960–1970 · *123*
LINDA SABIN

"We Had a Good Time" · 156

Five · Tension and Triumph, 1970–1979 · *165*
MARY FRANCES KEEN

"Beyond the Bedside" · 196

Six · All Eyes on Hopkins, 1980–1994 · *201*
MAME WARREN

Seven · A Different Vision, 1995–2005 · *233*
MAME WARREN

Chronology · 262
MAME WARREN

Acknowledgments · 288

Notes · 290

Who We Are · 295

Bibliographical Note · 297

Credits and Sources · 298

Index · 299

I always wanted to be a nurse. My father wanted me to go to college. He hoped I would change and decide to go to med school. "Why don't you be a doctor if you want to be a nurse?" Just as now, there was no idea then that nursing and medicine are two distinct professions and that nurses are not people who couldn't make it in med school.

Doctors had two functions: to diagnose and prescribe treatment. Nursing was more. It was broader.

Nurses were considered, erroneously, to carry out the prescription and orders of the doctor. We were never taught that. We were interested in the total health and well-being of the patient. We were interested in how that person was going to stay well after he or she got well. We were taught to be interested in how the family was going to function, how that person was going to function in the family after discharge, how the family was handling things. While we did carry out doctors' orders, the mission and the philosophy of nursing we were taught were just so much greater.

Betty Borenstein Scher, 1950

Foreword

The opportunity to write the opening remarks for *Our Shared Legacy*, which is energized by so many strong voices, is truly an honor. As the current president of the Johns Hopkins Nurses' Alumni Association, I am among a noble chorus singing a song with many different stanzas and one repeating refrain: *One must constantly strive to be worthy of being a Hopkins nurse*. Membership in this chorus is earned and cherished and carries with it a responsibility to preserve the history.

As a student in the early years of the accelerated bachelor's degree program, I became fascinated with the rich heritage of nursing, much of which took place on the very campus where I was studying. Nursing leaders who were nationally recognized pioneers had walked the halls of our hospital, blending the art and science of modern nursing care. I wanted to know and be able to recite this story.

Several years after graduation, I was asked to be part of an alumni committee appointed by the board of directors. At that first Monday evening meeting, it was immediately apparent that no task was to be taken lightly. No matter how small the effort, it must be performed sincerely and efficiently. I left that meeting feeling uncomfortable, having been grilled about my interests and intent; I was, however, intrigued with the level of loyalty and commitment to the association the board members had demonstrated. I remained active and joined the board, serving on various committees and going to monthly meetings, where my ideas were scrutinized, dissected, and sometimes accepted.

When I was elected vice president of the alumni association, I had the opportunity to "peel the potatoes" with the president, Sue Wright, who happened to be one of the board members who had questioned my worthiness at that fateful Monday evening meeting several years before. Sue taught me frugality, efficiency, and the importance of preserving history. During those two years we forged a friendship, but I was cautious never to be careless in her presence and I was aware that the bar was constantly rising. The day she turned over the gavel to me, without pomp and circumstance, Sue presented me with her Maltese cross pin, the treasured emblem of her success in the first Hopkins School of Nursing. I was shocked and moved to a sentimental place where I remain. Indeed, since Sue Wright has championed the concept of this book over many years, it seems unfair that she is no longer president of the association, with the honor of introducing it here.

DEBORAH BAKER
1992, MSN 1997

We alumni have many people to thank for archiving our history and writing it down. The list is long, but I would be remiss not to mention a few: Betty Cuthbert, Sue Appling, Phyllis Naumann, Linda Sabin, Fran Keen, Sue Wright, Betty Scher, and Pat Sullivan. The association is indebted to Mame Warren, who has worked diligently to collect and record oral histories that make these pages vibrate with many voices. Mame has crafted a book rich in content, pictures, and quotations that take the reader on a journey back in time. Each chapter invites the reader to understand the personal as well as the institutional and social aspects of our history, all of which have had a great impact on and made lasting changes in nursing training and education. Authors Linda Sabin, Fran Keen, and Mame Warren present their information in a factual but entertaining way. Beginning with Johns Hopkins' charge to create a modern training school for nurses, through the years of metamorphosis into the brief and transitional Nursing Education Program of the School of Health Services, and on to the triumph of the establishment and success of the university school, *Our Shared Legacy* sparkles with pride about what it means to be a Hopkins nurse. No matter when you joined our ranks, the Johns Hopkins Nurses' Alumni Association welcomes you and hopes you will find your place along this continuum.

Introduction

"It has been said . . . that every woman makes a good nurse. I believe, on the contrary, that the very elements of nursing are all but unknown." So wrote Florence Nightingale in her widely read *Notes on Nursing*, published in London in December 1859 and in New York early in the next year.[1] Within months the book had sold fifteen thousand copies and it was frequently translated and reprinted in later years. Not only is it considered to be the founding bible of organized nursing and nursing education, but it is also a masterpiece of nineteenth-century social reform. Its mere seventy-nine pages include discussions of sanitation of houses, proper diet, and personal hygiene.

At the time that Nightingale was writing, her friend Harriet Martineau, the British writer and social critic, observed that where "there are mothers and daughters there will be good nursing."[2] But Nightingale, as noted, believed that nursing involved far more than feminine intuition. For the proper training of nurses, she, along with Pastor Fliedner, in Germany, and Elizabeth Fry, earlier in her own country, believed that there was a need for nursing schools.

The school established by Florence Nightingale at St. Thomas's Hospital in London in 1860 was not the first, but it soon became the important model for the Anglo-American world.[3] As Nightingale wrote in *Notes on Nursing*: "I use the word Nursing for want of a better. It has been limited to signify little more than the administration of medicine and the application of poultices. It ought to signify the proper use of fresh air, light, warmth, cleanliness, quiet, and the proper selection and administration of diet—at the least expense of vital power to the patient."[4] Such was her credo for the school she founded, and it would be the philosophy of the first such training schools established on this side of the Atlantic, in 1873, in Boston, New Haven, and New York. Two years later, when the Johns Hopkins Hospital trustees began planning for a hospital in Baltimore, their chairman, Francis King, traveled to London to see the school at St. Thomas's and to consult with Florence Nightingale.

As Susan Reverby has pointed out, although Nightingale never set foot in the United States, she had a profound influence on American schools of nursing. Her model for the education of nurses "emphasized character, training and strict discipline, a distinct field of work for nurses separate from physicians, and a female hierarchy with deference and loyalty to physician authority."[5] It follows, then, that Nightingale resisted the notion

GERT H. BRIEGER, MD, PhD
Distinguished Service Professor
of the History of Medicine

Nurses were always considered second-class citizens. Nursing was not regarded as a profession. Many schools of nursing were put together without a lot of care about the curriculum or the faculty qualifications. Only fairly recently, now that nurses are nurse practitioners and highly skilled in many areas, have they been recognized by medicine, but that wasn't true until about twenty years ago. We were tolerated because we did a lot of the work and took care of the patients. We were there twenty-four hours a day. We reported to physicians about the condition of the patients. But that wasn't recognized as professional. That was true here and it was true in every other hospital in the country.

Ada Davis

of professionalization for nurses. She believed that nursing was a calling.

In 1873, not long before his death, the Baltimore merchant Johns Hopkins left $7 million to found a hospital and a university as well as explicit instructions on how the two were to be related. To the trustees of the hospital he wrote: "I desire you to establish, in connection with the Hospital, a training school for female nurses. This provision will secure the services of women competent to care for the sick in the Hospital wards, and will enable you to benefit the whole community by supplying it with a class of trained and experienced nurses."[6] The fate of that vision is the subject of this book. Like the university and the various schools that Mr. Hopkins envisioned would be connected to it, the School of Nursing would also produce leaders in its field for the twentieth century and beyond. As the centennial history of Johns Hopkins medicine notes, the nursing school, although not the first, soon became one of the leaders in nursing education. It quickly set a new educational standard, lengthened its program from two to three years, and treated its trainees as students rather than employees.[7]

When the first class was set to graduate in 1891, the physician-in-chief of the hospital, William Osler, told the young women that in the best of all worlds we might not continue to require the services of lawyers and ministers but that we would always need doctors and nurses. In a remarkable sentiment, Osler told these first graduates that if "the medical profession, composed chiefly of men, has absorbed a larger share of attention and regard, you have, at least, the satisfaction of feeling that yours is the older, and as older, the more honorable calling."[8] Such support from the hospital staff and its leaders has been an important theme throughout the history of the school. As the authors of this book have demonstrated again and again, the hospital directors, from Drs. Henry Hurd, Winford Smith, and Russell Nelson, to Robert Heyssel, have been eager supporters of their schools of nursing.

* * * * *

The history of nursing has witnessed a revival in the last two decades. No longer can we say, as Janet James wrote in 1984: "The history of nursing has been in a comatose state." James also noted that the profession had "had its past to itself and made the same use of it as other professions do, to enhance status and raise morale."[9] Any institutional history, such as this one, must plead guilty to such a charge, but it is only with a series of well-crafted histories of individual schools that historians will have the sources for more extensive histories of nursing education. Only then will they be able to discuss what was taught and what was learned. This history of nursing education at Johns Hopkins provides both primary and secondary historical sources, which will guide future nursing scholars to even more expansive material.

Medicine has become more than the story of doctors, nurses, and patients. The new histories of nursing include monographs, such as *The Physician's Hand* (1982), by Barbara Melosh, and *Ordered to Care* (1987), by Susan Reverby, as well as several collections of articles that focus on the rewriting of nursing history.[10] In tandem with these newer approaches came new social and cultural histories of American life and institutions. The history of nursing is now being written in the context of the histories of medicine, hospitals, women, the professions, occupational roles, and labor, and in the context of the shift from medical care to the broader rubric of health care.

Some of these newer themes appear in this book, but the authors have mostly limited themselves to the story of one school. The nursing school's relationship to the hospital and the medical school and its unsuccessful interlude in the School for Health Services are certainly well covered. It is only in recent years that the School of Nursing has assumed a full partnership in what is known as the Johns Hopkins Medical Institutions, a name that has persisted even though we no longer speak only about *medical care* but use the broader term *health care.*

Another theme that pervades this book is the relationship of the School of Nursing to the Johns Hopkins University. Despite the efforts of the early leaders of the School of Nursing, and even in the wake of the recommendations of the Goldmark Report of 1923—that schools of nursing are best located in colleges or universities—it took another six decades for the school at Hopkins to become an integral part of the university.

The Goldmark Commission, which included Dr. Winford Smith, the director of the Johns Hopkins Hospital, Dr. William H. Welch, the medical school's founding dean, and Adelaide Nutting, the second director of the School of Nursing, worked for five years. Named for the social worker Josephine Goldmark, the commission's secretary who wrote most of the report, the group studied twenty-three of the country's eighteen hundred hospital training schools and concluded that more university schools would be needed to train future nursing leaders. Some of the hospital schools, the commission found, were excellent, but too often these schools had low standards of admission and neglected education or confused it with basic ward-nursing services. In 1925 there were only twenty-five collegiate or university schools of nursing, with an enrollment of a mere 368 students. As the Flexner Report on medical education thirteen years earlier had also stressed, the Goldmark Report emphasized that the training of nurses was an educational endeavor and should be supervised by educators, not just practitioners.

Yale, the first university to respond to the Goldmark Report, established the first separate university department of nursing in 1924. This school grew out of the hospital training school in New Haven, one of the first three nursing schools in the country, opened in 1873.[11] Naturally, the Johns Hopkins Hospital School of Nursing, with equally strong academic values, should have quickly followed this lead; but, as the authors of this book so clearly show, many years had to pass and many ups and downs be endured before a university school became a reality at Johns Hopkins.

Medicine and universities have been allied since the Middle Ages. For medical schools in the last hundred years, this tie has proven to be one of their greatest strengths.[12] Just as the Johns Hopkins School of Medicine was an integral part of the university from its beginning, so too the leaders of Johns Hopkins nursing wished to realize the same benefits. But it was not to be until the 1980s.

Just as I began to write this introduction, the Johns Hopkins *Gazette* featured the story "Nursing Receives Largest Grant in Its History."[13] Thus, with a $2.5-million federal grant for cardiovascular studies, the School of Nursing continues to show one and all that it rightfully belongs in the university's sphere, where research is a cornerstone, along with teaching and practice.

*   *   *   *   *

As the proportion of older persons in our society grows, and as older persons live longer, we will undoubtedly require more and more nursing care. And with the uncertainties of the increasing threat of global epidemics, it is no wonder that there is widespread concern about nursing education and maintaining an adequate number of graduates. All of us who have studied medicine and worked in hospitals and clinics know well the importance of nurses, not only for the care of patients but also for the education of doctors and other health workers.

Historians of nursing Vern and Bonnie Bullough said it succinctly as long ago as 1969: "It has often been said that modern nursing could not have developed independently of modern medicine, but we feel it should also be pointed out that modern medicine could not have developed without the emergence of modern nursing."[14]

It has been half a century since an earlier history of the school, by Ethel Johns and Blanche Pfefferkorn, appeared.[15] That well-received book covered the years 1889 to 1949. The important support of the nursing school alumni in that effort, as well as in this one, shows clearly the continuing involvement in the activities and the welfare of the school by a remarkable and dedicated alumni group. The book you now have in your hands brings the story up to date, not only providing the history of one important school of nursing but also revealing the increasing complexities of medicine, nursing, and what has come to be called the medical marketplace. Were Dr. John Shaw Billings, the principal architect of the Johns Hopkins Hospital and School of Medicine, here to see the new School of Nursing, he doubtless would call it, too, "a model of its kind."

Nurses don't need to be asked how they fit in the hospital or how they fit in medical care. They need to ask themselves how they're going to meet the needs of the public as an independent profession. How they're going to set up practices, not how they're going to be employed in someone else's business. That's the next evolution.

Sue Donaldson

You don't really ever stop being a Hopkins nurse. You don't. No matter what you do, it's just there.

Cathy Novak, 1973

"Proud of Our Heritage"

Betty Cuthbert was a persistent, clear-thinking woman. She was very interested in the history of the school and also in the future of the school, which is a nice combination. She was very, very knowledgeable about decisions that had been made within the school. She kept so much memorabilia in her house, which was just packed to the gills. She always looked like somebody from the 1940s. She was a very attractive woman but her hairstyle hadn't changed. It turned gray but it went over and still had the little flip.

Sandra Stine Angell, 1969, BSN 1977

When they tore down the nurses' library, Betty Cuthbert took boxes of some of the important books and archives and stored those things at her house, keeping them for a time when she thought there would be a stronger nursing presence. The library really had some very important, historically significant things. If it hadn't been for Betty, a lot of those things would have been lost.

Betty was hoping for the day when somebody would value and take care of these things. She truly was, in a literal sense, the "keeper of the flame." Hopkins was her life. She was typical of a large group of people who, over the years, would come to Hopkins and quickly be taken up by everything that Hopkins represents, and it would be their lives.

Stella Shiber

I went over to Welch Library and found this roomful of memorabilia from early in the 1900s, when all the well-known nurses were here on the faculty. There were boxes of papers, memorabilia, notes, notebooks, and pictures from the very beginning of the Hopkins School of Nursing. Nothing had been categorized so I decided just to make lists of what was in each of the boxes: letters, papers, newspaper columns. I began putting them on the computer so I wouldn't get too far behind. I just recorded what was there. I was amazed at the amount of material there was. There were placards and medals given to nurses who had been in the Mexican-American War, First World War, and the Second World War too. Most of the alumni magazines were there. There was a lot of information in that, too. I got to know some of the early Hopkins nurses just from the memorabilia that were collected. It was a rich find.

Ada Davis

By and large, alumni are very proud of our heritage and those of us who are involved are really interested in the history. I've always found it interesting to dig into it and, of course, I work in the archives. When I hold a piece of paper that was written by Miss Wolf, it's just electrifying.

Lois Grayshan Hoffer, 1962

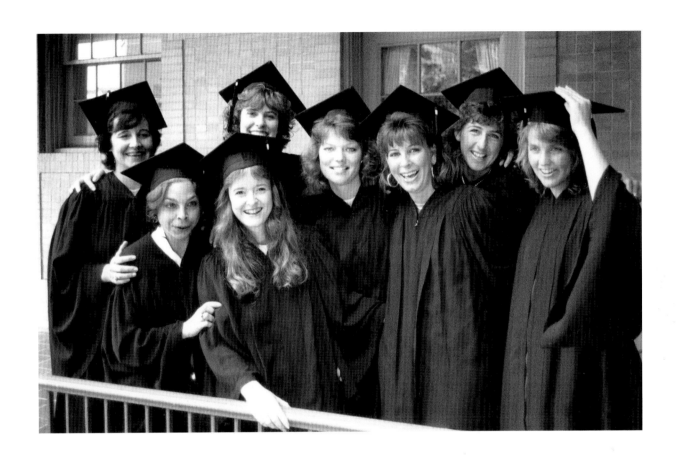

Conscious of the past, equal to the present, and reaching forward into the future—
that's the Hopkins way. That's our shared legacy. That's the challenge of your tomorrow.

Barbara Russell Donaho, 1956, graduation address delivered June 4, 1988

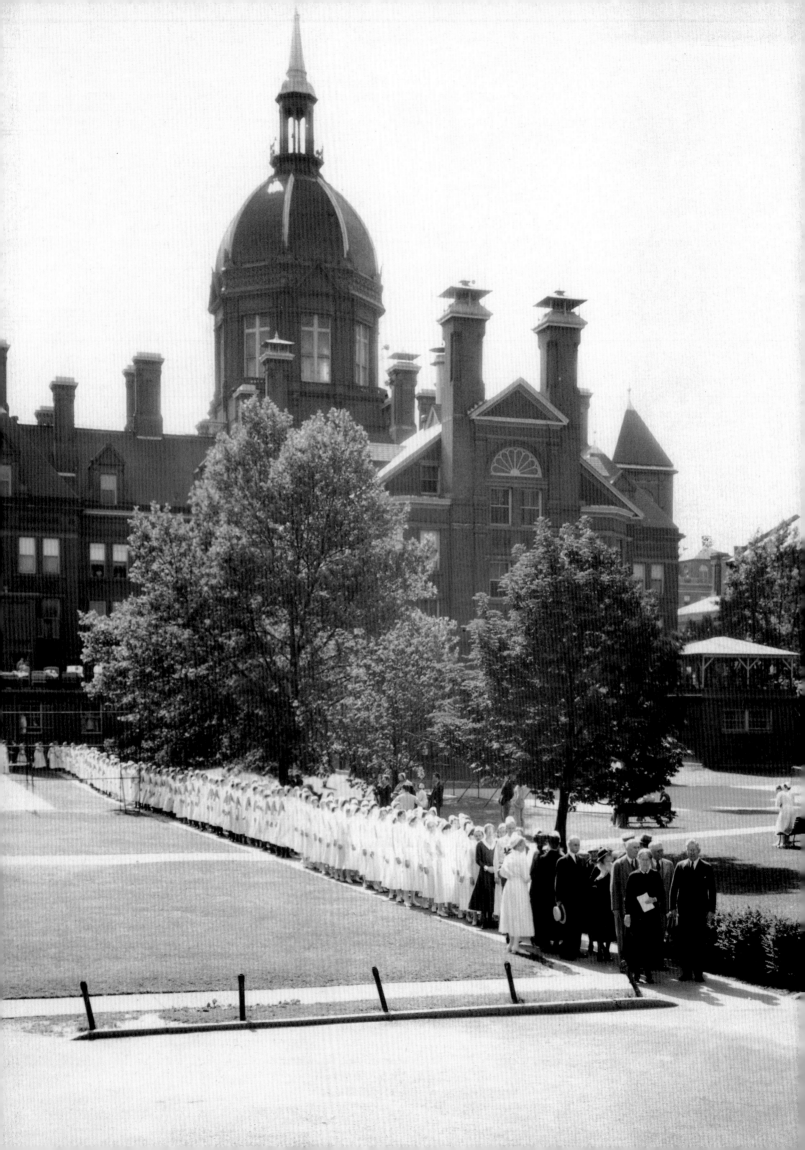

An Auspicious Beginning, 1889–1940 · LINDA SABIN

I

Superintendent Elsie Lawler and Winford H. Smith,
president of the Johns Hopkins Hospital, led a long
procession from a rear door of the Administration
Building toward commencement in the garden
of the Phipps Building in 1938. Trustees and honored
guests followed, then graduates in their formal white
uniforms. First- and second-year students, wearing
blue uniforms with white aprons, brought up the rear.

To the younger nurses particularly, there is just one word I want to say, and that is, in going out to practice your profession, do not try to give everybody the idea that you are the best nurses that ever happened because you graduated from this school. We have suffered here too much from that sort of a reputation. It is not peculiar to the training school for nurses. It is just as true, if not more so, of the medical school. Of course we think none of the other schools are quite as good as this, but let us try to keep it to ourselves, and let other people find it out for themselves, if it is so, without having to be told all about it so often.[1]

Hospital Superintendent Dr. Winford Smith's tongue-in-cheek admonishment in 1915 to members of the Alumnae Association of the Johns Hopkins Hospital Training School for Nurses of Baltimore City demonstrated his abundant pride in the success of his audience. After only a quarter of a century, the Johns Hopkins Hospital and its nursing school were setting standards throughout the United States for medical and nursing professions. Even more impressive, the achievements of the school's graduates were observable internationally.

This is a saga of two institutions and the individuals who shaped nursing education at Johns Hopkins since the nursing school's opening in 1889. The women who forged the program were recognized as standard-bearers. "We had some of the most notable nurses in the country here, at one time or another, beginning with the early nurses. They were in love with nursing and they were also young and adventurous," boasted historian Dr. Ada Davis. "Most of them are still remembered for the accomplishments they made and for what they left to nursing as a whole, not just Hopkins nursing but nursing altogether."[2] Dr. Paula Einaudi concurred. "They didn't just start the School of Nursing at this institution, they pioneered nursing as a profession. These women were giants. They set the tone for the profession. They made it more scientific."[3]

The Johns Hopkins Hospital community—administrators, physicians, and the hospital's board of trustees—recognized the symbiotic relationship between the School of Nursing and the hospital. This affiliation shaped the character of the nursing program for many years. The Johns Hopkins University was also a major influence because of its Schools of Medicine and Public Health, as well as its hospital connections. One of the ironies of this history is that by rigidly adhering to the original intent of the founding donor, the academic community became a major stumbling block in the progress of the nursing school after 1906.

Generations of students made their way to Baltimore because "they knew the quality of the university and of the medical school and the nursing school. They wanted to be part of this metropolitan and really global school known for its excellence, which never changed. It's always been known that way," Davis affirmed. "You go anywhere in the world and you say you've been at Hopkins or are a graduate of Hopkins,

Because Hopkins was such a famous, well-established diploma school with very loyal alums for so many years, it made it more difficult for the school to change. That's why the school came into the university model of nursing education later than the other top-tier schools. My sense was that Hopkins was clearly one of the top, if not the top, in the United States and in the world at its beginning. That made it more difficult for change to occur.

Elaine Larson

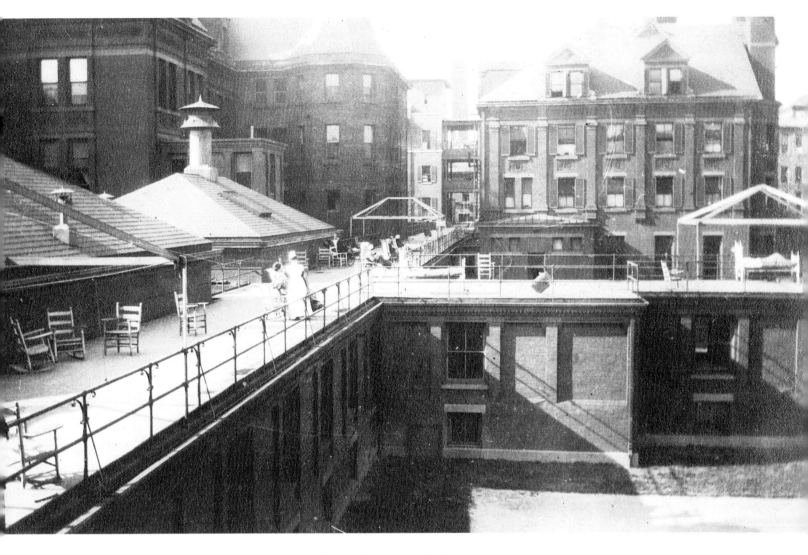

you're treated as something very special."[4] And the School of Nursing has earned its reputation, with countless students and alumni assuming starring roles in developing the stature and significance of the nursing profession in the United States and around the world.

The Johns Hopkins Nurses' Alumni Association has been a persistent and vital link among the school, the hospital, and the university since its founding just three years after the school began. Throughout its complex history, the association has had the courage to provide continuity for the vision of excellence established by the original leaders. Today its members remain devoted. "We have members of the alumni association who are in their nineties who would not think of missing the annual dinner. They come from all over the country. It's so uplifting to be among them and hear their enthusiasm and their activities since they graduated," Davis marveled. "Many of them have sent their children here, either to medical school or nursing school or to the university. The alumni all come together regardless of what program they were in at what level."[5]

Elevated bridges above the corridors that connected several hospital buildings provided an ideal setting for patients to reap the benefits of fresh air and sunshine. Nurses and nursing students regularly accompanied patients outside, sometimes escorting them to chairs, sometimes rolling out their beds. In an attempt to prevent contagion, the original hospital featured numerous detached buildings with separate ventilation systems.

My mother was a Hopkins nurse. She graduated in 1917. I always wanted to be a nurse. I just wanted to help people and be as kind and nice to them as Mamma was to me.

Constance Cole Heard Waxter, 1944

[The Johns Hopkins Hospital Training School for Nurses] is destined to be in the coming years scarcely less important and useful than the development of the more imposing science of medicine and surgery, of which it is rapidly growing to be the twin companion. Without careful nursing, medicine and surgery are crippled agencies in the preservation of health and life, and with careful nursing it is often possible to preserve both without their assistance.

Editorial in the *Baltimore American*, October 10, 1889

Opposite: Isabel Hampton arrived at Johns Hopkins with excellent credentials. The doctors, administrator, and trustee who selected her, however, considered her good looks her greatest attribute when they made her the first superintendent of nursing for the hospital and principal of the training school for nurses. "She entered the room looking like an animated Greek statue," Dr. William Osler wrote of their initial meeting. Although Hampton set the highest standards for the school, she gave her primary allegiance to the hospital. It was her successor who began the long campaign to separate the school from the hospital and establish baccalaureate nursing education in the Johns Hopkins University, a legally and fiscally separate institution from the hospital.

The motivation to establish nursing education at the Johns Hopkins Hospital was kindled in 1832, when, as a young man, Quaker merchant Johns Hopkins nearly died of cholera and learned firsthand the plight of persons needing nursing care during an epidemic. Mr. Hopkins survived his illness and, over time, his business interests flourished. He remained aware of problems with the care of the sick, however. In 1867 he investigated conditions in a Maryland hospital and discovered that the nurses were poorly prepared and lacked the skill to provide even minimal care. Circumstances had changed little since his experience with cholera years earlier.

That same year Mr. Hopkins, who was by then very wealthy, applied and received permission from the Maryland legislature to establish two corporations: The Johns Hopkins Hospital and The Johns Hopkins University. In 1873 he left instructions that were to be implemented with his will, in which he specifically included terms for a training school for female nurses to be connected to the hospital. "This provision will secure the services of women competent to care for the sick in the hospital wards, and will enable you to benefit the whole community by supplying it with a class of trained and experienced nurses," he wrote to the first trustees, who would set the will in motion later that year, when Mr. Hopkins died.[6]

Dr. John S. Billings served as a consultant to the board of trustees of the hospital. Billings was aware of Florence Nightingale's views on nursing. This knowledge, combined with his own experiences with American nursing programs, enabled him to guide the initial plans for nursing activities in the hospital. He reminded the trustees of the importance of finding the right persons to lead this new venture:

It should be remembered that our buildings and machinery are simply tools and instruments and the real hospital, the moving and animating soul of the institution, which is to do its work and determine its character, consists of the brains to be put in it. Whether it shall be a truly great Hospital and a charity such as was intended by its founder, is not a matter solely of arrangement and plan of buildings, it depends upon not more than half-a-dozen men and one or two women.... The most difficult thing in forming this Hospital is to find the proper and suitable persons to be the soul and motive power of the institution.[7]

On May 7, 1889, the first patients entered the Johns Hopkins Hospital, and just five months later, on October 9, 1889, the nursing school opened. On that occasion, Miss Isabel Adams Hampton, the first superintendent of the training school, described her vision for the graduates of the new program: "As the university and hospital are looked to from all quarters for what is best in science, so may it follow that as time goes on, and women go forth as graduates of the Johns Hopkins Hospital School for Nurses, this School may be looked to for what is best in nursing, and

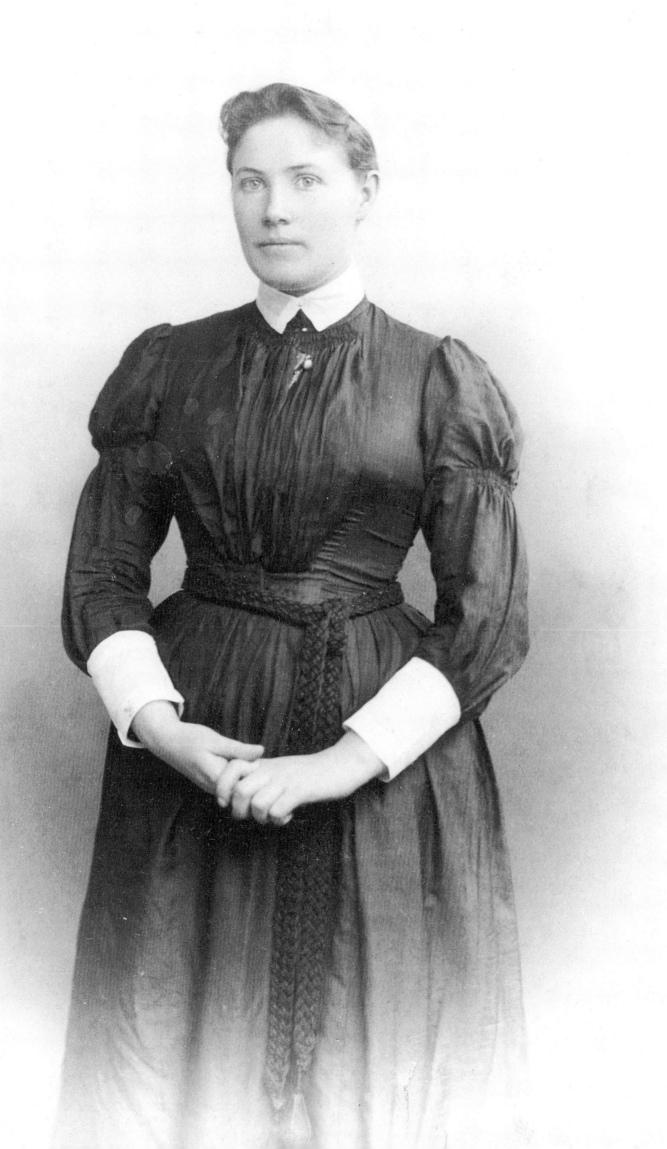

List of Officers and Employés of the Johns Hopkins Hospital. for 50, for 100 and for 150 Beds.

Title	Annual Salary	50 Beds		100 Beds		150 Beds	
		No.	Total	No.	Total	No.	Total
Resident Physician	1800 00	1	1800 00	1	1800 00	1	1800 00
House Physicians and Surgeons		2		4		6	
Superintendent	2000 00	1	2000 00	1	2000 00	1	2000 00
Apothecary	600 00	1	600 00	1	600 00	1	600 00
Apothecaries assistant	360 00			1	360 00	1	360 00
Engineer	1380 00	1	1380 00	1	1380 00	1	1380 00
Assistant Engineer (in winter)	600 00	1	600 00	1	600 00	1	600 00
Firemen (to work in grounds in summer)	300 00	3	900 00	3	900 00	3	900 00
Clerks	900 00	1	900 00	2	1650 00	2	1650 00
Storekeeper	900 00	1	900 00	1	900 00	1	900 00
Head Cook	360 00	1	360 00	1	360 00	1	360 00
Assistant Cook	240 00	1	240 00	1	240 00	1	240 00
Kitchen Help	180 00	1	180 00	2	360 00	3	540 00
Janitors	200 00	3	600 00	3	600 00	3	600 00
Messengers	120 00	1	120 00	2	240 00	2	240 00
Gardener	480 00	1	480 00	1	480 00	1	480 00
Stablemen and drivers	480 00	1	480 00	2	960 00	2	960 00
Painter	750 00	2	1500 00	2	1500 00	2	1500 00
Carpenter	780 00	2	1560 00	2	1560 00	2	1560 00
Laborers	300 00	2	600 00	3	900 00	3	900 00
Bath House Keeper	600 00	1	600 00	1	600 00	1	600 00
Superintendent of Nurses	1200 00	1	1200 00	1	1200 00	1	1200 00
Matron	600 00	1	600 00	1	600 00	1	600 00
Nurses, female (day and night)	180 00	10	1800 00	20	3600 00	30	5400 00
Ward tenders and Nurses, male (day and night)	360 00	3	1080 00	6	2160 00	9	3240 00
Head Laundress	360 00	1	360 00	1	360 00	1	360 00
Laundresses	180 00	3	540 00	6	1080 00	8	1440 00
Chambermaids and Waitresses	120 00	4	480 00	5	600 00	6	720 00
Scrubwomen	120 00	6	720 00	9	1080 00	12	1440 00
Sempstress	180 00	1	180 00	2	360 00	2	360 00
		58	22760 00	87	29030 00	109	32930 00
Resident to be fed		50		78		100	
* Non resident		8		9		9	

her graduates uphold their part of a grand work with all faithfulness."[8] Dr. Henry Hurd, the hospital's first superintendent, spoke of the relation of the school of nursing to the hospital: "Lest there be any misconception I ought to add that enthusiasm in work, devotion to duty, unresting fidelity to high ideals of efficiency, keen humanitarian impulses and love of scientific truth cannot and must not be considered obligations peculiar to nurses. The trustees and officers of the hospital accept similar obligations for themselves, and expect equal enthusiasm and devotion from all connected with the hospital in any responsible capacity."[9] Both Hampton and Hurd viewed the goals of the school and the hospital as strongly connected to hard work and excellence in performance.

As the first president of both institutions, Daniel Coit Gilman determined the direction of the university and the hospital. He came to Baltimore in 1875 from the University of California at Berkeley and introduced the idea of a research university based on the German model. He wanted to provide a style of higher education not then available in the United States, emphasizing graduate study for superior students. Gilman's plan for a program centered on laboratory research and graduate seminars was a dramatic departure from typical American college programs of the time. In Gilman's view, the focus of the Johns Hopkins University should be the outstanding men who would compose a strong faculty and provide a rich academic environment.[10]

Gilman took a great interest in the development of the hospital, its nursing school, and the medical school. Along with Drs. William Welch and William Osler, Gilman screened eighty applicants for the position of superintendent of nurses and principal of the training school before interviewing Isabel Hampton. Impressed by Hampton's handsome appearance, intelligence, and excellent experience, they quickly offered her the position.

The initial goals of the individuals who directed the university, hospital, and School of Nursing shaped many interactions and organizational issues for the next ninety years. Buoyed by the generous support of the original donor, they created institutions that would provide settings for momentous achievements in higher education; in medical research, education, and practice; and in nursing education and practice. The writings and activities of Isabel Hampton and her successor illustrated that these women considered the role of the nursing school to be one of innovation and leadership for the young profession. Their ideas and assertive attitudes set the stage for a struggle with the leadership in the hospital and university that would last for generations.

Isabel Hampton, a Canadian who had trained at Bellevue Hospital in New York, came to Johns Hopkins with experience as a practicing nurse and as a superintendent. The superintendent in this period was in charge of the nursing service for the entire hospital, while simultaneously

Opposite and above: Before the Johns Hopkins Hospital opened in 1889, a full budget was drawn up. As superintendent of nurses, Isabel Hampton, whose responsibilities were clearly defined, received a reasonable salary, but female nurses collected compensation equal to that of laundresses and seamstresses. Male nurses, however, were to earn twice as much.

From the beginning, nursing students at Johns Hopkins benefited from the practice of teaching at the patient's bedside. Physician-in-Chief William Osler consulted his notes as Elizabeth Boley, 1903, focused her attention elsewhere on the ward.

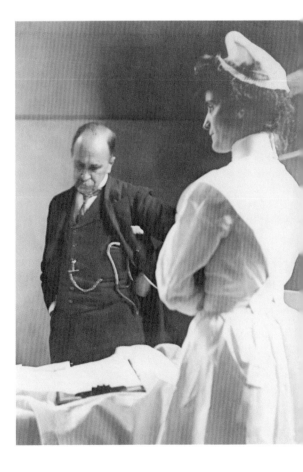

running the nursing school. To some, this would have been daunting, but Miss Hampton used considerable creativity to provide a comprehensive education for students while meeting the needs of patients. She was keenly aware of the issues she faced in 1889. In her address at the opening of the school, she described the relationship between hospitals and schools of nursing: "Up to this present time the usefulness of schools for nurses is recognized chiefly from three standpoints. They have solved the problem of how to properly care for the sick poor in our large charity hospitals and infirmaries, and have made it possible for private and church hospitals to give their patients skilled care. The rich can also secure the same services in their homes."[11] As an educator, Miss Hampton recognized the flaw in students exchanging service for education. She directed her energies to balancing the needs of patients and the hospital with students' need to learn. This skill would be called on as long as the hospital-sponsored nursing school existed because each of her successors faced similar challenges.

From the beginning, Hopkins physicians played a major role in the education of nurses. In the first year of the program, doctors gave regular lectures from November to June. Physicians provided expertise about the theoretical areas of physical disease and treatment, which was not included in the nursing texts of the time. Hampton augmented what the physicians presented and soon added nurses to the faculty, including Lavinia Dock, another Bellevue graduate.

In addition to lectures, students attended classes where they practiced skills and training sessions taught at the bedside. With Miss Hampton's encouragement, in 1891 students formed a journal club, which met every other Monday evening. Attendance was mandatory and students presented articles from American and British journals. All students had to complete final examinations before graduation. The average score for the first class exam was 86.4.[12]

Isabel Hampton eliminated the usual practice of that time of sending students out to work private duty in wealthy clients' homes—an assignment she saw as a pernicious practice with little educational value. She believed that students needed supervision, which was impossible to give when they practiced away from the hospital. She also initiated a cooking program to teach students how to prepare diets for patients.

Hampton's approach to the organization and structure of the nursing school reflected a strong religious and military slant toward the management of students and staff within the hospital bureaucracy. She had learned this method as a student at Bellevue, which had one of the earliest American programs espousing the philosophy of Florence Nightingale.[13] Students' uniforms were inspected daily before they went on duty. When eating meals in the nurses' dining room, students made requests to the head nurse who presided at each table and the head

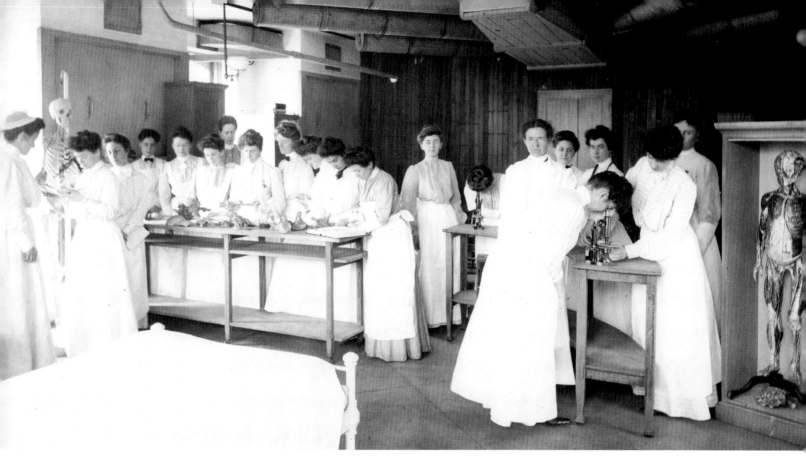

nurse then gave instructions to the waitress. Every part of the day and all routines were structured and regulated. Hampton expected unswerving loyalty and devotion to physicians and head nurses by students at all levels. Her approach to etiquette and ethics was strict; she expected a narrow chain of command, deference to superiors, and a quiet, meek attitude by the lowliest of students, especially probationers.[14]

During her tenure, Miss Hampton saw the program she established running well. She hoped to extend the course of study from two to three years, eliminate cash allowances for students, and shorten the students' workday to eight hours, but her role as superintendent ended with her marriage, in 1894, to Hunter Robb, an obstetrician/gynecologist on the hospital staff. Although some of her colleagues viewed her marriage as an unfortunate end to a brilliant career, Mrs. Robb continued to be active in nursing affairs for the next sixteen years. She and Dr. Robb moved to Cleveland and they had two sons.

In 1897 Mrs. Robb was elected the first president of the Associated Alumnae of Trained Nurses of the United States and Canada (now known as the American Nurses Association). She also served the American Association of Superintendents of Training Schools (now known as the National League for Nursing) on a committee that helped to establish the first postgraduate collegiate program for nurses at Teachers College at Columbia University. In addition, Mrs. Robb wrote two books and edited a third, which she had written before her marriage. Unfortunately, she died in a tragic streetcar accident in Cleveland in 1910, at the age of forty-nine. Her premature death leaves us to wonder what she might have accomplished with a full life span.

Many of the best teachers in the School of Medicine also taught nursing students. When this anatomy and physiology class met in 1905, Dr. Florence Sabin (wearing glasses and standing just beyond the student looking through the near microscope) had just been promoted to associate professor. It would be many years before instructors in the nursing school achieved similar academic standing.

Students in the classes of 1892 and 1893 formed the night nursing staff for the hospital in March 1892.

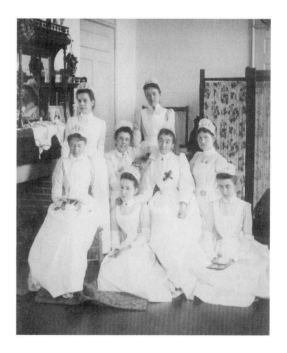

Nursing in this country was developed because of Isabel Hampton Robb and Adelaide Nutting, and also Lavinia Dock and some of the others who truly made an impact on nursing which we still see today. The two professional nursing organizations, the American Nurses Association and the National League for Nursing, both grew out of organizations started by Isabel Hampton Robb. It was Lavinia Dock who really pushed for baccalaureate education for nurses. Our students are indoctrinated with that. I think they feel they have a responsibility to keep it up.

Maureen Maguire

Adelaide Nutting had a strong belief in publishing. She was one of the founding members of the first nursing journal. She was adamant in her demand that nurses owed it to each other, to the profession, and to their patients to disseminate the information they learned and the knowledge they got. I have a strong conviction about that, too. I would go so far as to say that I think it's unethical not to publish or to disseminate in some medium the information you learn, especially if you're a researcher. You've spent a lot of resources learning that information. If you don't communicate it, everybody's going to have to reinvent the wheel over and over again.

Elaine Larson

Opposite, above: M. Adelaide Nutting, a graduate in the first class, became, at age thirty-five, the second superintendent of nurses and principal of the training school. Nutting achieved many important changes during her tenure but was unable to accomplish her prime goal: affiliation with the Johns Hopkins University.

Opposite, center and below: A well-appointed dwelling designed to accommodate fifty nurses was part of the original plan for the hospital. Known both as the Nurses' Home and the Main Residence, it was situated near the Wilmer Institute. The first floor included a parlor, a living room, and a small library.

Mary Adelaide Nutting became the second superintendent of nursing and principal of the training school after Isabel Hampton Robb's departure. Nutting was also a Canadian who, though two years older than her predecessor, had graduated in 1891 with the first Hopkins class. She was able to fulfill many of Robb's goals for the school, as well as to develop some of her own ideas to advance the program. Having gained approval for eight-hour workdays and the elimination of cash allowances for the students,[15] she then redirected the money saved to the educational program, added teaching staff, and led an effort to set up a scholarship program for students in need. Miss Nutting also negotiated the establishment of a preclinical period for the education of students before their assignment to care for patients on the wards. She gained administrative approval to lengthen the program from two to three years and began to hire full-time instructors. In 1899 she expanded class offerings to senior students by adding a series called Studies of Social Conditions.[16]

Adelaide Nutting was well versed in national trends in higher education, and she tried to mold the program in keeping with the newest ideas. She recognized the critical problem of students trading work for training and how it limited their education. Her retention of Isabel Robb's structured, militaristic leadership style, combined with her own natural reserve, led some of her colleagues and students to view her as cold or remote.

In 1907 Adelaide Nutting authored the first nursing research study on schools of nursing in the United States, *The Education and Professional Position of Nurses*, which was published by the federal government. While she was at Johns Hopkins, she met and developed a mutual interest in nursing history with Lavinia Dock, who had been one of her instructors. Dock, an independently wealthy woman with an excellent academic background and a passion for writing, was fluent in foreign languages and appreciated the lessons of history. The two women co-wrote the first four-volume history of nursing, which is still considered a classic. In order to complete the work, they traveled in Europe to document nursing's development from ancient times to the early twentieth century. Both women valued primary research and understood how it could benefit nursing as an evolving profession.

Throughout her career, Nutting was concerned with national and international nursing activities. During her years at Johns Hopkins, she served with the Committee to Secure by Act of Congress the Employment of Women Nurses in the Hospital Service of the United States Army Nurse Corps. The organization was established in December 1898, after the Spanish-American War. The committee, which included Isabel Hampton Robb, Georgia Nevins, 1891, and Ellen M. Wood, 1895, advocated passage of legislation to establish a standing nurse corps to avoid the usual frantic recruitment of large numbers of nurses when war broke out.

The Spanish-American War had been a disaster for the U.S. Army. The brief conflict had led to 968 battle casualties and 5,438 deaths from sickness—a death rate from illness of 67 percent, compared to 18 percent in the Civil War.[17] In spite of these statistics, the medical establishment and many military leaders were violently opposed to involving women in the military except in dire emergencies. The Dodge Commission was appointed to investigate the conduct of the War Department during the short-lived war. Basing its arguments on the achievements of trained nurses in the recent conflict, it urged the establishment of a women's nursing corps.

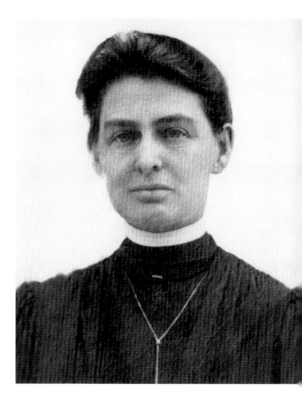

Nutting worked tirelessly to support the committee's goals because she understood the achievements and difficulties of her former students in the war effort. Her papers include writings by Hopkins graduates who served in the war and experienced the difficulties of the makeshift system that existed prior to the formation of the Army Nurse Corps. Agnes Ysobel Irvine, 1894, wrote to Nutting detailing her experience with U.S. Health Service relief after her arrival in Manila. There, Irvine and her colleagues immediately received seventy-four sick and wounded men:

It was a harrowing night. . . . Men covered with blood, in mud, in rags, fatigued. . . . How they did enjoy the beds, the food and the rest. . . . Three men died, two shot dreadfully in the pelvis, one through the trachae and lungs, the latter lived two days, the others died the next morning. The patience of the men was something to remember forever, there were no complaints, no groans, all were cheerful and ready to be dressed until the last and willing to help each other. Our hours were 6:30 A.M.–7 P.M.—with time for meals but with 74 patients requiring so much attention and only two nurses and five corpsmen.[18]

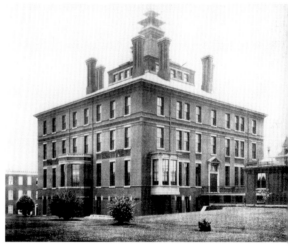

Many prominent women in the Daughters of the American Revolution and other groups joined with Nutting and her colleagues to lobby Congress, but they were faced with the sexism prevalent at the time. Distinguished physicians and military leaders opposed any introduction of women into the military on a regular basis. The primary arguments included the need to exclude females from rail and water transport, hospital trains, or boats. "Men are more serviceable than women on shipboard, less liable to exhausting sea sickness, requiring fewer facilities and less comfort, and can be used for more purposes when, as frequently occurs in such sea duty, there is no work with the sick," one officer claimed. He concluded that the expense, inconvenience, and risk did not warrant using the services of women in land-based hospitals. "They must have a separate dormitory, a separate toilet, a different mess, and some facility for cooking and laundry work. They will often be unemployed, for there are large numbers of cases in our

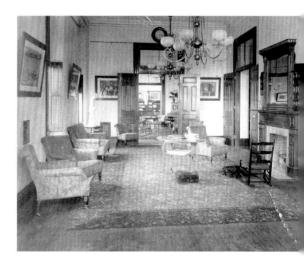

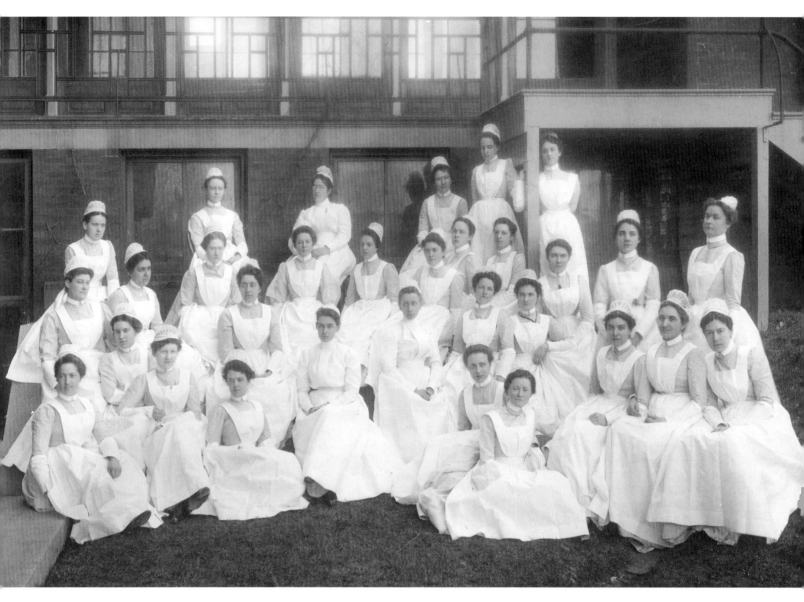

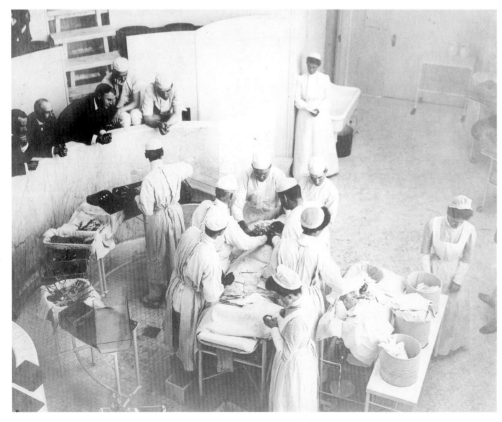

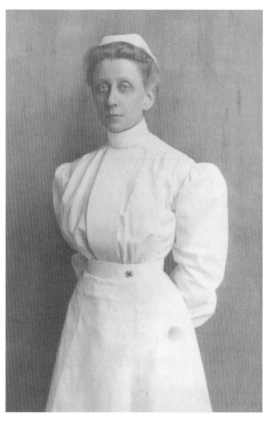

military posts which they cannot properly attend. . . . I can see much expense, idleness, risk of friction, and a certain disquiet about immorality, in this innovation, without commensurate gain."[19]

At one point Miss Nutting wrote to her Hopkins colleague Dr. William Welch regarding a letter from a physician in Philadelphia who strongly opposed the proposed bill to establish an army nurse corps. Welch replied that it was unfortunate that so many physicians still viewed nurses as unchanged since the Civil War. He admitted to Nutting that much of the medical profession still needed education about the value of the trained nurse.[20]

The efforts of the committee, combined with the findings of the Dodge Commission, led to the passage of the Bill to Provide for the Employment of Women Nurses in the Military Hospitals of the Army, which was part of the Army Reorganization Act of 1901. This bill established the Army Nurse Corps, which officially organized under the leadership of Dita H. Kinney in 1901. This was the first of what would become a long series of efforts to establish the professional status of nursing in society by people like Adelaide Nutting and Isabel Robb. In the future, nursing leaders from Johns Hopkins would tackle the battle for licensure, full rank for nurses in the military, and the creation of university-based education programs. Much of what early leaders learned in this first round of political action would be used repeatedly in the twentieth century.

Adelaide Nutting left Johns Hopkins in 1907 to take charge of a fledgling postgraduate collegiate program being established at Teachers College at Columbia University. In accepting this position, she became the first professor in the world in the field of nursing. Her career would continue for many years and her influence is still felt today. "Adelaide Nutting was frank and to the point. She made good, logical arguments. She gave good evidence," said Dr. Elaine Larson, the first person to hold the M. Adelaide Nutting Chair in the Johns Hopkins University School of Nursing. "To be cogent, logical, and evidence-based is very important for a profession like nursing, where we have a reputation of being caretaking, loving, and not so smart. [Adelaide Nutting] became one of my role models."

Georgina Caird Ross, yet another Canadian, succeeded Miss Nutting as superintendent. Miss Ross was a devoted student, colleague, and later a friend of Nutting's. She had graduated from Hopkins in the class of 1894, remained at the hospital after graduation as a head nurse, and been promoted to the position of second assistant superintendent in 1896. For the next eleven years, Georgina Ross had major teaching responsibilities in the school. Her tenure as superintendent lasted less than three years, however. She resigned following internal administrative problems and as a result of ill health.[21] She then settled in Potsdam, New York.

I was fascinated by the choice those women made, many of them counter to their upbringing, in choosing to be a nurse. It wasn't an exalted role at that time. You were thought a bit odd if you walked away from your family's inheritance and comfort to be a nurse. It was difficult. Nurses worked seven days a week, many hours a day. It was a calling and I guess that's what I was responding to. It felt like that to me. My biggest concern was whether I could do it. I just wasn't sure that I was that caliber.

Cathy Novak, 1973

Opposite, above: The group portrait taken in 1902 included an extraordinary assembly of students and nurses who would go on to distinguished careers. Bessie Baker and Ellen LaMotte were members of the class of 1902; their instructors (not wearing aprons) were Adelaide Nutting, 1891, Georgina Ross, 1894 (both center front), and Elsie Lawler, 1899, all of whom later took charge of the school.

Opposite, below left: Two nursing students and an alumna worked diligently on William Halsted's team during the surgery in 1904. Doctors and medical students crowded into the new amphitheater's seats, but nursing instructor Adelaide Nutting preferred to watch at ground level, although she stayed in the background.

Opposite, below right: In addition to her responsibilities as an instructor and administrator, Georgina Caird Ross took charge of the new six-month training for probationers in 1901. After Adelaide Nutting left for Columbia University, Ross served as superintendent of nurses from 1907 to 1910.

Elsie Lawler, a fourth Canadian and a member of the class of 1899, took over after Georgina Ross's resignation. Lawler already had several years of administrative experience at Johns Hopkins and other large medical centers when she returned to Baltimore in 1910. She would devote the next thirty years to nursing at Hopkins. Like her predecessor, Elsie Lawler had been a student loyal to Miss Nutting, and she wrote to her mentor promising to do her best to carry on Nutting's teachings.[22]

Miss Lawler and her staff had to cope with constant change throughout her tenure. She weathered a prewar building frenzy, difficulties touched off by World War I, the explosive 1920s, and the stark days of the Great Depression. She perpetuated the Robb/Nutting approach to structure and rank within the nursing system. Maravene Hamburger, 1937, remembered that one alumna, Sophie Packer, 1918, had an approach that differed from Lawler's.

The nurses who taught us were all unmarried, prim, and proper. I doubt if any of them had ever kissed a man besides their father. I don't think any of them ever had any dates. When one of my classmates, Ruth Jeffcoat, wanted to marry Russell Nelson, Elsie Lawler told her that if she got married she couldn't work in the hospital. She and Russell did get married and when she came back, she didn't have a job. There was one married nurse in the outside OB, Sophie Packer. Sophie Packer called Ruth in and offered her a job. Ruth said, "Well, I was told I couldn't work in the hospital." Sophie Packer said, "Elsie Lawler runs the School of Nursing. I run the dispensary."[23]

Elsie Lawler, 1899, led the nursing school longer than anyone before or after. Her thirty-year administration was marked by changes, mostly due to influences outside the school. Lawler did little to further the effort to bring the school into the Johns Hopkins University, a cause held dear by many alumni. Still, she was fondly remembered by many students who attended the school during her tenure.

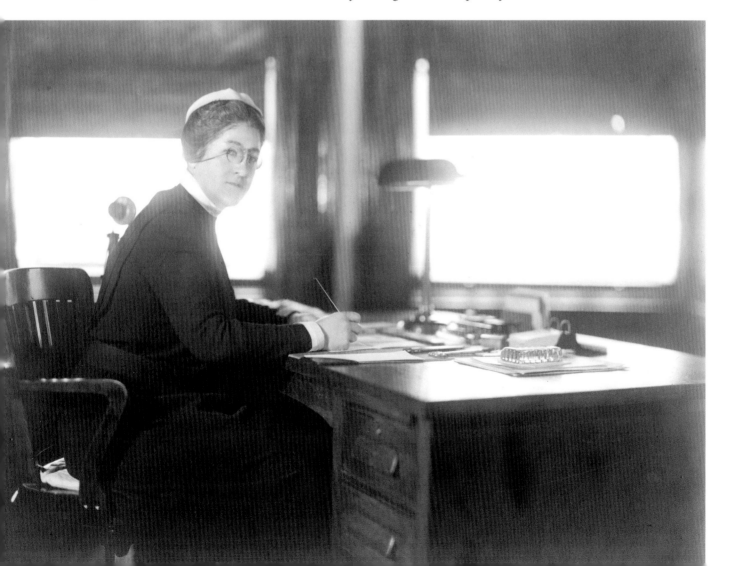

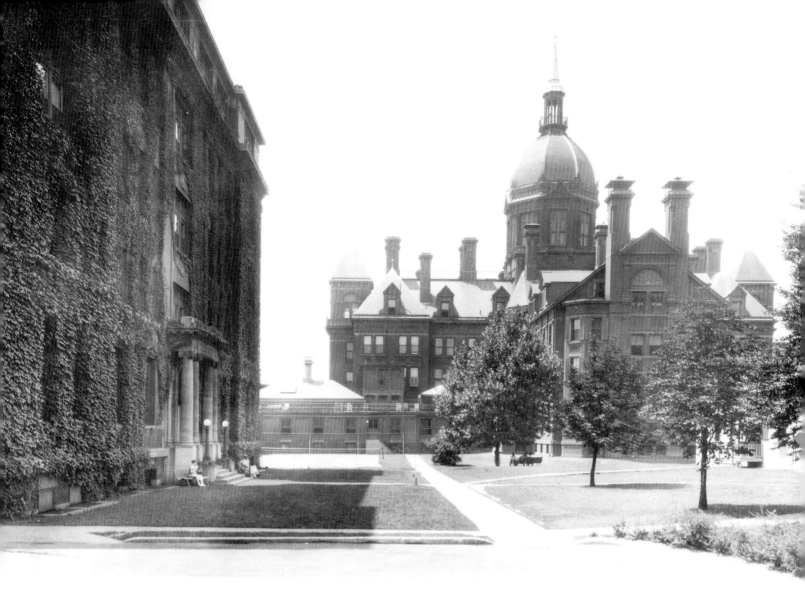

Lawler's administration left its mark on more classes of students than any other in the history of nursing education at Johns Hopkins.

During the first ten years of Miss Lawler's leadership of the nursing department, the hospital added four new buildings with new services and significantly increased the number of beds. Lawler inherited a legacy of tension between meeting the educational needs of students and the service needs of the hospital—a tension that intensified with each new development. When World War I broke out, a Hopkins medical unit organized, and thirteen head nurses and assistant head nurses from the active staff left to serve in the military. Two other administrative nurses, Anna Dryden Wolf, 1915, and Effie Taylor, 1907, also departed, to serve as senior instructors at the Vassar Training School and the Army Nursing School, respectively.

An abundance of applicants kept enrollment at its maximum throughout the expansion, the war, and the Depression and provided strength to the nursing program in its first fifty years. Miss Lawler had her share of administrative headaches stemming from growth in the hospital and the school. She made significant strides in several areas and met with frustration in others, in which progress was hindered by hospital realities. She responded positively to the creation of the advisory

During the early decades of the twentieth century the hospital underwent a building boom, including the construction of two new buildings on the southern side of the property, fronting Jefferson Street. The Harriet Lane Home for Invalid Children, seen on the left, was completed in 1912, and the adjacent Phipps Psychiatric Clinic opened the following year. This created a parklike setting until additional buildings filled in the area.

We got our caps in six months if we passed the probie [probationer] period. We worked seven days a week. Saturdays and Sundays, we worked six hours a day. During the week, it was eight hours a day plus classes. We might work seven to nine in the morning, four to six in the afternoon, and then seven to eleven at night. It was pretty much of a physical grind but we were all young and so we could take it. A few of my classmates developed health problems that may have been because of the physical stress.

Maravene Deveney Hamburger, 1937

board, in 1930, which increased consultation and communication with representatives of the medical school, private physicians, university leaders, alumnae, and hospital leaders. The members of the advisory board were charged with the responsibility of assisting in the advancement of the school.

Curriculum change was almost constant in the 1920s and '30s as the profession and the school refined the elements of a basic nursing education. In the 1920s obtaining dedicated classroom space for theoretical instruction and strengthening science courses were primary concerns. The preclinical or preliminary curriculum was also regularly refined to better prepare students to function in each major clinical rotation.

By the early 1930s every department in the hospital had an instructor-supervisor who planned the students' clinical experiences. Greater attention was paid to methods of rotation for students, although imbalances in clinical experiences persisted throughout the Depression because of staff shortages. Instructors began formal meetings in the late 1920s for the purpose of sharing teaching strategies and suggestions for student learning. Still, their practices were often limited by their lack of higher education. "Our instructors had no college, except for a few. Most of them were high school graduates. Elsie Lawler was a high school graduate. For me, it was a little bit of an intellectual letdown," admitted Maravene Hamburger, who, like several of her classmates, had a bachelor's degree when she enrolled in the nursing school and was accustomed to faculty with advanced degrees. "Somebody with a PhD has a different outlook than somebody with a high school diploma," she explained.[24]

In 1934 Miss Lawler and her staff determined that the theoretical content in the nursing curriculum had grown dramatically, to more than three hundred hours. When clinical practice was factored into the schedule, this theoretical load significantly increased the students' already long hours. Students were working fifty-four- to fifty-six-hour weeks, exclusive of classes. Administrators proposed a forty-eight-hour workweek. This change would require adding four more general staff nurses and thirteen ward helpers—a clear demonstration of the value of students' contributions to the hospital. The proposal was approved by the board of trustees immediately but not implemented for another four years.[25]

In the midst of war, a building boom, and the Depression, higher education was not Miss Lawler's primary concern, but in 1935 she did manage to establish the first relationship between the nursing school and the Teachers College at the Johns Hopkins University. After graduation, students with two years of college prior to enrolling in the hospital school were allowed to earn another thirty credits and receive a bachelor's degree. The Teachers College was predominantly an evening school, and the only division of the university that accepted undergraduate women. This was a significant step forward in recognizing the academic

I was a chemistry major at Goucher College and there were no jobs. This was 1934. So I decided to come over to Hopkins in nursing. I wasn't the least bit interested in nursing, but I figured in a few years I could make some contacts and maybe get a job in one of the labs.

I became engrossed in nursing. The operating room, the accident room, and the delivery floor were much more exciting than it would have been to work in a lab. The doctors at Hopkins were wonderful. I had no feeling for the patients, but from them I began to be interested. I wanted these people to get well. There were many dramatic moments in nursing in those years. We had typhoid patients. We had pneumonia patients who were really, really sick.

Maravene Deveney Hamburger, 1937

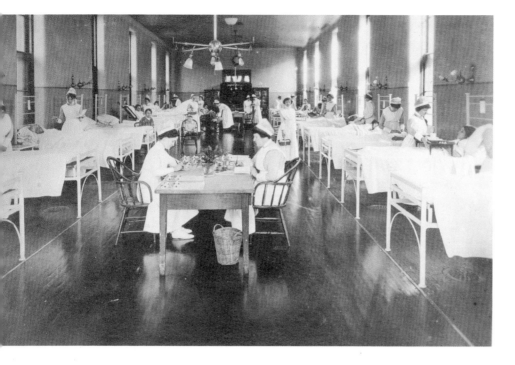

Students worked many hours in the hospital, usually seven days a week, rotating among services to gain exposure to various aspects of patient care. In ward F, Dr. Halsted's clinic, c. 1910, they tended surgical patients, made beds, made sure the bedside was spotless, delivered supplies, and kept medical charts.

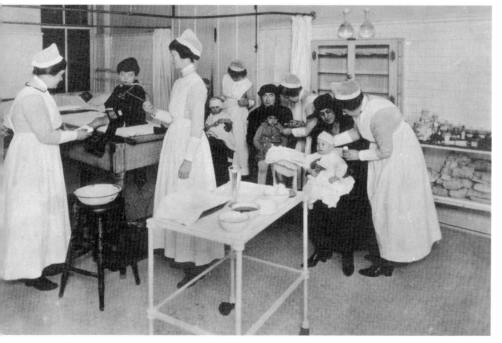

The outpatient department in the Harriet Lane Home was busy from morning to night, as parents brought in children with everything from infectious diseases and epilepsy to cuts, burns, and broken bones. Often, it was nursing students who applied or replaced bandages on young children, as in this scene, c. 1923.

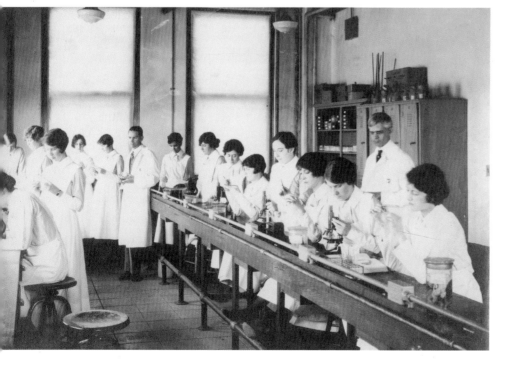

Classes were squeezed in between hospital shifts. Most of the students in this 1927 chemistry lab had discovered that fashionable bobs were easier to tend than long hair.

The reasons for becoming a university school of nursing have to do with people becoming educated and credentialed in a way that society says, "This is a professional person. This is a profession." The whole argument for graduate education is that if you're going to maintain that stature then you must be scholarly in what you do. Nursing must be an evidence based–practice profession. You have to be able to demonstrate what nurses do and what difference they make or you may not continue to exist as a profession.

Martha Norton Hill, 1964, BSN 1966

One of the most difficult things to accept and become adjusted to was the nursing school's discipline system, which was almost military. . . . Elsie Lawler, who graduated from Hopkins in 1899 and was director of the nursing school from 1910 to 1940, was certainly the product of and exponent of that rule of authority. She and I never really got along. . . . The way the system worked was that the nursing director had full and absolute power over everyone under her, without challenge. Next, under her, were her two assistant directors. Under them were the three or four head nurses in charge of different areas. Then came the senior students, then intermediates, then juniors, and at the bottom of the heap were the probationers. Orders were passed down from the top to those below, and unquestioning obedience to authority was the order of the day.

Maude Magill Bagwell, 1929

worth of nursing education at Hopkins, but it failed to address the key issue of a separate academic program within the university.

Elsie Lawler may not have been as farsighted or dynamic as Robb and Nutting, but she provided steady leadership during turbulent times that taxed the hospital and the school. A skillful administrator who worked cooperatively with physicians and hospital leaders, she understood her limitations and, at one point during her tenure, offered to resign so that a better-educated nurse could assume leadership. The hospital director, Dr. Winford Smith, refused to consider her offer because of her success in maintaining excellence in spite of great difficulties.[26] Perhaps Dr. Smith also appreciated her disinclination to rock the boat. "Miss Lawler," he commented, "has not been carried away by the enthusiasm of the moment for some newer ideas in nursing education."[27] Looking back, however, some long-time alumni activists consider Lawler to have "held back the collegiate school of nursing for many, many years." Betty Scher, 1950, clarified: "One of the reasons that she did not want a collegiate school of nursing was 'We are already turning out the finest nurses in the country.' The other statement she made was 'What are the poor girls to do who can't afford college?' She was looking out for them."[28]

Miss Lawler got along well with physicians and endeared herself to many of her students, but some found her rules oppressive. Maravene Hamburger felt overly restricted by regulations intended for younger students but enforced on all. "We had to be in at ten-fifteen every night, except for one night a week we could be out till twelve," Hamburger recalled. "There were a number of us in our class who had college degrees. If we had gone on to graduate school or med school, no effort would have been made to control our social life."[29]

Espousing the philosophy and standards of her predecessors, Elsie Lawler maintained the values passed to her by Isabel Hampton Robb and Adelaide Nutting. Like them, she revered the doctors she and her students worked with. There was a strict adherence to hospital rules and a distinct chain of command. Students and hospital nurses were required to stand when doctors entered the nurses' station or other rooms in the hospital. Miss Lawler never forgot the close relationship between the advancement of the school and the success of the hospital. Lawler retained the vision of nursing as a profession, however, and this shaped her efforts to advance the school. She also viewed excellence in clinical practice as a primary goal and fostered a full generation of Hopkins nurses who kept this ideal alive in practice.

Two crowning achievements came in the closing years of Miss Lawler's tenure as the leader of nursing at Johns Hopkins. In 1935 the entire Hopkins community came together to celebrate her twenty-five years of service as superintendent of nursing. In the same year she received an

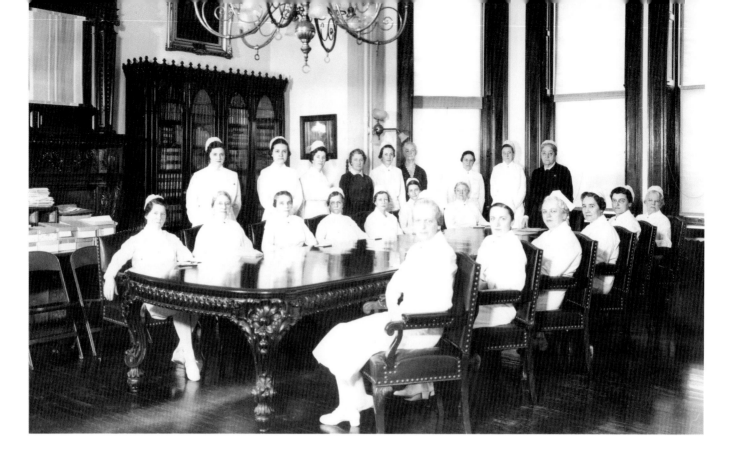

honorary master's degree from the Johns Hopkins University. And in 1939, just before her retirement, Lawler oversaw the fiftieth anniversary of the school, which by then was formally known as the School of Nursing.

Elsie Lawler retired in 1940 and traveled extensively in her first years of leisure. She settled in California, where she suffered a stroke in 1946. Miss Hester Frederick, 1912, traveled to California and brought Miss Lawler to Johns Hopkins for rehabilitation. Elsie Lawler remained at the Johns Hopkins Hospital in a room in the Marburg Building until her death, in 1962. The hospital's extended hospitality illustrated its gratitude for the thirty years Miss Lawler had served as superintendent of nurses. Her highest annual salary had been $5,000, plus her main-tenance, so she never owned a home or accumulated any material wealth. On her retirement, the board of trustees voted to give her an income of $1,000 per year.[30] This stipend, plus a small Social Security income and her savings, would never have covered the cost of a nursing home, and there were few facilities in that era that offered rehabilitation services. Most important, the hospital had been Lawler's home for more than half her adult life, and the institution was not then under the kinds of economic pressures common today.

While she lived in Marburg, Miss Lawler occasionally made appear-ances at graduations and other occasions. She met with nursing lead-ers in the community and enjoyed the fellowship of many women she had helped to educate. A colleague remembered that Lawler's successor, Anna D. Wolf, paid a visit to Miss Lawler's room each day at the noon hour and gave her a report on hospital events. Miss Lawler, although suffering hemiparesis, remained alert, oriented, and interested in the activities of the school and hospital.

By the time she retired in 1940, Elsie Lawler's staff had grown significantly and included nurses who would continue to influence classes in the years to follow. Most were alumnae. Seated around the table (clockwise from left) were Marie Hutchins, Mabel Hay, Mary Purcell, Louisa Kolb, Elizabeth Sherwood, Mildred Struve, Hester Frederick, Loula Kennedy, Kathryn Witmer, Hilda Miller, Bernadette Mullin, Chelly Wasserberg, and Sophia Packer. Standing, from left: Ethna Kurtz, Esther Weber Freadkin, Anne Hahn, Miriam Ames, K. Virginia Betzold, Christine Dick, Clarice Weymouth, Catherine M. Loeffler, and Elsie Lawler.

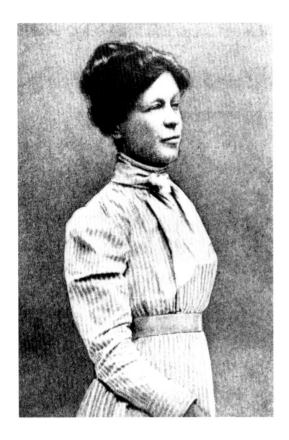

Lavinia L. Dock was the first instructor appointed by Isabel Hampton, her former colleague at Bellevue Hospital. Although Dock stayed in Baltimore only three years, she exerted a broad influence on academics at the school and on its early students, including Adelaide Nutting, with whom she later wrote a four-volume *History of Nursing*.

The Welch Medical Library opened in 1929, and various departments in the hospital had libraries tucked here and there. Most nursing students, such as Betty Liggett Cuthbert (left foreground, facing the camera reading a journal), 1943, and their instructors preferred their own specialized library in the Main Residence. Loula E. Kennedy (in black), 1903, a member of the faculty from 1921 to 1946, was the person most responsible for developing this facility, which was dedicated in her honor in 1949.

Three other nursing leaders served as faculty during this early chapter of the School of Nursing. Lavinia Dock taught for a short period in the 1890s with Miss Hampton and, later, Miss Nutting. She was an early international leader in nursing. In addition to her work with Miss Nutting, Dock wrote the first nursing manual on sexually transmitted diseases and an early text on pharmacology. She was also active in the women's suffrage movement and went to jail more than once for picketing. Miss Nutting credited Miss Dock with molding important aspects of the school:

There was one other in these early days, a woman of rare character and qualities, who as assistant and teacher filled a large place in the school for several years. Independent, fearless, loyal, Lavinia Dock exercised unconscious[ly] an influence which was both strong and enduring, and few connected with that early life had more to do in the last analysis with shaping ideals and giving direction to future activities than this beloved teacher. . . . She had an extraordinary way of driving directly to the heart of a matter, pulling out the essential facts in the situation, and showing us the right way to think about them and to deal with them. Her sense of justice was keen, but her sympathies were well nigh boundless.[31]

Loula Kennedy, 1903, a graduate of Goucher College, was the director of theoretical instruction for twenty of her twenty-five years at the nursing school. She had considerable impact on the development of the curriculum and student life. She advised students after initiating the idea of a yearbook and often worked with students outside the classroom. Kennedy also dedicated many hours and personal resources to developing a high-quality library for nursing students. During her retirement years that library, which was located in a renovated portion of the Main Residence, was named in her honor.[32]

In the clinic Hester Frederick, 1912, was a role model for students for more than twenty years. After graduating, she became an active member of the alumnae association and held a variety of leadership and clinical positions elsewhere, then returned to Hopkins as the director of practical instruction in 1919. She wrote a textbook on the fundamentals of nursing that was used in the program for many years. Except for a brief assignment in another hospital, Miss Frederick remained at Hopkins until her retirement in 1941.[33]

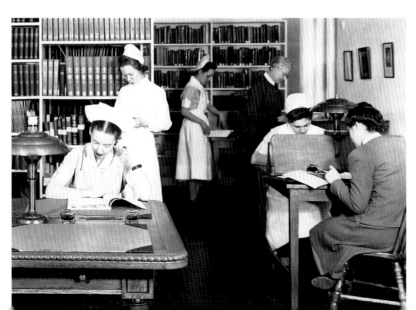

In 1907 Isabel Hampton Robb described the daily life of students at the opening of the school: the workday was twelve hours long, from 7:30 A.M. to 7:30 P.M. for days or the reverse for nights. Students were given time off for meals and a two-hour break for exercise, study, or rest sometime during the day. Each student got half a day off each week and a half day to attend church on Sunday. A two-week vacation was permitted each year. All classes were held in the evenings after day duty, except bedside teaching, which was done during the regular shift.[34]

Miss Hampton led discussions among the nurses at Johns Hopkins to select the style of uniform to be worn by the students in 1889. A meeting was called and students were invited to participate. The group selected a blue dress with white cuffs patterned after the uniform of the Blockley Training School in Philadelphia. A collar was later added to the basic pattern. The apron was copied from an English style offered by Miss Tillie Spencer. Miss Susan Read presented an organdy cap that was modified from the Philadelphia Episcopal Hospital cap.[35] Students wore black shoes and stockings and were never to wear these shoes outside of the hospital. The original cap covered the hair for cleanliness purposes. (In later years the cap was smaller but essentially unchanged.)[36] Students wore the Hopkins cap after their probationary period until the student cap was introduced in the 1940s.

Elsie Lawler remembered her first days as a student in an interview late in her life. She recalled bringing her probationary dresses with her to training because there was not a standard uniform until the student passed this period. She described her outfit as a gray washable dress with an apron (without a bib) and turnover white starched collar fastened in the front. After two months of probation, students received a blue uniform with a tight "Basque" bodice and a full skirt. Each student wore a full gathered apron with a bib and the graduate cap.[37]

Student life then was spartan and highly regimented. Elsie Lawler and her fellow students answered to everyone in the hospital with higher rank. A typical staff for a twenty-eight-bed unit was a head nurse (who might be a senior student), a temperature nurse, a senior nurse, three or four juniors (some of whom might be probationers), and a maid. Lawler remembered that her first day consisted of making beds and learning how to bathe a patient. Although the eight-hour day had been instituted by 1899, it was not adhered to because of the shortage of nurses. Students did maid's work on the maid's day off.[38]

Helen Wilmer Athey, who entered as a student in 1902, recalled different experiences. Probationers in her class had cooking duty for the Nurses' Home, where they learned how to cook for invalids in preparation for private duty cases after graduation. Next, they worked in the surgical supply room, and then gradually moved onto the wards by about the sixth month of school. Once there, Helen Wilmer got to

There is something about Hopkins, its record, its traditions, its thoroughness and excellency, its spirit, which grips one and forces a personal devotion that doesn't wane.

An anonymous alumna in the alumnae magazine

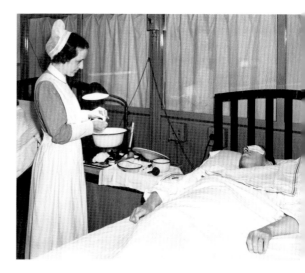

Students learned and practiced skills at the bedside. This student was applying hot compresses to the eyes of a patient in the Wilmer Ophthalmological Institute. She had to be careful not to soil her pristine white cuffs and apron, which were part of the nursing uniform until 1940, when the starched apron disappeared and more practical short sleeves relieved some stress.

Medicine was different. Patients were in the hospital longer for healing. You didn't have as much of this "in today and out tomorrow." Medicine has changed so drastically that patients get well faster. For instance cataract surgery, they would be lying in a bed for seven to ten days and so they needed a bed bath. I don't know whether nurses are even taught to give bed baths anymore. The care you give a person who's up and around and the care you give somebody who's lying in bed are entirely different.

Maravene Deveney Hamburger, 1937

Students used the kitchen of the Main Residence as a laboratory to learn how to select, prepare, and serve food for their patients. In 1901, when this photograph was made, cooking became part of the program for probationers, which also included housekeeping. In the 1950s the faculty eliminated cooking classes in favor of a greater emphasis on nutrition.

make beds, clean the units, and care for the doctors' washstands. The students' classroom for materia medica (pharmacology) and anatomy was located in the basement of the Nurses' Home. Residents or a department head taught practical nursing classes, which were held in the evenings in the basement of one of the clinical buildings. She reported that she and her peers often had to fight sleepiness during class after working all day. The students worked a seven-day week, with four hours off each Sunday. "In our day, convenience in arranging ward routine

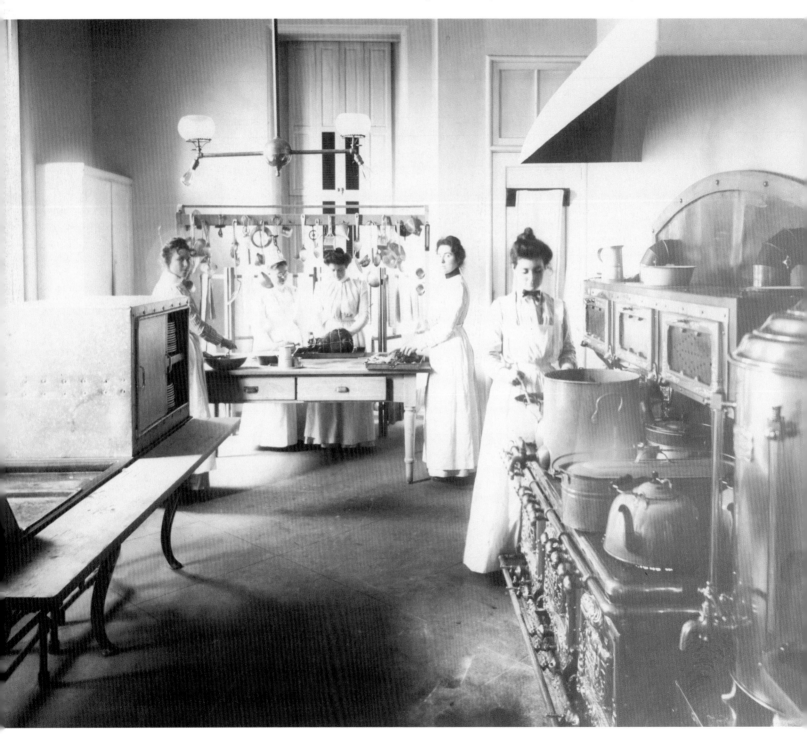

very often outweighed giving us a balanced training. Mine was almost wholly surgical and gyn with only the briefest glimpse of medicine," Mrs. Athey recalled.[39]

In 1941 Effie Jane Taylor, 1907, reminisced about her feelings when she came to Johns Hopkins from her home in Canada: "I will always remember the calm and peace which seemed to fall upon my whole being as I entered the great, dimly lighted hall of Johns Hopkins Hospital at one o'clock in the morning and looked for the first time upon the inspiring figure of Christ and read his compassionate face of welcome to a forlorn and anxious probationer about to enter a new world."[40] Miss Taylor went on to describe her anxieties about entering such a renowned program and her tardiness arriving because of severe weather in western New York State. She recalled how kind the staff had been to her that first night and how caring Miss Lawler was. She believed being at Hopkins was really a family experience in spite of all the hard work and effort. She felt she belonged right away. Miss Taylor created the initial psychiatric nursing service when Phipps Clinic opened in 1913 and went on to a significant career after her graduation.

In 1912 Anna Dryden Wolf, a graduate of Goucher College, came to Hopkins to become a nurse. She found the discipline in the program "terrifying" and felt the students were not expected to think for themselves. This impression was quite accurate if the detailed rules for students in this period are any indication. Students were instructed that all regulations had to be obeyed at all times. They were told how late they could study, when they had to be at meals, and how long they had to eat. Laundry had to be done with military precision, and all students were subject to criticism if any rule was not followed to the letter. Although Miss Wolf believed that the instructors were trying to impress upon the students the need for discipline in life-and-death circumstances, she thought such severe discipline instilled fear and hindered learning. (Wolf spent the rest of her career trying to establish educational systems in which fear was not a primary motivation.) The friendships she established with her peers and instructors at Johns Hopkins lasted her entire career.[41]

Anna Wolf described an average day in her 1912–15 era, which consisted of prayers at 6:50 after a 6:30 breakfast. Even before breakfast, student rooms had to be "slicked up, beds made," ready for inspection. Assignments were functional, with each student taking turns doing medications or treatments in addition to patient care. Responsibilities were heavy, especially on night duty, when a student was accountable for half a unit. Day assignments were accomplished between the busy periods in the morning and early evening, with a short break in the afternoon. Classes were in the evenings with instructors or physicians. Miss Wolf recalled having textbooks but few library resources.[42]

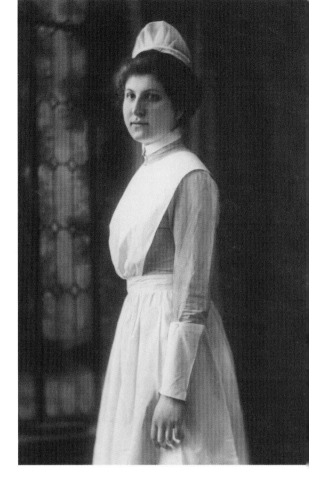

When Anna Dryden Wolf arrived at the nursing school, she already had a degree from Goucher College. After graduating in 1915, she went immediately to Columbia University to earn a master's degree. There, she met Adelaide Nutting, who became her lifelong mentor. Nutting galvanized Wolf's belief that nursing education should be separate from service in the hospital.

Adelaide Nutting was this giant, forward, visionary thinker. Elsie Lawler ran the school from 1910 to 1940. She was very old school and did not really push an agenda. She really listened to the docs. She had only a high school education, and a lot of students had college degrees when they came to the School of Nursing. She was running the school with an iron hand, was not very lenient in terms of bending rules, and really didn't move the school forward that much. Then you get Anna D. Wolf, who was another visionary, another Adelaide Nutting.

Paula Einaudi

*What is a nurses' home? It is a home where
two hundred and fifty young women, from two
hundred and fifty homes, where there were
five hundred varieties of parents, come to live
for three years. They grew up in those homes,
but in this home they experience a second growth.
The home is full of growing pains.*

Routine, 1932

Hampton House, named to honor the school's first
director, Isabel Hampton Robb, opened in 1926. All
rooms were singles and featured sinks with running
water. The new dormitory, primarily for students, was
on the west side of Broadway, leaving the Nurses'
Home available for hospital nursing staff. Hampton
House's large parlor provided plenty of room to
socialize, and there were recreational facilities in the
basement and on the roof level.

The construction of Hampton House, which opened in 1926 and was
enlarged in 1938, relieved severe overcrowding among students who
had been living in various structures around the hospital since the
Main Residence had become too small. One student who entered the
training school before Hampton House was completed recalled sharing living quarters with several classmates in an old building south of
the hospital on Broadway, where the students could just make out the
words "livery stable" on the front of the building.[43] Hampton House
made an enormous difference in nursing students' lives, giving them a
common dormitory experience and a setting for organized activities
that became a regular part of their school days, as well as for special
occasions like dances and formal teas. With a communal living area, a
new culture of student life began. Shared experiences promoted lifelong
friendships among generations of students who spent three formative
years in Hampton House.

After World War I, probationers' uniforms changed to pink dresses
with cuffs and white aprons. These students were known as "pinkies,"
and capping was introduced in this period. Students received their
Hopkins caps and began to wear blue student uniforms after the
difficult probationary period had ended.

Lucile Petry Leone, 1927, loved to recount a particularly memorable
anecdote from her student days. "I remember Miss Lawler making surprise rounds on old Ward M when I was head nurse (still a student of
course). She was stately in her black uniform with the white saucer cap
we students had seen only in two other places, the portraits of Isabel
Hampton Robb and Adelaide Nutting." On one occasion, a patient on
Petry's unit saw Miss Lawler and asked who that fine-looking lady
was. Before Petry could answer, another patient said, "Oh don't you
know who that was? That was Johns Hopkins' widow."[44]

By 1929 there were more theoretical classes and more nursing content in the curriculum. Clinical work continued to provide students
with challenging situations, however. Vivian Weinhardt William, 1929,
saved a vivid article describing a busy day on Ward E, a twenty-four-bed

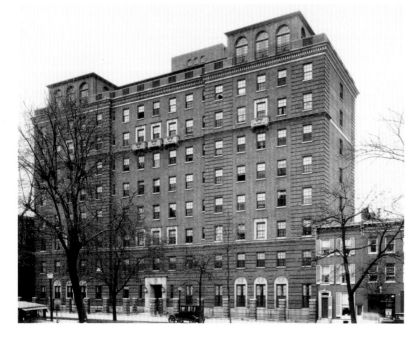

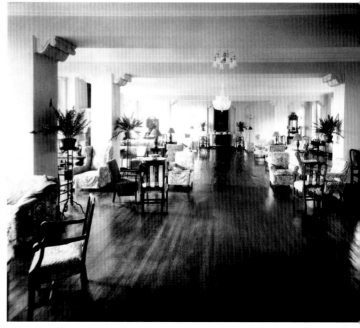

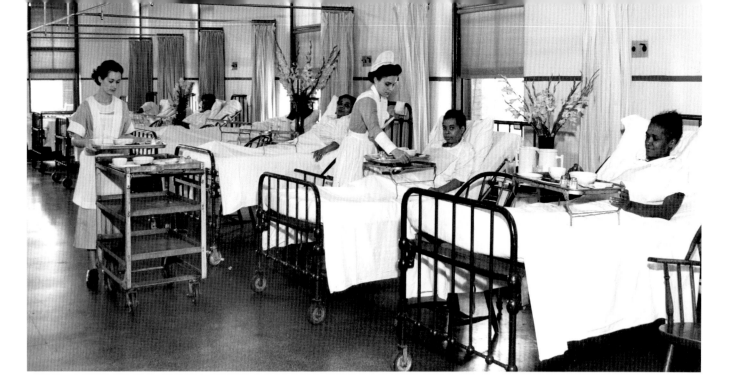

round ward, with twelve beds on each side and two adjacent back rooms with nine pediatric beds. On the day described, all the beds were full and all the adults were acute surgical cases. The patients needed morning care, which included baths and hourly temperature assessments. Four students, under the supervision of a head nurse and one senior student, were responsible for this care. The students came on duty at seven, and morning care was to be completed by nine, when the doctors made rounds. Each student was assigned by area to one side of the unit or to the pediatric patients. The students all had split hours, such as 7–11 A.M. and 4–7 P.M. or 7–9, 2–5, and 7–11.[45]

Miss Lawler had been superintendent for almost twenty years and was very experienced in selecting students by the time K. Virginia Betzold applied for admission. Lawler was not eager to have as a student a secretary with eleven years of experience; such an independent woman might not handle the restrictions and rigors of nurse's training well. However, Miss Betzold persuaded Miss Lawler that she could succeed, and she entered the school in 1930. At that time students worked a fifty-two-hour week, and most units had students as charge nurses. (Hospital expansion had stressed nursing resources in the 1920s, and then the Depression limited its resources to hire nurses.) Students had adequate classrooms and the instructors and doctors provided excellent classes, Miss Betzold remembered, but students had to do much of the cleaning and support work in the hospital. (She described making bandages, threading needles for surgery, and scrubbing equipment.)[46]

Student activities were few except for holidays, special hospital events such as the turtle derby, and occasional Hampton House activities planned by the students themselves. One long-held tradition was caroling in the hospital on Christmas Eve. Students would gather around the statue of Christ and walk with flashlights through the hospital grounds. Miss Lawler remembered: "In all my years at the hospital

In his 1873 letter to the hospital trustees setting forth the principles they were to follow, benefactor Johns Hopkins wrote that the hospital must provide for "the indigent sick of this city and its environs, without regard to sex, age, or color." The first ward "exclusively for colored people" opened with amenities similar to those in the white public wards. Some departments, such as the Harriet Lane Home, never separated patients by race. True integration at the hospital began in the 1950s and came gradually to various sections. The nursing student standing by the cart in the gynecology ward was a probationer who had not yet earned her cap.

The library was over in the Main Residence. The dining room was in one area of the basement and the practice ward was in another. Every morning before we went on duty we went to Hampton House for prayers. You had to be there at about five minutes to seven. I was always one who would wake up wide awake. One time we were going across Broadway. I guess I was talking a blue streak and Marie Lowe said, "Mary Farr, will you shut up?"

Mary Farr Heeg, 1941

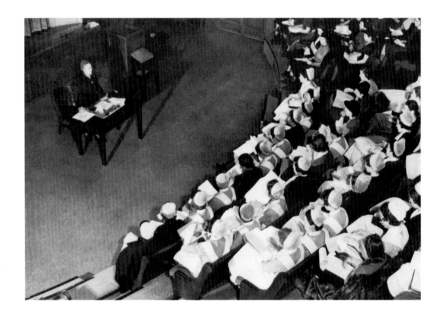

Right: Dr. Esther Richards, who graduated from the School of Medicine in 1915, was a prominent member of the psychiatric faculty. Many nursing students attended her lecture in Hurd hall in 1939, probably on her specialty, the behavioral and mental problems of children and adolescents.

Opposite, above left: First-year students took classes on preparing surgical dressings, an important skill in a time before such items were mass produced.

Opposite, above right: Nursing students rarely had holidays. Although they sang carols on the wards and tried to make things festive, in many ways, Christmas was just another workday.

Opposite, below: On May 23, 1924, Elsie Lawler addressed the largest graduating class in the history of the school. Its sixty members hailed from twenty-four states and three foreign countries. The day must have been chilly for the outdoor ceremony: many nurses and students wore capes and most guests wore coats.

There were eight ex-schoolteachers in my class. This was during the Depression and perhaps some of us saw war in the future. I was twenty-eight and a college graduate. We were housed in the Main Residence for six months, and my roommate was eighteen and just out of high school. She would get terribly homesick. Whenever she'd get really bad and decided that she just had to go home, I would get her busy cleaning the room or doing something. We were probationers for six months. Then we moved over to Hampton House and we had our own rooms.

Mary Farr Heeg, 1941

I missed only once in taking part in the carols. I am no singer but I made a good end to the procession, pushing the singers ahead and reminding them that they were singing carols and did not wish to make the impression of an approaching mob. In my last years at the hospital Miss [Mabel] Hay made a good assistant pusher."[47]

The turtle derby has been an enduring tradition at Johns Hopkins Hospital over the years. The event began in 1931 on the tennis courts and grassy area behind the administration building when two house officers, Edmund S. Kelly and Harold Finkelstein, learned that Ben Frisby, the head janitor of the hospital, had been collecting live turtles that lived on the hospital grounds. The two doctors were fans of racing and concocted a contest to "race" the plodding reptiles for the sake of good fun. Clinical divisions and academic groups entered turtles for a fee and watched them compete for a cup, which was actually a fancy specimen glass from the Brady Urological Institute. The first derby winner was Sir Walter, sponsored by Dr. Walter Dandy's neurosurgery group, with Rest Cure coming in second, and third place won by Ectopic. The event attracted house staff, nurses, students, and patients. What started as a day of fun became an annual event that everyone in the Hopkins community looked forward to.[48]

Graduation traditions evolved as the school and hospital changed, but the event remained the highlight of each school year. The earliest graduations were held in the rotunda of the hospital around the statue of Christ. As the classes grew and the need for additional space became an issue, the event was moved to the Phipps Garden following a solemn procession from the administration building. Speakers came from the medical staff and nursing leadership of each generation. Students proudly wore their official white uniforms with their Hopkins caps to symbolize the transition to graduate life.

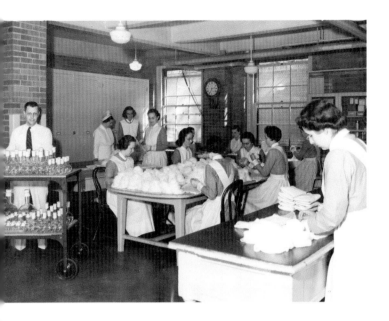

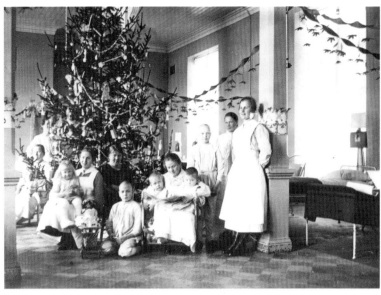

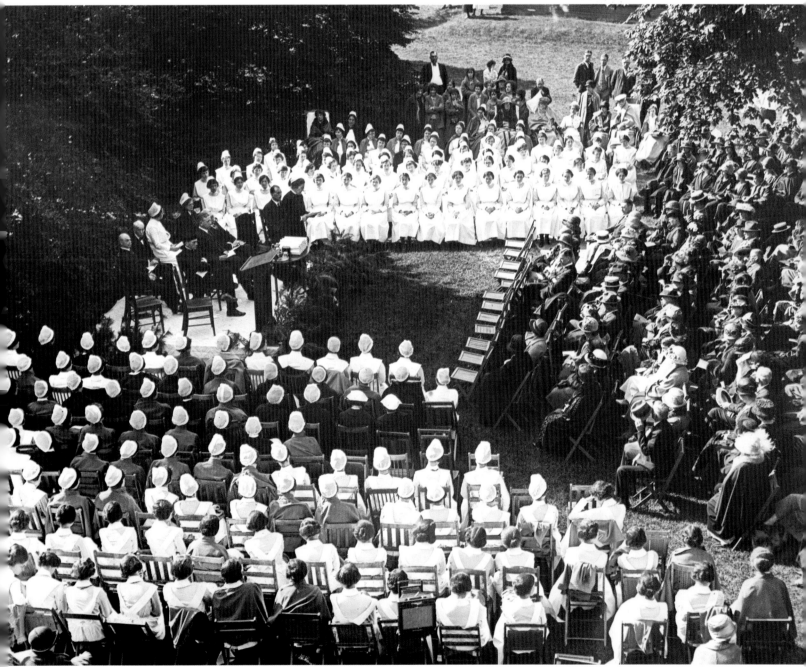

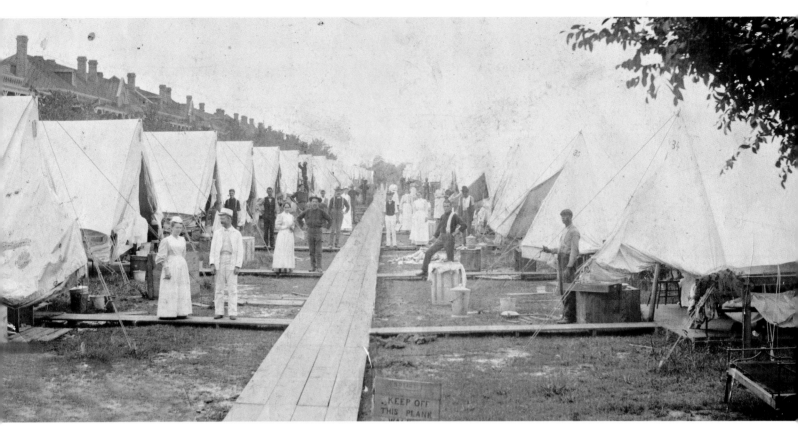

EXTRAORDINARY SERVICE
IN EXTREME CONDITIONS

*The school and the alumnae have steadily worked
together in the interests of nursing education,
and the improvement of professional life and
status. And this close cooperation between school
and alumnae is so essential to the true interests
of both that it should in every way be fostered
and encouraged. It is not the well-ordered
nursing service of the hospital but the alumnae
which stands to the world as the highest
achievement of the training school. The steady
progress of the school is vital to the health,
life and progress of the alumnae. That they
should individually and collectively be found
equal to the demands and to the opportunities
which are so insistently pressing upon them,
is the richest reward the school can ever have,
the public test and tribute to the worth of its work.*

M. Adelaide Nutting in a 1916 editorial
in the alumnae magazine

The first fifty years of the nursing school at Johns Hopkins produced leaders for the fledgling nursing profession during war and peace. A cursory view of professional organizational histories, biographical dictionaries, and institutional histories for hospitals and universities reveals a significant number of Hopkins graduates. Foreign service and international outreach were also prevalent during this early period. One of the symbols for the school's fiftieth-anniversary celebration was a world map showing where the graduates had scattered. Some of the earliest alumnae served as nurses in the Spanish-American War and on the committee that was formed to promote a military nursing corps and military status for nurses. Hopkins nurses provided valuable national and international leadership during World War I and its aftermath. Early records of the alumnae association are filled with letters, reports, and articles of rank-and-file graduates serving as pathfinders in every type of institutional and community-based practice.

When the school was less than ten years old the Spanish-American War broke out. Few stories of the graduates who served during this war period have survived. Yssabella Waters, 1897, who served with the Seventh Army Corps in Savannah, Georgia, wrote to her public-health nursing colleague Lillian Wald, in New York, that the temperature in the camp was 110 degrees in the shade, a condition that was "not conducive to letter writing when off duty—and we are not off duty much." Waters reported that she had been "in charge of a ward in Jacksonville in which there were forty-five typhoid patients." Her workdays were fifteen hours long. She was promoted to superintendent when the previous head nurse was sent home with typhoid fever. Waters and the fifty-seven nurses in her charge expected to leave for Cuba the next day.[49]

An article that appeared in the *Atlanta Journal* depicted daily activities of nurses in the military hospital in Fort McPherson, Georgia. Despite serious illnesses among the soldiers, there was a low death rate, and nurses were described as the "heroines" of the war. Seventy-five nurses were assigned to the base, including Charity Babcock, 1897. "The work of the nurses consists in the keeping of the beds tidy and clean, the personal supervision of each patient, the taking of the temperature of each patient every four hours, the feeding of the sick, the bathing and rubbing of all, requiring the plunging in ice baths of fever patients, and other duties too numerous to describe." The article continued:

The nurses are on their feet almost continuously while on duty. It is considered unprofessional to sit on the bed of patient and they are so constantly in demand by one patient and another that they get out but a few moments during the day to sit down. The keeping of a record of patients in a hospital ward is no small undertaking in itself. In the case of fever patients not only is the ordinary record kept, but a chart for each has to be made showing the rise and fall of the temperature during the day.[50]

The author was particularly impressed with the patriotic spirit of the nurses, noting that some of them had been making as much as $100 per month before the war. In the army, they gave up "comfort and pleasant surroundings to work for $30 a month and live on any fare." The writer also noted their fastidiousness: "One thing regarding the appearance of the nurses is especially noteworthy. No matter when you see them their costumes are always fresh and clean and look as if they had just come

Opposite: Florence Nightingale established the benefits of having trained nurses serve near the battlefront in the mid-nineteenth century. By the century's end, graduates of the Johns Hopkins nursing school were involved with the United States military as it fought the Spanish-American War. Charity Babcock, 1897, volunteered with the American Red Cross the year after she graduated, and soon found herself serving in a hospital of tents, a long way from Baltimore.

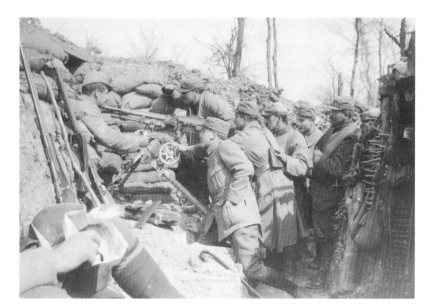

By the time the United States entered World War I in 1917, more than a hundred nursing alumnae were already in Europe serving with the Red Cross. Doctors and nurses established hospitals as close as possible to the trenches, where thousands of European soldiers had been fighting since 1914.

from the ironing board. And they keep their wards and patients as tidy as their own persons."[51]

Charity Babcock worked twelve-hour duty, either days or nights, under contract at Fort McPherson for $30 per month and board, caring for men ill with typhoid and yellow fever.[52] She received a certificate of recognition for her service.

The most serious challenge facing the first generation of Hopkins nurses was World War I. Within weeks of the outbreak of hostilities in 1914, nurses from Baltimore were recruited for the American Red Cross mission, later dubbed the Mercy Ship. This vessel carried ten units of doctors and nurses to Europe, with two units being sent to each of the five countries already at war. Alice E. Henderson, 1907, was recruited to direct Unit B, which was sent to Pau, France, in October 1914. Vashti Bartlett, 1906, was also a member of Unit B. Each unit had twelve nurses and three surgeons. These nurses were part of a group of pioneers in relief work during modern war. They all practiced under primitive conditions in makeshift hospitals. Much of what the American Red Cross learned from this first effort to provide medical care to war victims during 1914–15 was used to help nurses and physicians in 1917, when the United States entered the conflict.[53]

Unit B set up in the Palais d'Hiver (the Winter Palace, which had been a casino) in Pau, where facilities were available to care for 166 patients. Miss Henderson wrote back to headquarters that she'd had little idea of what war really was about until she saw "a train of wounded come from the front, the men so dirty, so ragged, so tired, so sick, yet not one of them ready to admit that he is either hungry or exhausted or that his wound is more than a scratch."[54]

Nurses in this first wave treated men with sloughing bedsores, advanced tetanus (the first groups of European war recruits, who had not been immunized against tetanus, fought on manured fields), and infected wounds of all descriptions. The nurses ascertained which uniforms would be most serviceable when water was scarce, and they learned the hard way which equipment was vital or unnecessary. The Mercy Ship nurses served in Europe from August 1914 until December 1915.

Many early Hopkins graduates came from Canada (which entered the war in 1914), so there were Hopkins nurses involved with the war from the beginning. Gertrude Muldrew, 1904, joined the University of Toronto's base hospital in 1915 and served in France, Malta, Gallipoli, Solonica, and England, for which work she was honored by King George and the Royal Red Cross. She was promoted to matron and by 1918 was in charge of a Canadian general hospital in England that had a capacity of fifteen hundred beds.[55]

In 1916 Jane Delano, director of the American Red Cross Nursing Service, recruited Clara Dutton Noyes, 1896, to become the director of

You forgot all about nursing etiquette.
You forgot many things that you had been taught.
You only remembered that it was no place for
any but those who would roll up their sleeves and
dig in and work, and work, and work. It was
work, eat, sleep. One day was the same as the
next. You forgot the days of the week. You thought
not so much how many you could nurse as how
many you could keep from dying.

Gertrude H. Bowling, 1915

Opposite, *above*: The American Red Cross hospital at Tumen, Russia, cared for refugees and soldiers wounded in the Russian Revolution. As in World War I, large public buildings were often transformed into hospitals to accommodate the vast numbers of casualties.

Opposite, *below left*: During much of 1919, Vashti Bartlett, 1906, served with the Red Cross in Vladivostok, where she tried to establish order from the chaos of war for hundreds of orphaned Russian children.

Opposite, *below right*: Vashti Bartlett, the offspring of a prominent Baltimore family, epitomized spirited alumnae who wanted to use their nursing skills around the world. From Newfoundland to Belgium, from Siberia to Haiti, she found time to take and collect photographs as well as care for patients.

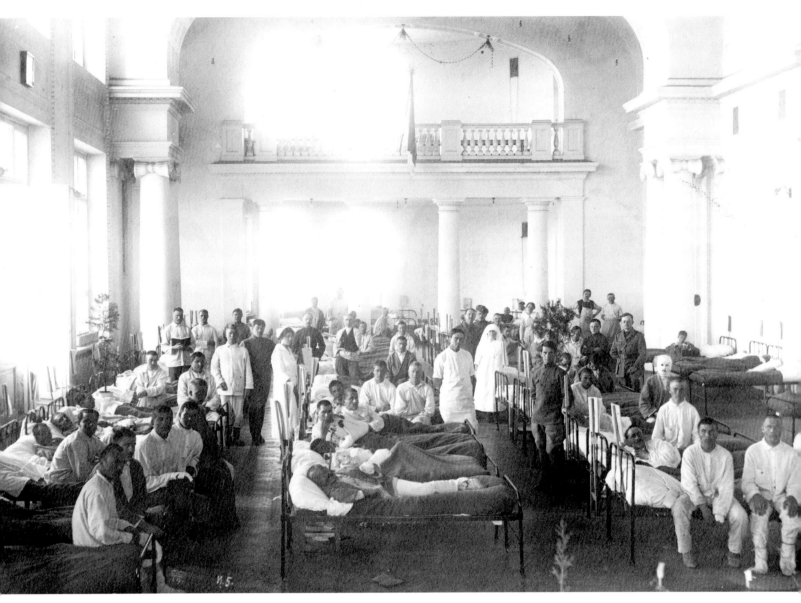

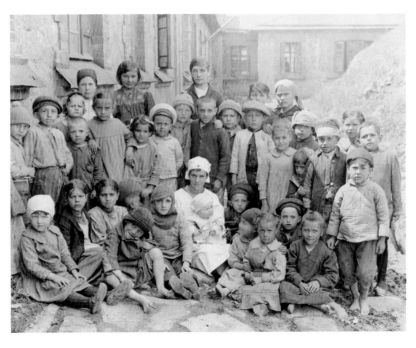

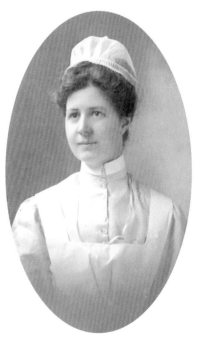

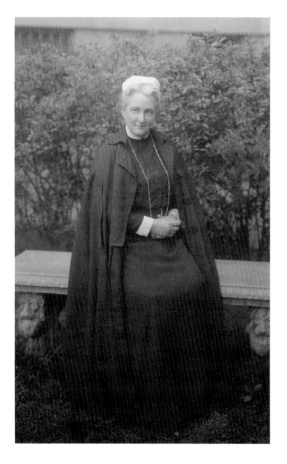

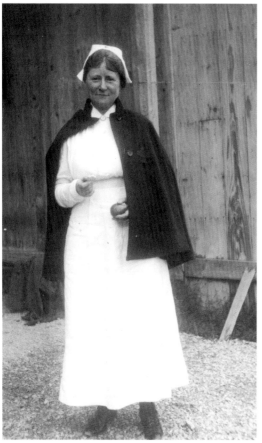

the Bureau of Nursing. Noyes was superintendent of the Bellevue and allied hospitals nursing school in New York when Miss Delano contacted her, and she reluctantly agreed to go to Washington and oversee the recruiting, equipping, and educating of all nurses entering the American Red Cross. At the time, the Red Cross was the entry route for all nurses wanting to serve in the military. All Red Cross nurses were army reservists. This meant that Noyes oversaw all the activities of American Red Cross nurses serving in Red Cross facilities, as well as all nurses serving in the U.S. Army and Navy. She led the Washington staff in daily operations and wrote and spoke extensively about the need for Red Cross nurses in the war effort. She also worked for standardized procedures and treatments to be used within the American Red Cross Nursing Service.[56]

After the United States entered the war, a major portion of the medical treatment for victims came from units organized by hospitals from around the country. These units served the U.S. Army as base hospitals during the war. Base Hospital No. 18 was staffed primarily with personnel from Johns Hopkins, and Bessie Baker, 1902, was the chief nurse. She had sixty-four nurses under her supervision, thirteen of whom had been active staff members at the Johns Hopkins Hospital before the war. Miss Baker had been assistant superintendent for the nursing school. All other staff members were either former head nurses or assistant head nurses. Baker was described as a nurse with a good sense of humor, twinkling brown eyes, and a high level of energy and enthusiasm in all her clinical activities.[57]

Dr. John M. T. Finney was the medical director of the unit. In later years, Finney wrote about his impressions of the Hopkins nurses under his command:

Too much cannot be said in praise of the nursing staff. Under great difficulties and very trying conditions they all, from Miss Baker down, acquitted themselves with great credit. It was surprising how quickly they adapted themselves to the changed conditions, uncomfortable surroundings, lack of ordinary conveniences, petty annoyances of one sort or another, and the thousand and one unpleasant things that they had to put up with. . . . They were a splendid body of women—well trained, uncomplaining, never hesitating to do what needed to be done, regardless [of] whether or not it strictly belonged to the province of a nurse. Their work was done under great difficulties; the weather was cold, damp and rainy much of the time, the accommodations were poor and many of the bare necessities of life were lacking, to say nothing of the comfort and luxuries. Quite a number of nurses made the supreme sacrifice and gave up their lives for the cause.[58]

The Hopkins unit arrived in France in late June 1917 and was assigned to Bazoille on the Meuse River, where they set up a hospital in a chateau that could accommodate a thousand patients. One Hopkins nurse wrote

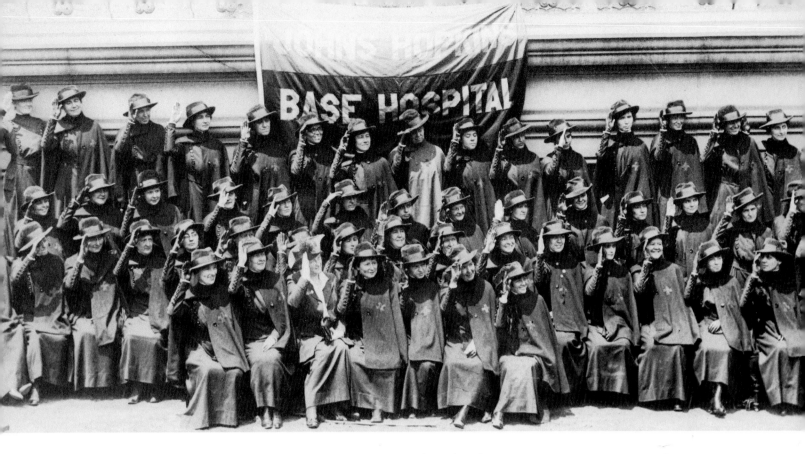

back to headquarters about her patients: "They are mostly boys from little towns and from every walk of life. . . . To us they are just sick and lonely boys whose life we could make a bit more cheery."[59]

The nurses in Base Hospital 18 dealt with clinical problems similar to those of their predecessors in 1914, except that the assaults by the allies were much heavier and casualties from them could overwhelm the best of hospitals. This group of nurses also had to cope with a new problem: the victims of poison gas attacks. One night after eleven o'clock, some two hundred fifty blindfolded, gassed men dressed in tattered uniforms arrived at the hospital. The young men had to lead each other as they groped to find their way, blinded and suffering from blistered skin and lungs. Most of the more seriously injured men died within two to three weeks from untreatable pneumonia. After one gruesome experience, Bessie Baker wrote: "As the long line of stretchers continued to be moved in hour after hour, each one holding what seemed to be a case more helpless than the last, we can only pray for the end of such brutality."[60]

The problems of sickness and disease compounded the victims' injuries and placed the nurses at risk. The winter of 1918 was cold, and there was no heat in the hospital or the nurses' sleeping quarters. Many nurses developed chilblains (frostbite) and joked about forming a "Chilblain Club." Although they kept their sense of humor, Miss Baker was concerned; she would find nurses soaking their feet in cold water in their rooms, just to warm them up enough to go back on duty. "There came a time," she wrote, "when we began to believe stories about people freezing in their beds."[61]

Grace Baxter, 1894, and Alice Fitzgerald, 1906, also served overseas during the war, but their service was quite different from that of the

Nurses in Base Hospital No. 18, which included many Johns Hopkins nurses and doctors, posed for the camera before they set sail for Europe in 1917, after the United States declared war on Germany. Their departure left the hospital and the school severely short-staffed.

Opposite, above: Clara Dutton Noyes, 1896, was superintendent of Bellevue Hospital in New York when she was asked, in 1916, to head up recruiting and assigning nurses for the American Red Cross. By the war's end, she was responsible for more than twenty-one thousand nurses. Noyes became president of the American Nurses Association in 1921.

Opposite, below: Bessie Baker, 1902, was assistant supervisor for the nursing school when she was named head nurse for Base Hospital No. 18. She and her nurses faced extreme conditions, from both contagion and unforgiving weather conditions.

Members of Base Hospital No. 18 arrived in France on June 28, 1917, and set up a permanent base at Bazoilles-sur-Meuse. With colleagues in several other base hospitals situated there, they treated more than twenty thousand sick and wounded patients before the war ended.

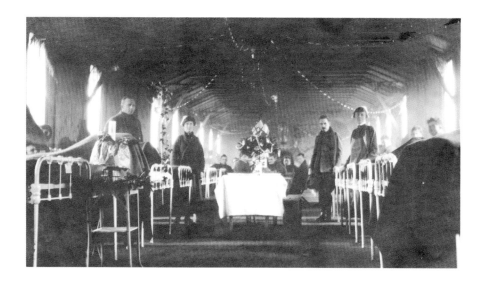

Poisonous gas posed a new threat to medical staff as well as their patients. Nurses were fitted with gas masks, an effort to protect them from the horrible effects they had seen in many of their patients.

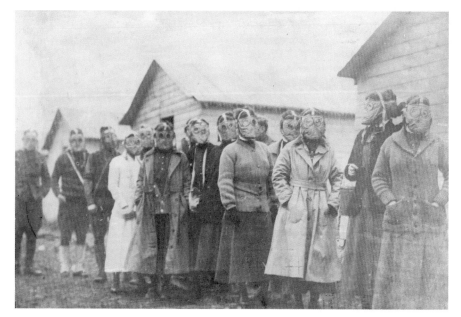

Opposite, above: During the war, Grace Baxter, 1894, supervised nurses at the American hospital for wounded Italians. Born in Italy, she returned there after graduating from nursing school.

Right: Before the war, Baxter was in charge of Croce Azzura, a nursing school in Naples, where she utilized instructional techniques she had learned at Johns Hopkins. The nurses she trained were soon in demand by Italian doctors.

Opposite, below: Alice Fitzgerald, 1906, also was born and raised in Italy. Like many of her contemporaries, she entered nursing school in her late twenties and went on to a career with the American Red Cross.

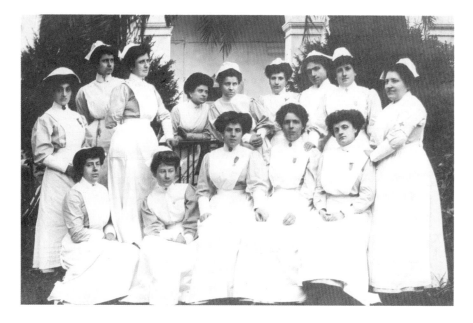

members of Base Hospital 18. Miss Baxter was born and grew up in Florence, Italy, a child of English parents. After graduating from Johns Hopkins, she returned to Italy and practiced for several years. During this period she wrote articles on Italian nursing activities for the *American Journal of Nursing*. She went back to Hopkins to study pediatrics and then returned again to Italy, this time to Naples, as the matron of nurses at Gesu' Maria Hospital. She directed a school called Croce Azzura, which prepared many leaders for modern Italian nursing. In a letter about her efforts in the school, she told how she used the textbooks and her notes from classes at Hopkins to fashion an educational program for her students.

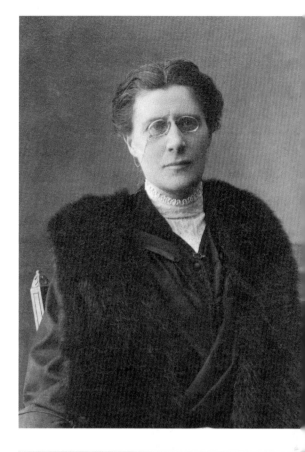

One of Baxter's early difficulties was finding time to train students on the wards while having to leave the rest of the patients in the hands of untrained servants. Once she had prepared them, her students took over the rest of the wards and were highly esteemed by the Italian physicians.[62] Like her American counterparts, Grace Baxter struggled to raise standards in her nursing program. In the beginning, she had to accept women into the program who did not have the kind of educational, moral, or intellectual qualities needed in the profession. As the program developed such persons dropped out or ceased to apply at all. Doctors quickly learned the difference between the educated and the untrained nurses in the field, and they sought out Baxter's graduates.[63] Baxter also inaugurated Red Cross training in Italy. During the war, she accepted the position of superintendent of nurses at the American Hospital for Italian wounded. Afterward, she turned her attention to the care of the poor in Naples, initiating a dispensary and a district-nursing program in Naples.

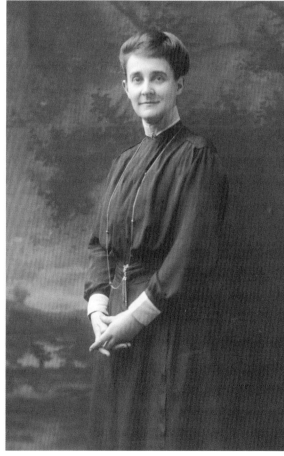

Alice Fitzgerald, 1906, also was born and raised in Florence, Italy. Educated in Switzerland and Italy, she spoke Italian, French, German, and English fluently. She entered Johns Hopkins at the age of twenty-eight and practiced in Italy after graduation. She served as a volunteer in the great earthquake at Messina in 1908. The next year she returned to the United States and practiced as a supervisor and nursing administrator in several facilities. In 1915 she was selected by a committee in Boston to serve as the Edith Cavell Memorial Nurse in the British Army.[64] Miss Fitzgerald sailed for England in early 1916 and served with the British Army for one year, then transferred to the American Red Cross and served in various hospitals for the remainder of the war.

For twelve years after the end of the war, Alice Fitzgerald traveled internationally for the American Red Cross and the Rockefeller Foundation, teaching nursing and organizing nursing schools. She wrote regularly for nursing journals and reported her experiences to colleagues at home. Fitzgerald demonstrated a spirit of adventure and a

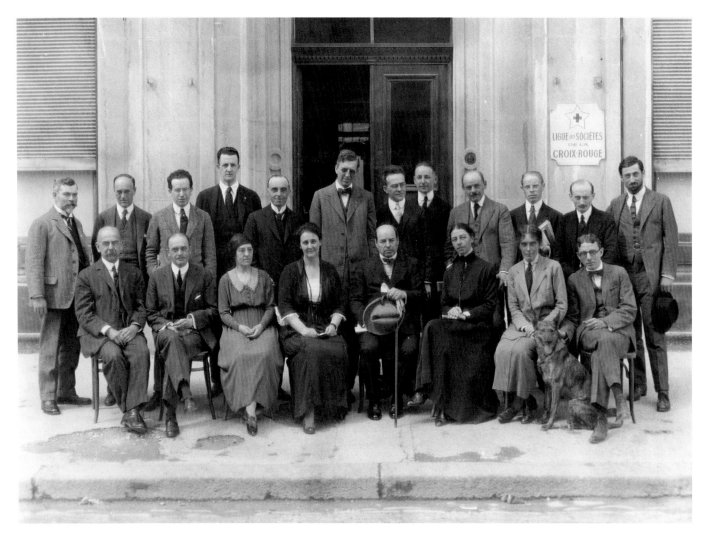

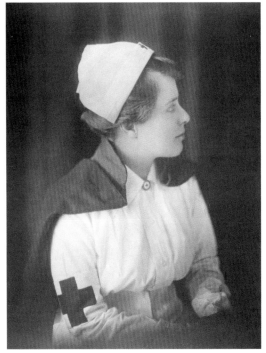

cross-cultural practice that helped her be a pioneer from Europe to the Philippines to Thailand.

Many other Hopkins alumnae served in World War I and some made extraordinary contributions after the armistice. Katherine Olmstead, 1912, served in Romania with the American Red Cross in 1917 and 1918. She entered military service with experience in public-health and tuberculosis nursing. (She is credited with pioneering public-health nursing in Wisconsin.) She served in the war as part of a small staff (twelve doctors and twelve nurses) in a makeshift hospital that had to move because of hostilities. Describing the last months of her time in Romania, Olmstead wrote:

There are countless refugees. Quite a number of refugee girls are helping around the hospital and the Boy Scouts are generally helpful. I went out this morning to look up a badly burned baby who had not been brought back to the hospital and I found a family of six children under ten, the father a prisoner in Germany, the mother evidently ill with typhus. Every child was stark naked, huddling beside a queer little plastic stove; typhus evidently does not take the children. . . .

We are living in a huge corridor affair in one wing of the hospital. In the evenings we play cards if we can get warm enough; usually we are so cold and hungry that we crawl into our straw bunks and forget everything as soon as possible.[65]

Olmstead's tenure in Romania ended when the Germans ordered the medical staff out of the country. (The medical staff escaped through Russia on a train they themselves drove.) Olmstead returned to the United States and served as the executive secretary of the National Organization of Public Health Nurses. In 1921 she was appointed assistant to Alice Fitzgerald, director of nursing for the League of Red Cross Societies; in 1922 she succeeded Fitzgerald and served for six more years. During her tenure Katherine Olmstead directed the establishment of many schools of nursing. She was decorated by several nations, and her awards were later donated to the Hopkins School of Nursing. While in Europe, she studied cooking at the Cordon Bleu. And even though she established a restaurant in Sodus, New York, which she ran as the Normandy Inn until her death in 1964, she served on the executive board of the New York State Nursing Council for War Service during World War II and also continued to teach Red Cross home-nursing and nutrition courses.[66]

Ellen LaMotte, 1900, was a prolific writer who also pioneered in the field of public health and tuberculosis care before the war. During those years she penned many articles and also a book on tuberculosis nursing. She served in France with the French Army in 1915 and 1916; afterward she wrote a book about her experiences. LaMotte then traveled to the Far East and discovered a nascent disaster related to the abuse of opium, which inspired her to write a series of articles on that subject. She continued her career as a writer, receiving several awards for her campaign to alert the public to the dangers of opium.[67]

LaMotte's book on her experiences in Europe was an unvarnished account of the grim realities of war:

When he could stand it no longer, he fired a revolver up through the roof of his mouth, but he made a mess of it. The ball tore out his left eye, and then lodged somewhere under his skull, so they bundled him into an ambulance and carried him screaming, to the nearest field hospital. The journey was made in double quick time, over rough Belgian roads. To save his life, he must reach the hospital without delay, and if he was bounced to death jolting along at breakneck speed, it did not matter. That was understood. He was a deserter, and discipline must be maintained. Since he had failed in the job, he must be saved, he must be nursed back to health, until he was well enough to be stood up against the wall and shot. This is war.[68]

Emotional problems, depression, shell shock, and suicide were not addressed openly in this era, so the opening of this book, which alluded to these issues, revealed the writer's courage as well as the horrors of war.

Opposite, above: When prominent members of the League of Red Cross Societies gathered in France in 1920, Alice Fitzgerald, 1906, its director of nursing, sat on the right of the man holding a cane.

Opposite, below: Katherine Olmstead, 1912, succeeded Alice Fitzgerald as director of nursing of the League of Red Cross Societies in 1922. During the war, when this portrait was made, she served with the American Red Cross in Romania, where she experienced heartbreaking and life-threatening adventures.

Ellen LaMotte, 1900, wrote graphically about the terrible conditions she witnessed during World War I in *The Backwash of War*, as well as articles about public-health issues relating to opium abuse.

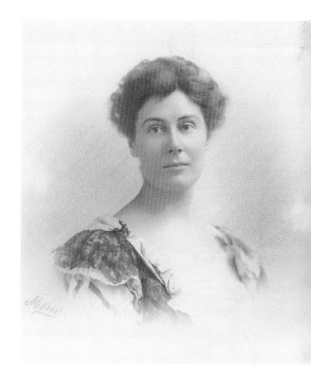

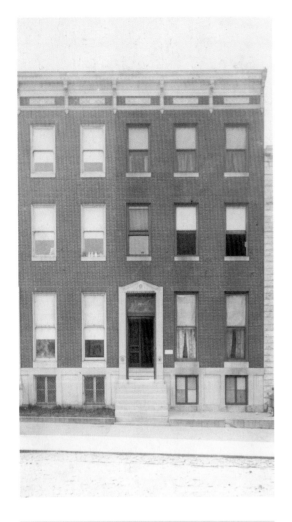

The book also gave evidence that may explain why LaMotte never practiced nursing after the war. She was a creative writer who saw the world from a point of view unconventional for a nurse. Another example is revealed in a comment about her patients: "Five men here, lying in a row, all [with] ptomaine poisoning, due to some rank tinned stuff they'd been eating. Yonder there, three men with itch-filthy business! Their hands all covered with it, tearing at their bodies with clawlike nails! The orderlies had not washed them very thoroughly—small blame to them!"[69] Compared to her peers who were writing for the general public, Ellen LaMotte was far more honest and graphic about her feelings about the consequences of armed conflict.

At the same time these and many other alumnae were blazing new trails abroad, still more graduates were entering private duty as their field of practice. The development of the Nurses' Club and the Johns Hopkins Nurses' Registry enabled Hopkins graduates to pursue more effectively the primary form of employment for nurses during the first fifty years of the school's history. The club was the result of the care Charlotte Ewell, 1893, gave to a young girl in the girl's family home. The girl's father, George W. Grafflin, wanted to show his appreciation, so he offered Johns Hopkins nurses a small house at 219½ East North Avenue free of charge to ease a housing shortage for private-duty nurses. The alumnae association agreed to manage the home and named it the Nurses' Club. Dr. Henry Hurd loaned the association money to establish the facility, and Dr. William Osler installed a phone

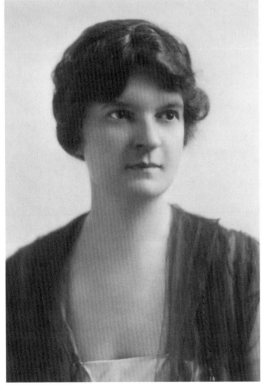

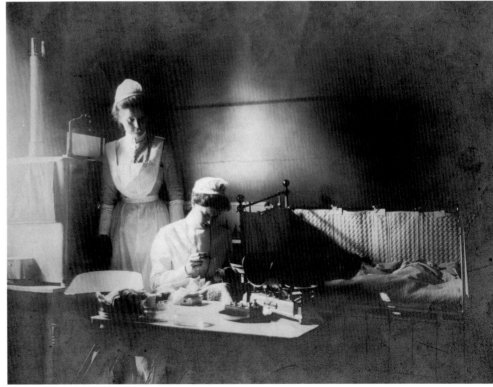

and paid telephone charges for a year. The building opened on July 4, 1895, with a reception provided by Dr. Osler. The group issued information sheets informing the public of the availability of graduate nurses to provide care in every type of case. Fees were 75¢ per hour before 6 P.M. and $1 per hour after 6 P.M. for short-term duty and $3–$4 per day for extended care. By 1897 a formal nurses' registry had been organized. By 1900 more than six hundred patients had been cared for and by 1927 the number of cases covered exceeded two thousand.[70]

In addition to pioneering efforts in education, private duty, and military service, early graduates of the nursing program at Johns Hopkins led the profession in public health. Mary Lent, 1895, began practicing as head nurse with the Instructive Visiting Nurse Association in Baltimore in 1903 and later became the superintendent of that organization. She led the association to provide innovative services to tuberculosis patients (Katherine Olmstead, her niece, came to work with her), and she created instructive programs in preventive health hygiene and home nursing for several population groups in the city. She also began a program that provided health screening for all athletes playing sports in Baltimore. During World War I, Lent traveled throughout the country for the U.S. Public Health Service and organized public-health nursing zones for direct services to populations in need. Covering more than twelve thousand miles in less than two years, she organized nursing activities in thirty-seven geographical zones with a directed a staff of two hundred nurses. This effort was needed because large concentrations of troops and their families, as well as the organization of war industries, created unhealthy situations all over the country.[71]

Mabel Wilcox, 1911, traveled to rural Kauai in the Hawaiian Islands to establish a public-health practice. She started as a tuberculosis nurse under the Territorial Board of Health, receiving a salary of $125 per month, and expanded her duties to include most of the prevention activities characteristic of the public-health services she had known in Baltimore. Wilcox recruited nurses in the Hawaiian territory for service during World War I and later served for two years in France as an American Red Cross nurse. After the war she returned to Kauai—her service to the region spanned thirty-six years[72]—to coordinate all public-health nursing services for a large multicultural work force on the island. She became a recognized community leader and innovator.

These and other early graduates of the school were members of an emerging profession. They addressed issues related to the public's perceptions of nursing, established professional relationships with physicians and military leaders, and helped define the role and status of the nurse in the early twentieth century. As a group they were outstanding; individually, they provided diverse and much-needed contributions to the profession.

Some of Anna Wolf's classes were devoted to the development of the alumni association. She started from the very beginning and told us how and why the alumni association was formed—not only to keep the group together but to have an association that could help to support nurses, a lot of them single women, who had no health insurance. That's how they got the endowed bed. It wasn't a bed in a certain unit. It was a hospital bed, which could be used by a student or graduate nurse if they had to be admitted to the hospital.

Then they also had a sick benefit fund, which was used to help to care for nurses when they went home from the hospital and to pay for their medical bill or maybe even their food and clothing and lodging because they were not working. There was no such thing as insurance for nurses. This fund was available to any of our alumni and many of them did have to use it. It made the difference as to whether they had medical care or they didn't. So that was very forward thinking from a group of women who had to look out for their own futures. These two funds were maintained for years and years until the board said, "We really don't need this because now most everyone has health insurance."

Betsy Mumaw McGeady, 1955

Opposite, above: In 1895 the nurses' alumnae association's clubhouse opened at 219½ East North Avenue with Ethel Barwick, 1893, as registrar and housekeeper. By 1898 the house had become too small for the number of nurses who wanted to live there; work on an addition was completed in 1899.

Opposite, below left: Carolyn Van Blarcom, 1901, was a crusader in maternal-infant nursing. Her campaign to prevent ophthalmia neonatorum, a form of conjunctivitis, led to her position as an officer on the Committee for the Prevention of Blindness.

Opposite, below right: When she worked at Johns Hopkins Hospital after graduation, Van Blarcom toiled diligently to be sure that babies' eyes were kept clean. Here she gently put silver nitrate drops into an infant's eyes as a nursing student observed her technique.

If I ever win the lottery, I'm going to give the School of Nursing a chunk of money and name it the Adelaide Nutting School of Nursing. This woman was truly a giant. In 1903 she was writing about the importance of an endowment. She knew that the nurses were not given the power they deserved within the structure of the hospital. By 1914, for the hospital's twenty-fifth anniversary, she was going to the alumnae and saying, "It's our twenty-fifth anniversary. We are still not given the recognition or the power that we deserve if you look at what it is we are getting done for the hospital. You want them to listen? There's only one way to make them listen: if we have the power; if we have our own endowment." She set a million dollars as her goal. In 1914, can you imagine how much money that was? So, it took a long time.

Paula Einaudi

The step from the undergraduate instruction of nurses in the Training School to a Post-Graduate School which shall fit graduate nurses to be teachers in other schools is not a long one. I confidently anticipate that such a school will develop in connection with this school at no distant day.

Dr. Henry Hurd, speaking at the opening ceremony for the Johns Hopkins Hospital Training School for Nurses, October 9, 1889

Not long after the school opened, Isabel Hampton learned of a movement among other nursing schools in the United States to organize alumnae associations to provide mutual support to graduates and to help them continue their education through sharing and programs. She convened members of the first two classes on June 3, 1892, in the Nurses' Home, with Georgia Nevins, 1891, acting as temporary chairman. Helena Barnard, 1892, was elected president; Adelaide Nutting, vice president; Georgia Nevins, secretary and treasurer; and Susan Read, corresponding secretary. The group set up a plan to develop bylaws, program meetings, and annual sessions in which to share information. Little did Miss Hampton or these original members know how significant this group would become to the future of nursing at Johns Hopkins.

The original constitution of the Alumnae Association of the Johns Hopkins Hospital Training School for Nurses of Baltimore City noted that "Vigilando" was the motto of the organization. Vigilando means that Hopkins nurses must watch, guard, defend, and protect patients, literally, "ever watchful" or "I stand guard." Members designed an alumnae pin in the shape of a Maltese cross in blue and black enamel on a background of gold with the letters *JHH*.[73]

In 1901 the alumnae association began publishing a quarterly magazine, which provided educational articles and news of the hospital, students, and graduates. From the earliest issues, attempts were made to provide continuing education through thoughtful articles about innovations at the hospital or among graduates. The *Johns Hopkins Nurses Alumnae Magazine* quickly became a vehicle for communicating among colleagues who were working all over the world.

At the school's twenty-fifth-anniversary celebration in 1914, Adelaide Nutting made a prophetic presentation. She totally agreed with Dr. Henry Hurd, who had stated almost ten years earlier that schools of nursing, like schools of medicine, needed to have independent endowments. Miss Nutting had lived with the dilemma of students who financed their education through long hours of work. She knew the difficulty of the school not having a separate budget for its educational program. Fully aware that without endowment funding, the school was vulnerable to changes in hospital finances, she called on graduates to establish a fund for the school to ensure future standards of excellence.

Miss Nutting had noted the rapidly changing trends in higher education, and she viewed nursing as an ideal profession to participate in this evolution by establishing nursing education in university settings. She recognized the need for women to bring financial resources into universities if they wished to be included. In particular, she knew of the large donation that wealthy women had given years earlier to the Johns Hopkins University, which helped to establish its School of Medicine; their contribution, Nutting knew, had enabled women to enroll in the medical

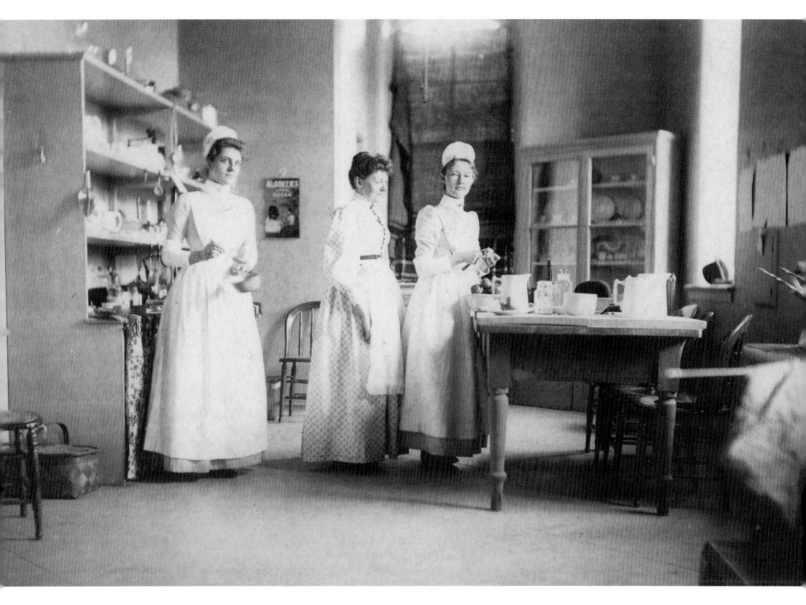

school. Miss Nutting called on alumnae to lead the effort to fully endow the nursing school so that it could make the transition into the Johns Hopkins University. The tradition that she began continues today.

What Miss Nutting perhaps did not recognize at that point was how difficult it would be to separate the valued service rendered by nursing students in the hospital in order to transform the students into participants in higher education. Nor did she appreciate how difficult it was going to be to convince the brilliant men in the Hopkins institutions that this change would be beneficial. That struggle continued for years.

Adelaide Nutting agreed to chair the Endowment Committee in May 1915, and she chose her members carefully. They began meeting in December, and in early 1916 they sent a questionnaire to over seven hundred graduates asking for "expressions of faith in the undertaking and suggestions for carrying it out."[74] The group quickly recognized the

Susan Read and Georgia Nevins, both members of the first class to graduate, were elected founding officers of the Alumnae Association of the Johns Hopkins Hospital Training School for Nurses of Baltimore City at its first meeting, on June 3, 1892. (Their cooking instructor, Mary Boland, stands between them.) The association's purpose was "the promotion of unity and good feeling among the Alumnae, and the advancement of the interest of the profession of Nursing, and also of providing a home for its members, and making provision for them if ill or disabled."

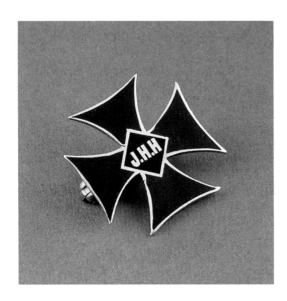

The alumnae association chose "Vigilando" as its motto and a pin in the design of a Maltese cross in blue and black enamel on a background of gold with the letters *JHH*. For many years, the alumnae pin was the only jewelry nurses could wear while on duty, except for inconspicuous collar or cuff pins and a wrist or chain watch; no bracelets or rings, except wedding rings, were permitted.

The secretary would be very glad of instructions or suggestions for further effort in behalf of the endowment. She would like to call attention to the fact that only a very small percentage of our graduates have contributed to the Fund, which now amounts approximately to $12,200.

At a committee meeting held this morning Miss Lawler compiled the amount which we might have in our treasury had all our graduates given a penny a day for the past five years. It would be $16,425.00, and with the few large sums we have been given, we should have nearly twice the amount at the present time. Let me urge every graduate to give something, no matter how small the sum, as it is the pennies which make the dollars.

Yssabella Waters, 1897, in the alumnae association's 1920 annual report

value of the alumnae magazine as a vehicle for informing graduates of the need for an endowment. Miss Nutting returned to Baltimore for the next annual meeting of the association to share what she had learned across the nation about interest in philanthropy for educational ventures. She encouraged the group to continue to search for sources of donations.

In the early 1920s a report of the Committee for the Study of Nursing Education, commonly called the Goldmark Report, was published. This study concluded that the outstanding hospital schools of nursing should convert to university programs as soon as possible to prepare leaders for education, administration, and the practice of public health. Miss Nutting, Dr. William Welch, and Dr. Winford Smith were on the committee. The principal author of the report was Carolyn Gray, of the Frances Payne Bolton School at Western Reserve University.

Miss Gray was invited to Johns Hopkins in 1924 to survey untapped nursing-education resources in Baltimore. After a six-week study she submitted a plan to the training school committee, which consisted of Miss Lawler, several physicians, and Dorothy D. Filler, 1920. Miss Gray proposed two programs for Hopkins: a five- and a three-year program. The five-year plan proposed that students spend two years at the Johns Hopkins University and the three-year plan added only public health to the current curriculum. There was much interest in this plan, which excited the Endowment Committee. Soon thereafter, however, Johns Hopkins University President Frank Goodnow offered a competing plan, which proposed eliminating the two university years—because he wanted to do away with the bachelor's degree entirely (this never happened). As the planning dragged on, the clock kept ticking, and nothing was ever decided about the Gray plan.

In 1922 Miss Nutting met with George E. Vincent of the Rockefeller Foundation to ask if the time had come for the alumnae committee to make an appeal for the Johns Hopkins nursing school endowment. Vincent later informed her that the foundation board was unwilling to enter the field of direct financial aid to specific schools of nursing. The board reversed itself a year later, after the publication of the Goldmark Report, and granted $500,000 to the new Yale University School of Nursing. The real problem, Miss Nutting realized, was that the foundation's leaders in New York understood that, at that time, physicians at the Johns Hopkins Hospital and administrators and trustees at the Johns Hopkins University were opposed to a university program for nurses.

The Endowment Fund, as it was called, began modestly with small donations, but Miss Nutting set a goal of $1 million, an enormous sum in that era. Although the fund never grew as quickly as hoped, the principal accumulated steadily during the 1920s. Efforts of the Endowment Committee led to the organization of a special training school committee, with Elsie Lawler, Anna Wolf, Effie Taylor, Amy P. Miller, and Drs. Welch and Smith as members. In 1928 the committee issued a report to the trustees of the hospital about the nursing program, calling for an academic program organized along university lines. They wanted the school to come under the purview of the university and become an integral part of the medical school.

The medical advisory board of the hospital rejected the proposal because the School of Medicine was a graduate program and nurses did not meet this standard with their quest for a bachelor's program. The board also stated that nurses did not require a broad liberal arts background to be competent in their field. Finally, it expressed the belief that a nurse prepared in the program as proposed would not be any "better fitted" for nursing than those in the current diploma program.

The board did approve the organization of the Advisory Board of the School of Nursing, which would meet monthly and have eleven members representing the medical advisory board of the hospital, the board of the School of Hygiene and Public Health, the director of the hospital, the director of the nursing school, the president of the Johns Hopkins University (ex officio), two members of the alumnae association, and two at-large members from the community who were interested in the school. This was the first time the alumnae association had gained a voice in a policy-making body in the School of Nursing.

Although the Endowment Fund did not reach the levels hoped for initially, resources from the fund made a major difference to the school during the Depression.[75] Alumnae used the interest earned from the fund in the early 1930s to underwrite the beginning of public-health nursing at the school and to pay faculty salaries for the program. In 1936 the Endowment Committee recommended that the sum of $136,000 be turned over to the hospital. The fund was to be known as the M. Adelaide Nutting Endowment Fund for the School of Nursing, and the income it generated was to be used to improve educational work in the school. The committee kept just over $7,000 to use as a working fund for adding to the endowment.

The Endowment Fund continued to be a focal point for the alumnae association throughout this period, providing a link for supporting nursing education at Johns Hopkins. Work on the fund also enabled the alumnae association to contribute to the development of the curriculum because its resources were needed by the financially limited hospital. One can only wonder what might have happened had Miss Nutting's trip to the Rockefeller Foundation in the 1920s produced a grant to the school. But the time was not yet ripe; the rest of the Hopkins community was not ready for Miss Nutting's vision. Although her dream was delayed, the foundation to provide a legacy for future generations was in place. The goal of an independent university-based school for nurses at Johns Hopkins would not be forgotten.

Adelaide Nutting was in the first graduating class of the diploma School of Nursing. Then she went to Teachers College, Columbia University. They had a program preparing superintendents of nurses and she was one of those first graduates. She's well regarded in the nursing literature. When I was going to school I heard about Adelaide Nutting.

Medea Marella

Although Adelaide Nutting left the Johns Hopkins administration in 1907, she remained a commanding presence. At Columbia University's Teachers College, Nutting headed the Department of Home and Institutional Economics, where she eventually became the first professor of nursing in the world. With that prominent designation, she often returned to Baltimore to champion the cause of university-based education for nurses.

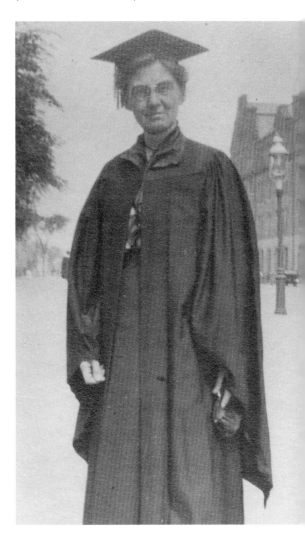

LINDA SABIN

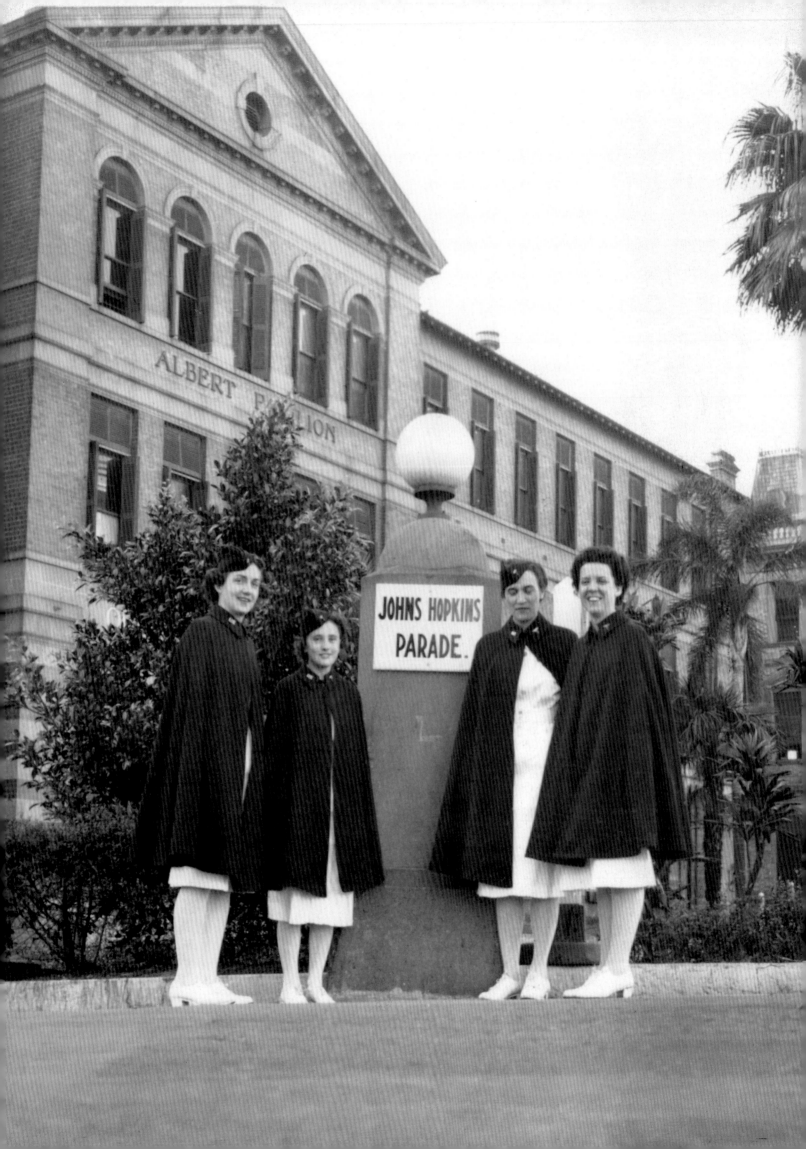

Rapid Change, 1940–1950 · BY LINDA SABIN

2

Johns Hopkins nurses and doctors left their mark on
the Royal Prince Alfred Hospital in Sydney, Australia,
in 1942, when members of General Hospital No. 118
treated World War II casualties there. Margaret
Wheeler, 1942, Florence Smith, 1939, Emma Chapman,
1929, and Mary Farr, 1941, posed proudly by the
standard proclaiming their presence.

PROSPECTS FOR THE 1940S might have been brighter, a new decade bringing fresh hope of further recovery from the Great Depression, had not war again been ravaging Europe. By the end of 1940 Hitler had already invaded much of Europe, bombs were decimating large parts of England, and anxiety in the United States was growing by the day. Before the end of the year, the Johns Hopkins Hospital was again organizing a hospital unit in preparation for war. This conflict would have an even greater impact on the hospital and the school than World War I did in 1914. The realization that another world war was possible was in everyone's mind, yet hope remained that this aggression might be stopped without American involvement.[1] Recognition of the coming risk inspired the mobilization of resources to organize the Nursing Council on National Defense. By July 1941 funds to support a significant increase in nursing enrollments and an expansion of nursing education began to flow. The profession both benefited from and struggled with transformations World War II brought, and those changes had lasting effects.

A COMMANDING PRESENCE

Anna Dryden Wolf returned to her alma mater on November 1, 1940, to inaugurate the next nursing administration. She was the fifth chief of nursing and the first director not born in Canada. As she began her tenure, Miss Wolf was the best-educated and most seasoned administrator to run the program in its history.[2]

Anna Wolf was born on June 25, 1890, in Guntur, Madras Presidency, in Southern India, one of four children and the youngest girl. Her father, a Lutheran clergyman, headed a boys' school and served as an officer for a foreign mission board. Her mother was a teacher for Indian girls. In 1893 Wolf and her siblings returned to the United States to live with relatives in North Carolina. Her new family lived in conditions even more austere than those she had known in India, and this experience left its mark. Her mother returned to the United States in 1900 and moved the family to Lutherville, Maryland. The Wolf family's appreciation for education and devotion to duty as well as their strong religious faith marked Anna Wolf throughout her life.

In 1912, when she entered Johns Hopkins to become a nurse, Wolf already had a degree from Goucher College. Her older sister was a physician, and their father encouraged his youngest daughter to consider going into medicine, but she was determined to pursue nursing. She thought she did not have the science background for medicine, and she was interested in helping people more personally while giving patient care.[3] In her later years, Wolf credited the rigidity, the demands of patient care, and the intimidation she experienced while a student in the hospital as the source of her resolve to move nursing into a purely educational setting. She came to believe that a university would provide

Opposite: Just four years after graduating from Johns Hopkins, Anna D. Wolf was named dean of a new school of nursing at the Peking Union Medical College in China. For her faculty, she chose fellow alumnae Lillian Wu, Kathleen Caulfield, Bertha Sutton, Faye Whiteside, Mary Purcell, and Sophie Booker, all members of the classes of 1918 and 1919, whom she had taught when she was an instructor at Johns Hopkins, from 1916 to 1918.

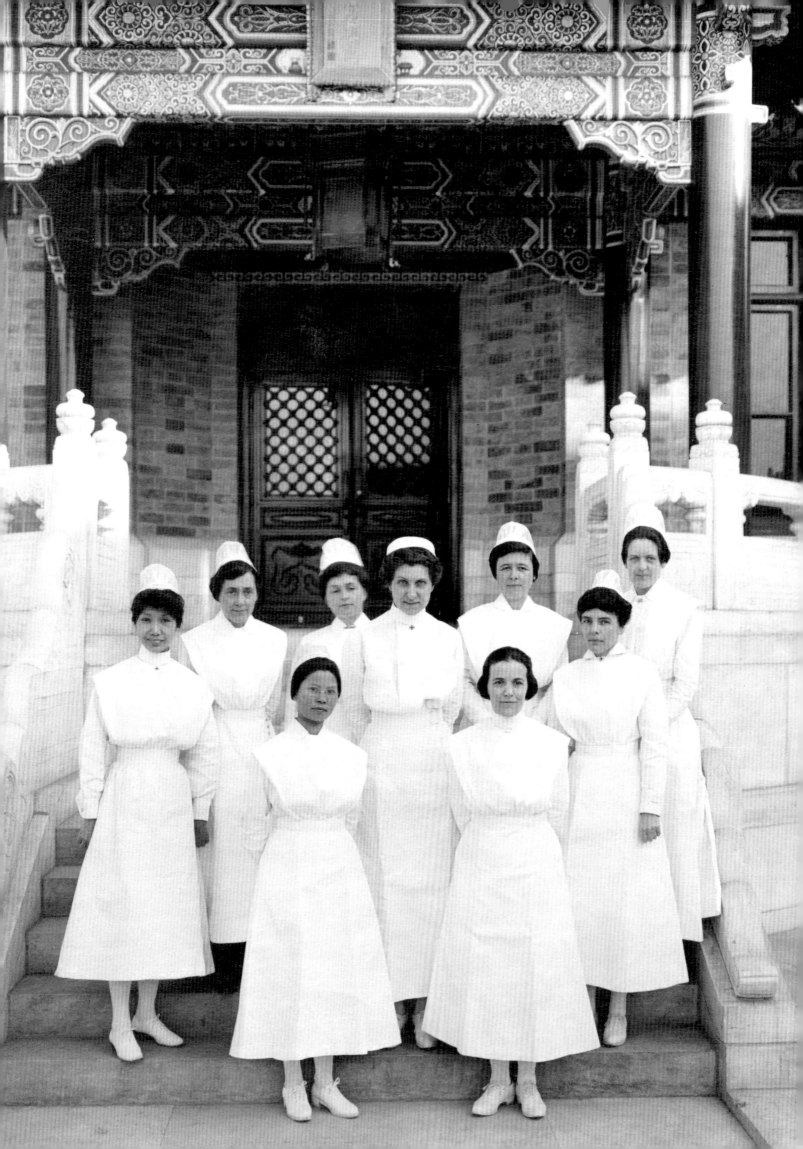

a superior environment for student learning because patient care and the needs of the hospital were the primary concerns in a traditional training program. (Her subsequent experiences with Adelaide Nutting solidified Wolf's views.)

After graduating from Johns Hopkins in 1915, during Miss Lawler's tenure, Wolf went immediately to Teachers College, Columbia University, to continue her education. While there, she studied with Adelaide Nutting, who became her lifelong mentor. She agreed with Miss Nutting's views about the need for financial endowments for schools of nursing. As a result, Miss Wolf brought renewed vigor to the drive for a university-based nursing program at Hopkins when she became its director in 1940.[4] Her background and value system enabled her to work unceasingly for a cause she believed in. This determination would both help and hinder her in her work at Johns Hopkins.

Anna Wolf was a tall woman, standing five feet ten inches, with broad shoulders, erect posture, and a commanding presence. She possessed leadership qualities before entering nursing school, and her strength as a leader grew with her education and experience. In 1916, after earning her master's degree, Miss Wolf returned to Johns Hopkins to serve as an instructor and as assistant superintendent of the training school. In the summer of 1918 she took a leave of absence from Hopkins to serve on the faculty of the Vassar Training Camp, but she returned in the fall and served in the great flu epidemic of 1918.

In 1919 Anna Wolf left Johns Hopkins to serve as dean of the new school of nursing being launched by the Rockefeller Foundation at the Peking Union Medical College in North China. A new medical school and hospital were under construction, and planners wanted to open a nursing school. The school opened in 1920 and Miss Wolf organized the nursing service and the curriculum. In 1922 an affiliation with Peking University was established, with an eye to attracting educated Chinese women. Although the school of nursing was not fully controlled by the university, strong ties to the school made the nursing program an innovation. In later years Miss Wolf recalled her time in China as among the most productive in her career.

Miss Wolf developed a thyroid problem in 1925 and had to undergo surgery in Peking. She then returned home to visit family and to rest. Once recovered, she began to take doctoral courses at Teachers College but was interrupted by an invitation to go to Billings Hospital at the University of Chicago as superintendent of nurses. Initially, Miss Wolf addressed the needs of the nursing service in the hospital by organizing a nursing team that utilized graduate nurses to provide bedside care along with students. This practice of using graduates to care for patients in the hospital was considered an innovation in the mid-1920s.[5]

As an associate professor, Wolf turned her attention to developing courses in teaching and administration in nursing schools. She was hopeful that she could stimulate the development of a collegiate program in nursing at Chicago because the alumnae of the Illinois Training School had given the university a large endowment fund for that purpose. By 1930, with the onset of the Great Depression and a reduced endowment, it became apparent to Miss Wolf that her efforts would be unsuccessful.

Miss Wolf moved on to the New York–Cornell Medical Center in 1931 as the director of nursing and the School of Nursing. She took over right after the merger of the New York Hospital and Cornell University, which actually merged four clinical facilities: the New York Hospital, Cornell Clinic, Manhattan Maternity, and Lying In. She began work in October 1931, and the new 1,000-bed hospital opened in 1932. Wolf successfully led the merger of nursing staffs, raised standards, and upgraded the curriculum in the nursing school. She recruited outstanding faculty and developed the curriculum to the point that it was considered college caliber.

Wolf was unable to persuade the medical board at Cornell that a bachelor's program was appropriate. When she left her position in 1940, she believed that she had failed in her efforts, that she had been let down by people she had trusted, and that her tenure in New York had come to an unsuccessful conclusion. Two years after her resignation, however, university affiliation at Cornell was approved, and many credited Wolf's groundwork and the quality of her curriculum for this acceptance.

Miss Wolf found both the University of Chicago and New York–Cornell to be conservative institutions with medical staffs that were reluctant to upgrade nursing-education programs. Some of her fiercest opponents at Cornell were Hopkins-trained physicians. In later years she reflected that she knew what she was getting into when she decided to return to Johns Hopkins; she had no illusions but was hopeful that times were changing.

Anna Wolf received two invitations in the 1920s to come back to Johns Hopkins, but the timing of those offers, as well as conflicts with her personal goals for nursing, prompted her refusals. When Elsie Lawler retired, however, Wolf accepted Dr. Winford Smith's invitation to consider the position as superintendent of nurses and principal of the School of Nursing—with several conditions. She made it clear to Dr. Smith before her employment that she would push for a university school, and he replied honestly that this would be acceptable to him but that he was not in sympathy with the effort. She appreciated his honesty. Miss Wolf's conditions for employment, which she sent in a letter to Dr. Smith, reflect her wisdom as a nursing administrator and educator.

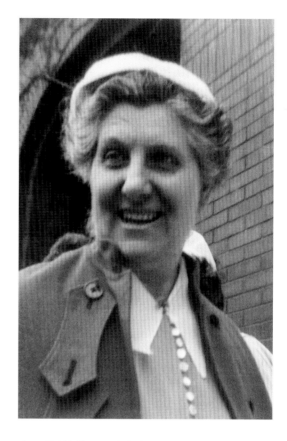

Anna D. Wolf succeeded Elsie Lawler as superintendent of nurses and principal of the School of Nursing in 1940. She returned to Baltimore determined to move the school from the hospital's control, where it was regarded as a bottomless font supplying well-trained workers, to the university, where nursing might be deemed a profession paralleling medicine. From the start, she met resistance from both the hospital and the School of Medicine.

A TIME PROFITABLE TO US

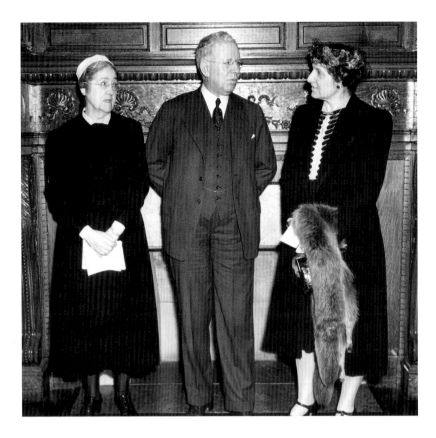

Commencement Day, 1940, symbolized the changing of the guard at the school. As usual, hospital president Dr. Winford Smith attended, but on that day he was flanked by both Elsie Lawler and Anna D. Wolf. The two women could not have been more different. Whereas Lawler had been compliant and easily controlled by the hospital administration and trustees, Wolf was assertive in her management style and aggressive in her resolve to bring about radical changes.

After giving very thoughtful consideration to your invitation to become Miss Lawler's successor as Superintendent of Nurses and Principal of the School of Nursing, I am honored to accept the appointment if the premises as stated may be acceptable and the following specific conditions may be met:

1. Re—general administration
It is my understanding that I shall be directly responsible to you or your successor for the administration of the school of nursing and nursing service with the hospital and out-patient departments unless conditions change as authorized by the Board of Trustees. My interpretation of this is that the administration of the school and services will not be subject to the dictation of the Medical Board but that matters relative to the several clinical departments as may affect the nursing school and nursing care of patients will be brought to my attention through individual contact.

It would be my intention to carry out the established administrative policies and practices relative to the nursing school and nursing service until such time as study may reveal that recommendations for change may be advantageous.

2. Re—School of Nursing and Nursing Service
It will be my earnest purpose to further in all respects the best care of patients and to cooperate with the medical staff and all others in this great responsibility. Because of my conviction that our school of nursing should maintain its eminence and its leadership in nursing education my efforts in regard to the school's program will constantly be directed toward this end. It is very much hoped that a

closer relationship to the university may be effected and that greater academic recognition of the nursing curriculum be granted.

These two primary assumptions should be interdependent and not contradictory.

3. Re—budget

It would seem highly desirable to establish a budget system differentiating education and service requirements and costs.

It is urged that the establishment of an endowment for the school of nursing be made a primary objective so that the progress of the school may be assured.

After further study of the salaries given the nursing staff, I am very deeply concerned over the low rates which obtain. Although funds may not be available to increase these at the present time, it is earnestly hoped that gradually there may be improvement in the salary scales.

As vacancies may occur in the two positions of First Assistant Superintendent of Nurses and Director of Theoretical Instruction which I understand are anticipated but I trust may not occur until some time mutually agreeable after my appointment, I request the prerogative of appointing two highly qualified associate directors, one of nursing service, the other of instruction or similar titles for whom salaries of at least three thousand dollars ($3,000.00) per annum plus full maintenance be available.

At as early date as possible effort should be made to reduce the hours of all students to a forty-eight hour week including class which I know has been a matter of deep interest and concern to Miss Lawler and her associations and which has been precluded because of budgetary implications.

4. Re—personal conditions of appointment
I respectively request that:

A. The title of my position be Dean of the School of Nursing and Director of Nursing Service or Director of the School of Nursing and Nursing Service. The former title is preferable to me and I believe is more indicative of actual functions than the latter. It is in harmony with educational and service titles and seems altogether appropriate.

B. My salary be six-thousand dollars, ($6,000.00) per annum plus full maintenance as presently provided the superintendent of nurses. (This is what I now receive at the New York Hospital). In the event that conditions would make it advisable after a year or more in residence I request the prerogative of living outside the residence with an allowance of at least one hundred and fifty dollars ($150.00) per month in lieu of maintenance.

C. I be allowed eight week's vacation, with salary, per annum, which might be broken if more convenient and more efficacious; necessary time for participation in extra-mural professional activities; and illness time and allowance for health service and hospitalization as may be granted members of the nursing staff in accord with policies already or as may be established.[6]

Anna D. Wolf came in 1940 and she made it clear, right from the get-go, that she wanted to change the Johns Hopkins Hospital School of Nursing into the Johns Hopkins University School of Nursing. She said, "If we want professional status, we have to have a baccalaureate degree. We'll never get the prestige that we want if we don't start off with that as a minimum." Johns Hopkins was an all-male institution, and they thought they would be lowering standards by letting in these nursing students and going against the mandate of the university by admitting women to the undergraduate program.

Paula Einaudi

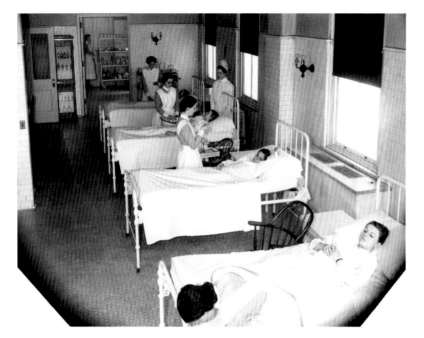
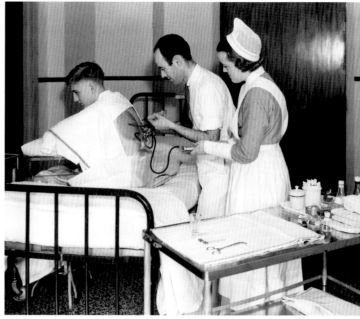

The era of probationers was coming to an end. In 1941 the term was changed to preclinical students, but at the beginning of Wolf's administration probationers were easily recognized because they had not yet earned their caps. These new students were learning to work with patients on the practice ward in the old surgical building while an instructor monitored their progress.

Above right: As their clinical skills increased, nursing students worked alongside house officers as they performed simple and complex medical procedures. Here the chief medical resident on Osler 6 drained a patient's chest while a student intently watched.

*My first experience with rounds was in Brady.
I was a probie without a cap. I got off duty at nine
o'clock and I just kind of hung around and then
I saw the doctors. I stood at the edge of the room.
I tried to blend into the wall. I wanted to hear
what they were saying. Dr. Young saw me there,
welcomed me to rounds and brought me up front.
I stood there and listened for the whole time and
I was fascinated. As rounds occurred at other
times during my nursing career, if I had something
to do on the ward I would always do it slowly so
I could hear what they were talking about.*

Frances Schlosser Scherer, 1944

Clearly, Miss Wolf accepted the position of director with an understanding of what was needed in nursing service and education at Johns Hopkins. She also knew how to structure working relationships with doctors and trustees. She attempted to set up arrangements so that she could achieve her goal, which was to fulfill the challenge Miss Nutting had set forth years before. Anna Wolf saw that evolution into a collegiate school of nursing was possible if a strong relationship could be forged with the Johns Hopkins University. She had, however, learned in her previous position that acceptance of the bachelor of science in nursing degree for nurses would be hard-won. She was fifty years old and had just finished nine arduous years hindered by the Great Depression and her frustrated attempts to move the New York–Cornell Medical Center nursing program into Cornell University.

Miss Wolf began her tenure at Hopkins doubtful that physicians or university administrators and trustees would be any more supportive than they had been in New York, although she was hopeful that support for her vision of university education could be built. At Hopkins, Dr. Smith was a supportive administrator who shared Wolf's goal of giving the students a solid education. But Wolf understood Nutting and Robb's dream that the School of Nursing needed to be conducted by an institution of higher learning. To achieve that status and be secure in the collegiate setting, the school would need solid funding in the form of an endowment.

The new nursing director found a large and dedicated nursing staff; some were open to change while many others were satisfied with the manner in which Miss Lawler had directed affairs. Wolf recognized that following Miss Lawler, who had led the program successfully for thirty years, would be demanding. Nursing service had been maintained with high standards, and exceptional clinical facilities provided educational experiences for a qualified, loyal student body. Wolf also found an existing relationship with the university through the Teachers College

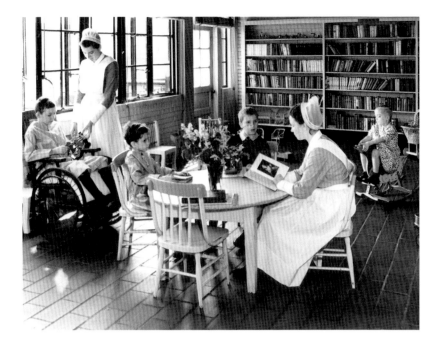

The Harriet Lane Home for Invalid Children was a favorite assignment for many nursing students. Their young patients were sometimes extremely ill, but they were often well enough to visit the play room, where attention was paid to children's emotional as well as physical needs.

(later called McCoy College, and then the Evening College) at the Johns Hopkins University.

Outstanding clinical opportunities and an exceptional medical staff—including many who taught in the School of Nursing—meant that recruiting students was not a problem. Hopkins attracted students from all over the country and abroad, and its graduates were in great demand as leaders, even though the program was not based in a university. In fact, the excellence of the school would be one of Anna Wolf's major obstacles in achieving a university-based program. The faculty of the School of Medicine and attending physicians were not concerned with or impressed by changes in the nursing profession during the 1940s. They could not understand why the skilled practitioners who completed the nursing program and ran the hospital would ever need additional education. Thus, the School of Nursing was hindered in its progress because of its success.

Miss Wolf was surprised to find that most of the nursing staff and all but one of the nursing leaders in the hospital were from Hopkins. She was also dismayed to realize that the traditional militaristic approach to the daily operations of the hospital had remained unchanged since her own student days. She quickly ended the practice of nurses standing when doctors entered the nurses' station, as well as the practice of probationers and junior students standing whenever a head nurse or senior student entered the nurses' station. Her view, based on her own experience, was that each nurse had too much to do giving patient care to take the time to stand and observe military etiquette. She also eased social rules and curfews for students, pointing out that these young ladies were going to take care of the lives of their patients, so they ought to be able to take care of their own.[7]

The new director discovered that nurses were performing many duties not related to nursing, such as recording, checking, and submitting payroll slips each week for all the workers on a unit. She negotiated

Our preclin program was accelerated—usually it would have been six months—it was four months. I liked it very much except for chemistry because I hadn't had chemistry in high school and I didn't have it in college. Dr. Katherine K. Sanford was the instructor and she took us along pretty fast. I thought, "If I come here and fail and all those girls from Podunk Center can make it and I have to go home and say, 'I couldn't get through it ...'" But eventually I did. I think we started out with eighty-eight and we ended up with sixty-eight in my class. There were quite a few who dropped out in the preclin. There was an old operating room and we had all these seats that medical students had used. That's where we had a lot of our classes. It was rather primitive and we all sat alphabetically. Everything was very well organized and I think that was Miss Wolf and the rest of her staff.

Ethel Rainey Ward, 1947

the elimination of some of these extraneous obligations and encouraged the addition of support personnel on the units wherever possible. Once the push of World War II began, Miss Wolf was able to place additional persons in the nursing office to relieve supervisors and instructors of some paperwork tasks. (This became critical once the cadet nurse program began and enrollment climbed quickly.)

Faculty issues immediately drew Wolf's attention. She encouraged her teaching staff to form an organization with bylaws and specific functions, marking the first time that the faculty was recognized as being responsible for development of the school. The organization and its bylaws were approved by October 1941. During the same period students established the Student Association, to encourage greater student participation in the advancement of the school and to improve their relationship with the faculty. Students created committees and wrote bylaws and an honor code for student conduct. This association affected student life positively and inspired many characteristics of student culture throughout the era of the hospital-based program.[8]

The nursing curriculum, which had undergone several changes during the 1930s, lacked any strong integration of theory and practice when Wolf assumed the directorship. Through the new faculty organization, she appointed a curriculum committee in 1941 to begin a review. Under Wolf's direction, the faculty found that the program of study was outdated, noting that the emphasis on clinical service was overwhelming. Students were working a fifty-six-hour week, which included forty-eight hours of clinical experience and eight hours of class. They had two six-hour days per week, and one was Sunday, when they also were expected to attend religious services. Many days, students worked split shifts, with morning duty, a break for several hours—which often included classes—and then evening duty. Assignments were given according to the needs of the nursing service and there was little consistency. Some students had months of night duty while others had little;

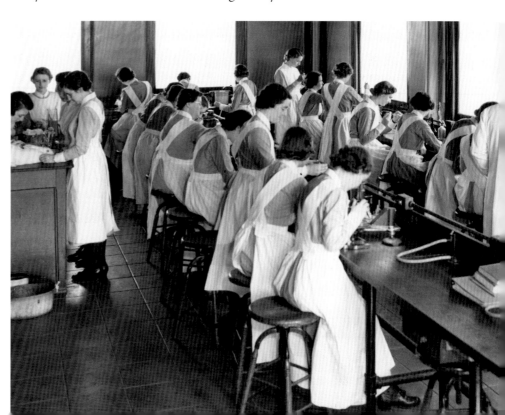

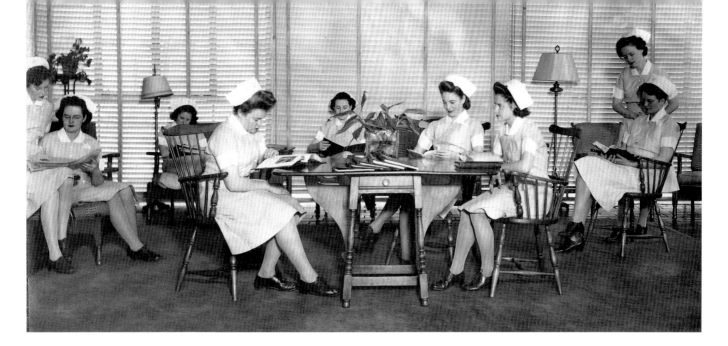

a student might spend a major portion of her time in one area and have scant experience in others. No effort was made to correlate clinical experiences with theory; if theory ran concurrently with practice, it was by coincidence rather than design.[9]

Undoubtedly, the Depression years and the pressing needs of patients had taken their toll on the educational program.[10] Wolf's primary worry was that students were graduating with uneven experience, because they were kept in areas where they functioned well, without concern for their educational needs. Miss Wolf persuaded the faculty to set up specific theoretical rotations based on a predetermined number of weeks to better coordinate clinical experiences.

On March 27, 1941, while plans to revise the curriculum were getting under way, Miss Wolf submitted a "Memorandum Concerning a University School of Nursing," to the Advisory Board of the School of Nursing. The detailed document described her view of how the program at Hopkins could be structured within the university. It included basic and graduate study plans and provided the reader with many pertinent suggestions for implementation.[11] The proposal was still under consideration when Pearl Harbor was attacked on December 7, and the matter was shelved for the remainder of the war. (Many of Wolf's ideas would reappear later in her tenure, once the war had ended.)

With the declaration of war, nursing schools were encouraged to shorten their programs to thirty months, at least for the war's duration. The new curriculum, when completed, reflected the demands of the times, but it was established on a rotation basis, which helped students receive a more balanced clinical education and more correlated theory.

On December 8, 1941, Miss Wolf called students into the large parlor in Hampton House for prayers. Most of the students were too young to remember the hardships and suffering of World War I, but she remembered those years well and knew prayer would be essential in the months to come. Mary Kuntz, 1943, recalled that the room was filled with students and faculty praying together and that everyone was in

Everything changed dramatically at the school and the hospital during World War II including students' uniforms. Long sleeves and starched aprons disappeared. Even though the new uniforms were easier to maintain, they still had to be kept immaculate, even during leisure hours—which were few. With many members of the faculty and hospital staff away at war, the responsibilities of nursing students increased, and emphasis on classroom education was minimal. Still, students crammed when they could, and the "fishbowl" was a favorite gathering spot.

The Welch Library was a great place. You had to go there to get your reading done, and there were no photocopiers, so you had to sit there and read and take notes. So that became a social center as well. I almost never studied in my room. I would retreat to Welch or there was a library then with a reading room in the Main Residence, and then there were several other nooks and crannies and places you could find. There were other libraries in the hospital.

Martha Norton Hill, 1964, BSN 1966

Opposite: For more than half a century, nursing students had no classrooms devoted to their needs. Instead, they usually were instructed in medical school laboratories, often by members of the medical faculty. Anna D. Wolf was in the midst of changing the curriculum when World War II interrupted her plans. Students explored bacteriology, including probing a large white rabbit, in the pathology building, c. 1938.

We were admitted in September of 1941 and the world was unsettled. We were all just learning the basics of bed making and baths and classes when along came December 7 and we found ourselves at war. There was, of course, a lot of buzz going on about what's going to happen. In that spring of '42, they sent a couple of units of doctors and nurses from the hospital. That meant that the student nurses were just about running things because there were very few graduate nurses left on the units. Of course, we didn't have the fast-paced nursing that they have today. Ours was a little more leisurely. The patients stayed longer with us. Most of those who went were the nurses from the floors and some head nurses.

Constance Cole Heard Waxter, 1944

When Miss Wolf pushed for a collegiate school of nursing, one of the things they told her was that nurses don't have the intellectual ability that meets the Hopkins standard. So she got people who had their degrees from other perfectly good schools because she wanted to show them that, yes, our students can match brains with anybody. Look, they've already done it.

Betty Borenstein Scher, 1950

tears, including Miss Wolf.[12] Wolf knew from her experiences in the previous war the potential suffering that lay ahead for her staff and students—and she also realized that her plans and dreams for the future would have to be postponed.

Miss Wolf anticipated the direction of political and military affairs when she addressed the graduating class the previous May:

We confront today not dissimilar circumstances to those she [Elsie Lawler] faced in the first decade of her service. Our opportunities of expressing that same faith in our profession and in our school are at hand. Are we ready and willing to give our most and best or are we content to express our service in narrow, selfish ways? . . . With the increased demands upon our profession for service in defense activities we can anticipate even more serious inroads upon our work which as in 1917 and 1918 placed unprecedented responsibilities upon students and almost superhuman burdens on graduates. . . . Our school must continue to meet the demands of the public through the preparation and graduation of as large groups of students as possible, however, our standards of quality of matriculants must not be lowered—in fact, it seems imperative that even stricter requirements be imposed if increased responsibilities obtain.[13]

While the war forced her to delay action on many of the goals stated in her contract with the trustees, Miss Wolf was wise enough to understand that adjustments caused by the conflict just might facilitate change at the hospital. It was obvious that students would play a critical part in the maintenance of normal activities at the hospital as graduates left for military service. Miss Wolf later reflected that the war in some ways came at a "time profitable to us," because enrollments grew dramatically. Hopkins could still be very selective, however, picking the better-educated, more mature students.[14] Thus, Wolf did not abandon hope for a university program. In the meantime, the curriculum would have to be restructured for wartime needs. First, in 1941, a six-month exemption was offered for those with two years of college who maintained a B average during their first year and a half in school. By 1942 the program was accelerated so that all students received theoretical material and basic nursing practice in thirty months.

The National Nursing Council for War Service determined that graduate nurses needed to be released for military and Red Cross service, so it rationed professional nursing care given to patients in hospitals. Two hospital units from Johns Hopkins Hospital were organized at the request of the U.S. Army. General Hospitals 18 and 118 went overseas in 1942, to various locations in the South Pacific, India, Burma, and the Philippines. Sixty graduate nurses went with these hospital units; twenty-three were members of the nursing faculty. More than seventy additional nurses had left Hopkins for other military duty by 1943, thus placing the nursing service and the school in dire straits in terms of personnel.[15]

Accelerated recruiting efforts stimulated a sharp rise in the number of incoming students in 1942. Establishment of the Cadet Nurse Corps by the U.S. Public Health Service in 1943 brought about the largest classes to be admitted in the history of the school. Standards remained high among the recruits, with a majority having a bachelor's degree or at least two years of college; in 1943–44, the number of high school graduate recruits began to grow.

During the summers of 1941, 1942, and 1945 preclinical programs were taught at Bryn Mawr College in Pennsylvania; in 1943 and 1944 the courses were offered at Goucher College in Baltimore. (These accelerated summer programs were fashioned somewhat like the training camp for student nurses at Vassar College, where Miss Wolf had served on the faculty during World War I.) The Bryn Mawr program, sponsored by the American Red Cross, required students to have completed two years of college, whereas the Goucher program allowed high school graduates to participate. Johns Hopkins had the largest number of students and also provided instructors in each of the programs.

Hampton House overflowed with extra students who had to share previously private rooms, and the Main Residence was filled; some students were even housed on closed hospital units or in nearby residences.[16] In 1943 Hopkins received federal funding for temporary housing for nurses to be erected between the Main Residence and the Harriet Lane pediatric clinic, and Hampton House was enlarged by adding two floors on the Monument Street side of the building. The increase in students allowed the institution to continue providing full services throughout the war period. As K. Virginia Betzold reflected,

Anna Wolf was awesome. She was a rather large woman and I think when you have someone of stature and that nature, you respect them. We had senior interviews with her. A bunch of us had decided we'd like to go into industrial nursing because that paid well and it would be fun to do. Miss Wolf let me know that I either stay at the hospital and work or else join the service. Those were the only two things that were acceptable for a senior to do. Having gotten married six months before I finished, staying at the hospital was the only thing to do because the services weren't taking married women at that point.

Constance Cole Heard Waxter, 1944

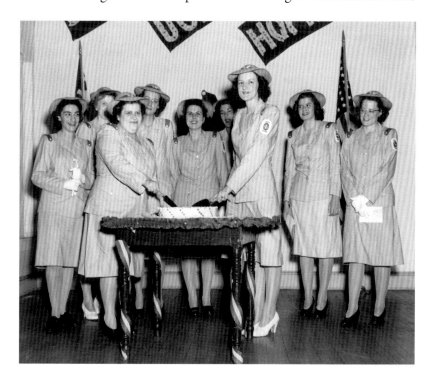

On July 3, 1944, members of the U.S. Cadet Nurse Corps, directed by Lucile Petry, 1927, celebrated the first anniversary of the organization. Enrollment swelled during the war, and many students were older and had bachelor's degrees or some years of college when they arrived.

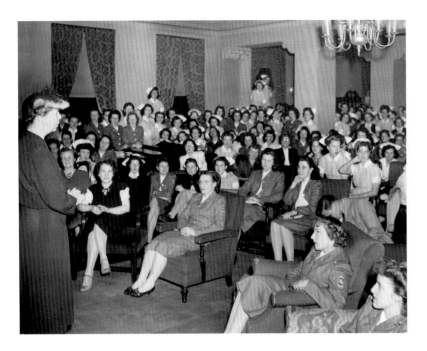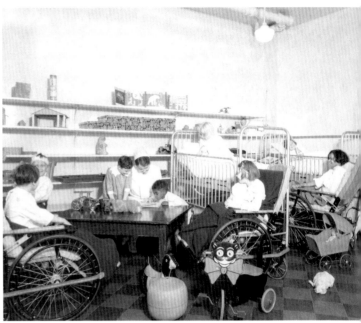

Cadet nurses were right up front when Eleanor Roosevelt spoke at Hampton House in 1945. She had just returned from the South Pacific and was able to report to members of the audience on the welfare of their peers.

Above right: Nurses working in the Department of Pediatrics knew the benefits of encouraging their young patients to live as fully as possible while they were in the hospital. An innovative development furthered their efforts beginning in 1944, when the Play Activities Program, which later became the Child Life Program, began.

The lounge area was always the best-looking part of Hampton House. Eleanor Roosevelt came for tea in the lounge in the lobby of Hampton House. I remember us just gathered there. Eleanor Roosevelt was very gracious and humble. She thanked everybody. Her presence was amazing. We heard about her visiting some of our friends in Walter Reed. Miss Wolf contributed a lot to the war effort so I think Eleanor Roosevelt was appreciative of that.

Ethel Rainey Ward, 1947

The fact that we were able to recruit large numbers of students for our own school and had many senior cadets from numerous schools around the country for the last six months of the three year program made it possible to care for patients without limiting [hospital] admissions or curtailing the medical school activities. The Hospital Administration and Medical Board came to rely more and more on the School of Nursing and its students. When the war was over and our student enrollment got smaller and smaller, it was a different situation.[17]

Miss Wolf recognized that students were being used for service with limited educational content and that they had little choice of where to serve their last six months. Joan Verlee DeYoung, 1945, remembered that Miss Wolf apologized for this situation in a professional-adjustments class during her last year in school.[18] Wolf tried to alleviate the situation by employing auxiliary workers whenever possible.

The students did get to participate in innovative activities during this period. In 1944 the Play Activities Program, which later developed into the Child Life Program, was begun in the Department of Pediatrics. Students learned of the need for healthy play among sick children who were hospitalized. This was the first program of its type and signaled a significant change in the philosophy of caring for acutely ill children.[19]

Concerned by the problems created in the curriculum after the Goucher training summers, when a significant number of high school graduates entered the program, Miss Wolf convinced the Advisory Board of the School of Nursing to take a bold step in 1944. After hearing Miss Wolf's argument for a better-prepared student body, which she based on prewar admission data, the board voted to make a baccalaureate degree from an accredited college program the requirement for admission to the School of Nursing at Johns Hopkins.

Wolf's rationale for the change was that more than 80 percent of the students entering the program between 1938 and 1942 had at least two years of college. She believed that experienced students would be less likely to drop out and would learn more quickly because of their maturity.

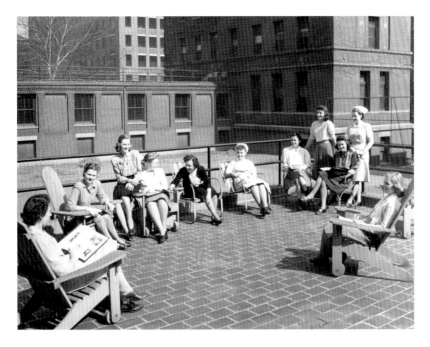

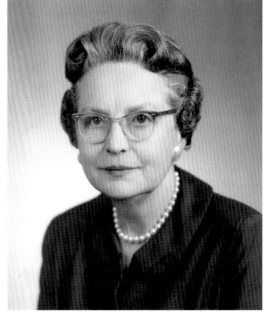

She also envisioned the possibility that university administrators might accept a graduate program, since that was their primary focus and they seemed so resistant to undergraduate study for nurses. Miss Wolf wrote to Miss Nutting, full of praise for the support she had received from doctors on the board. With this new policy in place, the class of 1947 was the first to arrive with all members holding a bachelor's degree.

The major flaw in the plan lay in the opposition that prevailed in the School of Medicine. The majority of its faculty was engaged in clinical medicine, applied biological science, or other types of pure scientific research. At the time the nursing profession had few journals, no noted clinical research, and very limited educational or behavioral research activities; the idea that nurses could do research seemed unrealistic to medical leaders. Miss Wolf recalled being asked point blank by one opponent of her plans, "What can a nurse research?"[20]

The timing of the decision to change entrance requirements could not have been worse. Just as the war was coming to an end and the number of entering students was dropping, this new policy limited enrollments even more. The goal was to admit 100 students per year; the school never achieved that goal while the degree requirement was in place. To make matters more difficult, nurses from the base hospitals and in other military service did not return in the numbers anticipated by Miss Wolf and the advisory board.

What none of the leaders at Hopkins could know was that nursing was about to enter one of its most challenging periods. After the war, everyone expected that nurses would return to work from war duty and that conditions at the School of Nursing would improve with a new generation of students. But the national nursing shortage in hospitals climbed to over forty thousand vacancies by 1948. Long hours and low pay eroded the popularity of nursing among potential students; in 1946 a young woman could earn almost twice as much as a seamstress ($1.33 per hour) as she could as a registered nurse in a hospital (74¢ per hour).

K. Virginia Betzold, 1933, joined the faculty of the nursing school the year after she graduated. In 1945 Anna D. Wolf chose Betzold to manage the nursing school's day-to-day activities, a position she continued into the next administration. Like Wolf, Betzold was a resolute advocate for university-based education for nurses.

Above left: By 1946 life was returning to normal and members of the classes of 1947 and 1948 found time to relax on the roof of Hampton House. Three years before, two upper floors had been added to the west wing, a reminder of the high number of students graduated during the war.

Loula Kennedy, 1903, began teaching at the nursing school in 1921 and quickly became a mentor to students. She retired in 1946 but continued her interest in the nurses' library, which held remarkable treasures, thanks to her diligence in developing it.

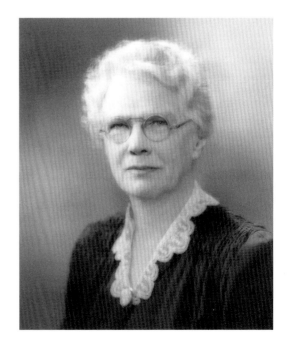

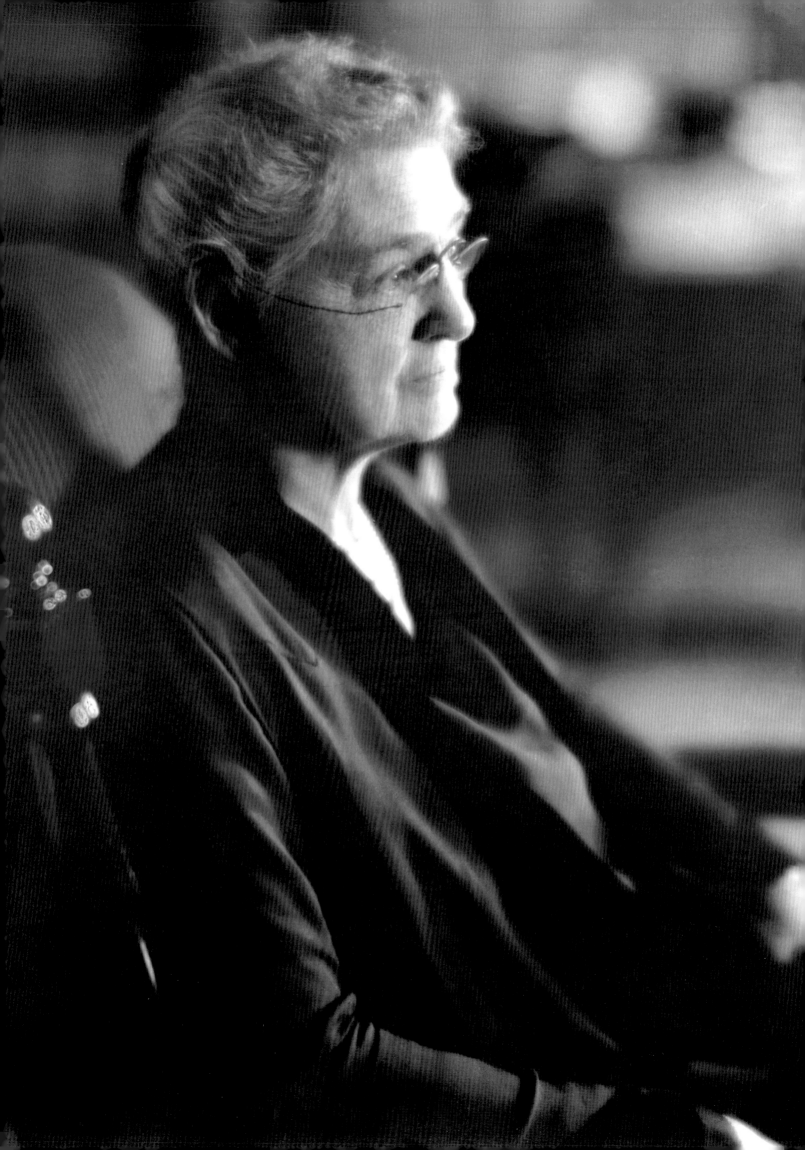

Nurses who had served in the war did not return to their previous jobs for a wide variety of reasons, including marriage and the desire for more autonomous positions, more reflective of the freedom they had experienced in the military. In addition, the number of young women graduating from high school was down because the birthrate was lower during the Depression than it had been in the 1920s.[21]

In 1945 Miss Wolf reorganized her leadership team, eliminating the associate director position for both the school and the nursing service. She placed nursing service management under the direction of Faye Whiteside and management of the School of Nursing under K. Virginia Betzold. Miss Wolf still controlled both areas, but she delegated day-to-day details to Whiteside and Betzold. (In this era, when students performed much of the bedside care of patients, the associate director for nursing service was intimately involved in the daily routine of the school.) This division was significant because it made a clearer distinction between the two functions, and Miss Wolf hoped thereby to facilitate a transition to a university-based program.

The postwar years were hard on the director and on those who worked with her. Clinical staff and faculty changed after the war as people married and left. The increased use of auxiliary personnel created problems in nursing service, and the shortage of students hindered Miss Wolf's plans to shorten student hours. Wolf had dug in during the war and tried to capitalize on the extra boost to nursing that the conflict had brought, but the simultaneous loss of the Cadet Nurse Corps (which survived only until 1948), federal aid to nursing schools, and nurses who never returned after the war caused serious shortages in the hospital and in the School of Nursing.

The late 1940s was also a period of loss for Miss Wolf and her staff. Several longtime faculty members retired, including Loula Kennedy, who had taught in the school for twenty-five years. Dr. Winford Smith, who had directed the hospital since 1911, retired. Although he did not support the baccalaureate concept, he believed strongly in the obligation of the hospital to support nursing, and he and Miss Wolf had enjoyed a productive relationship during the war years. Dr. Edwin Crosby followed Dr. Smith; Crosby was much younger, but he remained at Hopkins for just six years before moving on to his next position.

Then, in 1948, Adelaide Nutting, Miss Wolf's longtime friend and mentor, died. Wolf lost a correspondent of more than thirty years who shared a mutual vision of excellence for the Johns Hopkins School of Nursing. In addition, many staff members who were also friends left after the war. These losses compounded Wolf's difficulties. And late in the decade there were financial problems for the hospital. All of these changes increased the load and responsibilities for a leader who was approaching sixty years of age.

With a faraway expression in her eyes, she quietly spoke of the work of Florence Nightingale. At that moment it seemed to me that there was some great bond between those two women who have made such a profound impression upon nursing. They were of kindred spirit. It appeared as if Miss Nutting felt a keen responsibility for continuing to promote the great visionary efforts and far-reaching ideals of one whose work in nursing was revolutionary and far in advance of the times. Miss Nutting loved to speak of the historical background of nursing; of the forces which reacted upon the general trends in social, economic, professional and industrial living, and of their effect upon the quality of nursing carried on in our communities ... after a brief pause, Miss Nutting said, in her clear, firm voice, "History is the past, the present, and the future."

Jessie Black McVicar, 1930, recalling a visit with M. Adelaide Nutting in 1940

Opposite: M. Adelaide Nutting maintained an abiding interest in her alma mater throughout her life. On the occasion of the school's twenty-fifth anniversary, in 1914, she called for the establishment of a committee to work toward creating a $1-million endowment. She chaired the campaign for ten years because she understood that without adequate funding, Johns Hopkins University would never accept nursing as an academic discipline. The alumnae association voted in 1929 to rename the effort the M. Adelaide Nutting Endowment Fund for the Johns Hopkins Nurses' Alumnae Association, but at the time of her death in 1948, neither the endowment goal nor the dream of baccalaureate education for nurses had been achieved.

*All of us finished our clinical work at different
times in 1944. We had nurses graduating nearly
every day from July to the end of the year, since
those who had done college work were given six
months credit. Though we had three official
graduation days that year they were all dull by
comparison with the pagan rite we always
observed when a girl finished her clinical work.
We did this at the end of her last shift by tearing
her blue student uniform off her back and
sending her blushing and ragged, clothed in a
patient's gown, to her dormitory room, never to
wear a student uniform again. From then on
she would wear a snow white uniform and the
organdy Hopkins cap as well as the blue Maltese
Hopkins pin. It was a very satisfying activity,
a kind of catharsis for all the rage we may have
felt during our student days, rage about indignities
and hard work and no pay. The screams of
laughter and scuffling in the corridors on the way
to the elevators meant that someone had come
through alive, a graduate nurse!*

Frances Schlosser Scherer, 1944

In 1946 the Special Committee for the Consideration of a University School of Nursing formed. This body was made up of Dean Alan M. Chesney, School of Medicine; Dr. Richard Telinde, chairman of the Department of Gynecology, who also served on the medical board of the hospital; Anne Hahn, 1929, and Virginia Betzold, 1933, of the School of Nursing; and Mildred Struve, 1926, from the hospital nursing service. Having met for three hours every other Saturday for eight months, the committee recommended expansion of the existing relationship with the Johns Hopkins University through McCoy College. Under the new plan, students with two years or less of college credit would complete the hours prescribed and be granted sixty credits for the thirty-two-month course of study in the hospital training program. Students who had already earned accredited bachelor's degrees could receive a BSN degree when they finished the hospital program.[22] The plan was a compromise based on the judgment that any student with a baccalaureate degree or high grades for two years of college work would merit a degree when finished.[23] The Advisory Board of the School of Nursing approved the proposal, although Dr. Richard Mumma of McCoy College pointed out that no school ever gave a degree to a student who had never attended any of its classes. The authorities at the university praised the expanded relationship, but Miss Wolf and her team knew it was simply a stopgap measure in their effort to separate the school administratively from the hospital and convert the school's focus exclusively to education.

Dean Francis Horn of McCoy College wrote a short article for the alumnae magazine in April 1948 explaining that the program was unorthodox but acceptable. He attributed acceptance of the plan by the university to its recognition that Hopkins' "sound program of nursing education is the equivalent of upper division college work." Dr. Horn also pointed out that the two institutions would work closely on this program to produce high-quality graduates.[24]

In that same issue of the magazine, Miss Wolf reported that the board of trustees of the hospital had voted to reduce matriculation requirements for the nursing school to high school preparation in order to address recruitment problems. She noted that the school would

Faculty, family members, and students chatted at a graduation reception in Hampton House, c. 1948.

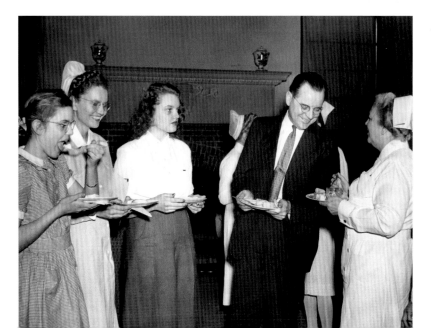

continue to give preference to students with two years of college but that it would no longer specifically try to attract college graduates. Putting these decisions in the most positive light possible, Miss Wolf pointed out that this new program, with support from both institutions and with the Hopkins reputation, would attract a larger number of students with college backgrounds. She was ready to compromise because it was "unlikely" that a baccalaureate program in Hopkins' all-male undergraduate university would be approved.[25]

Non-nursing members of the committee were pleased because this unorthodox solution addressed the shortage of student applications, kept the issue of nursing education at the baccalaureate level in McCoy College, and did not threaten either the undergraduate programs at Homewood or the medical school. In addition, it required no new funding or additional faculty from any Hopkins institution. But while the assumptions about the quality of the nursing school were well founded, the world of higher education in nursing was changing dramatically, and standards elsewhere were being rigidly enforced.

In 1948 the Russell Sage Foundation released a report that had a swift impact on nursing and nursing education. *Nursing for the Future*, written by Esther Lucille Brown, the outcome of a national study requested by the National Nursing Council, called for sweeping changes in nursing education for the second half of the twentieth century. Anna Wolf was on the advisory committee for the study, which rated nursing schools as excellent, good, or poor. The report suggested closing the poor schools immediately and having the excellent or distinguished schools affiliate with universities or colleges to produce the professional nurse needed in the future. The report also urged the federal government to consider giving added support to help nursing with this major transition. This approach would prepare nurses for all types of practice then evolving outside of hospitals.[26] Miss Wolf presented the findings to the advisory board of the school:

For us at The Johns Hopkins Hospital School of Nursing, Dr. Brown's book reflects in large part the ideology of professional nursing education long advocated by our great educational leader Mary Adelaide Nutting, an ideology which has been shared by many Hopkins Alumnae. To place our school upon a sound financial basis, our Alumnae Association, largely because of the inspiration of Miss Nutting, established the endowment fund for the school. . . . Valiant efforts by the several committees in charge of this great project have been met by whole hearted responses from many alumnae and friends. . . . We in the Johns Hopkins Hospital will have to go much further if we attain in the future professional status for our school, as Dr. Brown defines such status.[27]

Miss Wolf also commented on the new agreement with the university, which would permit graduates of the program with two years of

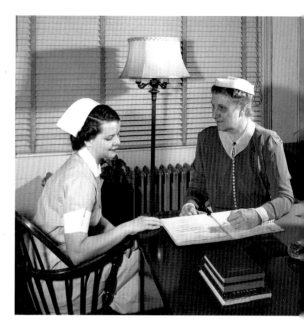

As students prepared for graduation, they knew that if they wanted it, there would be a job for them at Johns Hopkins Hospital. Still, they were expected to make an application, and part of the ritual was an interview with Anna D. Wolf. For many like Betty Stehly (at left), 1951, it was probably the first time they had ever been in the director's office.

I'd read about all the superintendents, as they originally called them. Each had her own particular accomplishment and legacy, which was a little bit different from the other's. Wolf's, particularly during the war years, was most impressive. To guide a school through that time couldn't have been easy, and yet she had a vision. I really admired that. She had a vision for how it could be done and that vision prevailed, certainly with a lot of help, but nevertheless I just understood what kind of backbone it took not only just to be the superintendent of that program but also to have a role on a national level like she did.

Cathy Novak, 1973

Beginning with the class of 1947, Wolf was able to persuade trustees to require that all incoming students have a baccalaureate degree. Her hope was that mature students would be more successful and that the university might be amenable to accepting nursing as a graduate program. The policy remained in effect for only a few years.

One of the things that has been the hallmark of Hopkins nursing right from the start has been really good teaching. Whether it's Adelaide Nutting pushing for lots of science early on, whether it's nursing faculty getting chemistry in the curriculum in the 1940s, they were always pushing the envelope and making sure that those undergraduates were prepared first, in terms of science, in terms of anatomy, and second, in terms of really delivering care in the best way possible. If you're a patient at the hospital, that's what you care about.

Paula Einaudi

We were so impressed by Dr. Dandy, going into the operating room with him, oh my, we thought there couldn't be anything more exciting. He was very helpful and kind to us, although most of us were kind of frightened of him, thinking, "Got to be very careful to do the right thing." Dr. Blalock was a great guy. And you know, even though we always felt rather overwhelmed by these people, the truth is they were kind to us and very accepting of the students. People that had never met the doctors as we did didn't realize how wonderful it was to have the help of a very fine, dedicated doctor.

Frances Schlosser Scherer, 1944

Opposite: Students in the 1940s were exposed to extraordinary strides in medicine that were taking place at Johns Hopkins. In 1944, Alfred Blalock performed the first "blue baby" operation. By 1947 there was so much interest in the procedure that on February 28, he led his surgical team in one of the first closed-circuit operations televised at Hopkins, with an enormous camera looming overhead. Nurse anesthetist Olive Berger assisted.

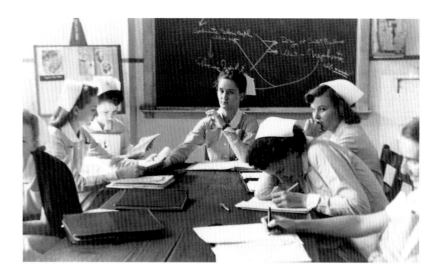

college credit to earn their degrees without requiring additional credits. She warned that this arrangement would not pass the test of time, because it was educationally unsound. She recognized the compromise that had been made and knew it had to be changed; but when?

During this postwar period, Miss Wolf was offered two prestigious positions that would have taken her away from Johns Hopkins. First, she was invited to become the director of the nursing service with the American Red Cross. (She had been a Red Cross volunteer nurse since World War I.) A second and identical offer came from the Veterans' Administration. A physician Miss Wolf consulted about her possible options encouraged her to remain at Hopkins because the university program was "just around the corner." She believed him and stayed, hoping the university program would offer more "promising" possibilities. This was one of many episodes in which Miss Wolf confided in Hopkins leaders and was encouraged that progress was being made in achieving her goals when really very little was going to happen. She described her experience as having people say "yes, maybe, or perhaps," but they were not really willing or able to achieve what she hoped for.[28]

Miss Wolf depended heavily on her faculty and nursing staff during the 1940s. Her relationships with her nurses reflected her age and background as well as the times. Although she eliminated many practices when she arrived, she remained a formal person in her collegial relationships. She seldom said thank you or praised her staff; perhaps she believed they were all just doing their duty. She required all faculty members to belong to the National League for Nursing Education and encouraged her staff to be active in professional associations. She always advocated for nurses seeking further education and personally helped many of them rearrange duties and obtain leave to complete degrees.

Former faculty members recall heavy workloads with many students and patients to oversee. Large lecture halls with more than a hundred students were common, and classes had to be taught using whatever was at hand. Doris Diller, 1932, remembered using patients in Hurd Hall to demonstrate procedures or discuss postoperative care. During the war, Diller said, faculty meetings were sporadic, and each

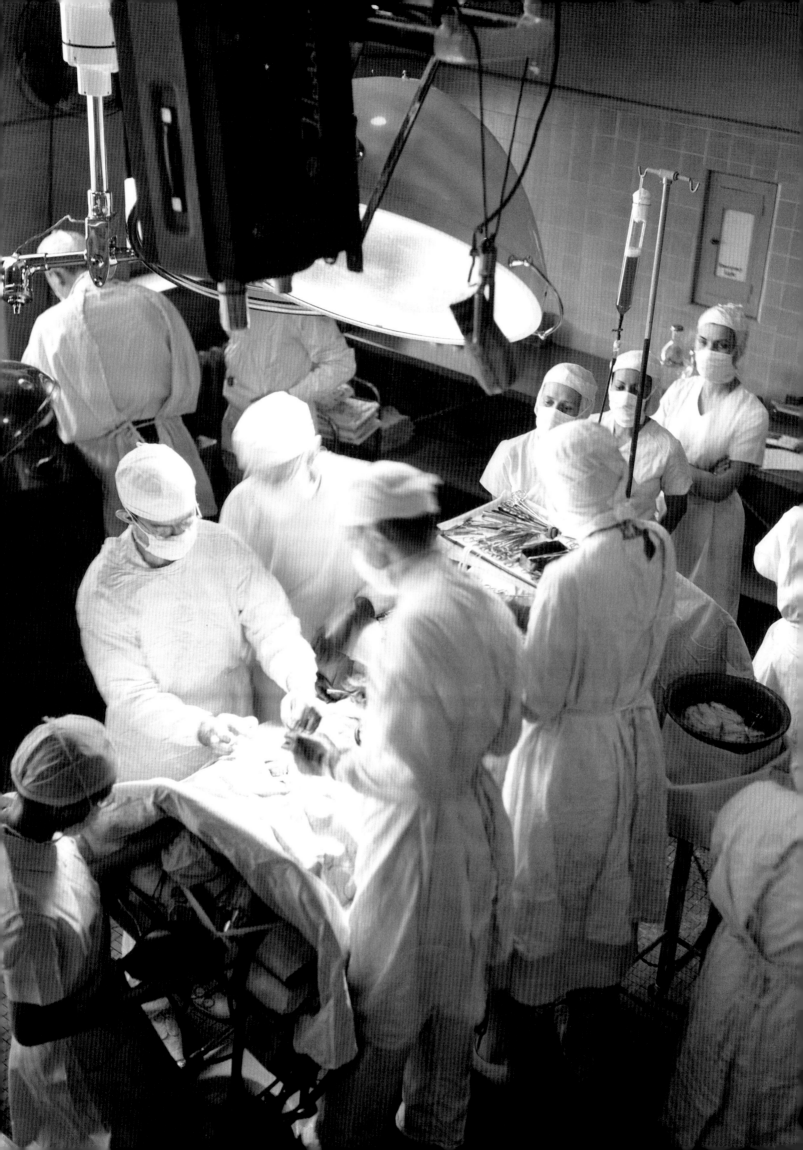

We had instructors who were so superior. Miss Grainger in preclin. I once said I thought that Ken Kesey, when he wrote One Flew Over the Cuckoo's Nest *and created Nurse Ratchett, had Miss Grainger in his vision. She was thin, straight, erect, austere looking, and plain talking, but she was not emotionally or philosophically like Nurse Ratchett. We literally trembled before Miss Grainger.*

I learned not to be afraid of Miss Grainger. We were in our first clinic to do bedside care. I got this cardiac lady. When you made her bed you couldn't put the bed flat. The woman was in the bed, her two arms clutching the bedrails. The bed looked a mess.

Miss Grainger, of course, waited till you were through. You could see her little feet under the curtains. Well, Miss Grainger came in and here's this woman and her knuckles were white. Miss Grainger came in and she looked at me and she looked at this lady. She took one hand and put it on one of the lady's hands. She took her other hand and put it on the lady's forehead. I could literally see the tension drip out of that woman. At that moment I thought, "How can you be afraid of somebody who can do this?" I stopped being afraid of her. We became good buddies. She had a great sense of humor— we just had to stop being afraid of her.

Miss Grainger gave us a list of ten things that we always had to check before we left a patient. I can't remember all ten but number one was "Is the patient safe?" Number two was "Is the patient comfortable?" Number three was "Did you do this effectively?" One was "Did you do it with the least expenditure of time and energy?" Another was "Did you leave the room set up so that the next person has what she needs to do the next treatment?" Way down on the list was "Did you do it safely for yourself?"

Miss Grainger also taught us the best definition of love I've ever heard. Love is the unselfish interest in another person. She said, "Love your patients but don't become their friends. They don't want you to be a friend. They want a capable professional." That's another thing you never forget.

Betty Borenstein Scher, 1950

nurse was left to her own devices to produce the content and clinical experiences needed by the students.[29]

Although Miss Wolf tried to change the militaristic tone of daily work in the hospital, her background and experience led her to make specific decisions and then expect her staff to carry them out—which might or might not have pleased them. Those who worked with her, however, never doubted her commitment to her nurses, her students, and the educational mission of the hospital. Her elegance, determination, and creativity enabled the nurses to cope during a very stressful period in their lives.

Miss Wolf never lost touch with her predecessor, writing to her frequently; after Miss Lawler's stroke, she encouraged Hester Frederick to bring Miss Lawler back to Hopkins. Wolf's life as director during the hectic 1940s also involved many allied responsibilities and time-consuming activities. Problems arose and had to be dealt with humanely rather than rigidly. Wolf also broke the marriage barrier for students, permitting wartime marriages because she was concerned about the young women's happiness and the possibility of their losing a loved one in the war. She implemented this change over the objections of the faculty. She also helped students who wanted to enter training even though they were married, which had not been done before. Betty Cuthbert, 1943, described Miss Wolf's sensitivity and caring when Cuthbert's husband was killed during the war. Wolf also took special care of her students who developed illnesses such as tuberculosis during their training and helped them finish their programs on individual timelines. She maintained a large correspondence with Hopkins graduates all over the world and passed many of the letters on to the alumnae association for publication in the magazine. In the midst of change and struggle, Anna Wolf was able to maintain a quiet determination to achieve her goals and to persist when others might have despaired. She was a woman of strong faith who left a legacy of advocacy for her students and cherished the dream of university affiliation for the school, an ambition she had first embraced as a student at Hopkins and Columbia.

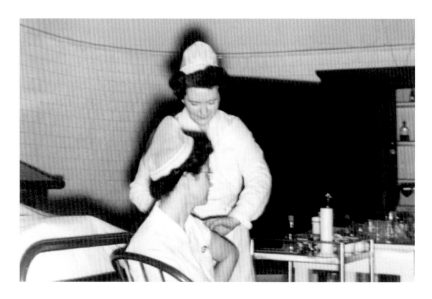

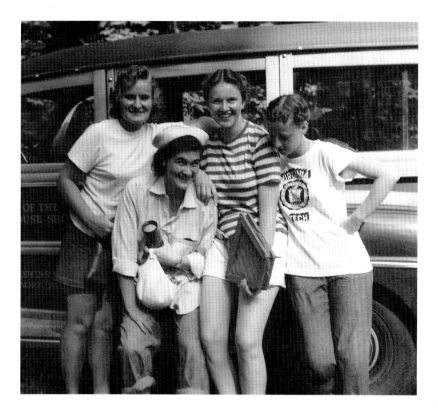

Betty Borenstein (wearing a sailor's cap), 1950, drove her friends Betsy, Boggs, and Kitty to the nursing students' retreat in Sherwood Forest on the Severn River. They were among the first to take advantage of the wood-sided station wagon, purchased by the alumnae association's Gate House Shop Committee to ease access to the cottage.

Students admitted during the turbulent 1940s coped with shortages, long clinical hours, and the pressure to work without the usual staff support while maintaining high morale and a strong sense of family. They lived in overcrowded circumstances and worked in excess of fifty hours a week but kept their sense of humor. They organized the Student Association shortly before the war began and sustained several student groups, which provided social life within Hampton House and the other residences.

When traveling was permitted, an old wood-sided station wagon was available for students to drive to a cottage designated for their exclusive use in Sherwood Forest, near Annapolis. Generations of Hopkins nurses have cited those escapes to Sherwood Forest as true lifesavers for exhausted students. In 1945 Mary Goldthwaite, 1916, reminisced about her first visit to the cottage, when she was a student and it was still brand new.

We put down our suitcases, looked about, then looked at each other. Simultaneously, we turned to open the double doors leading out onto the porch, the only doors that had screens. A glorious breeze spread through the house and we went out onto the porch where we could look down at the broad, sparkling Severn River.

The breeze and the view were too much. We sat down on the edge of the porch, swung our legs over the side and gazed over and through the trees at the bathers, the small boats with their white sails, and a few gay colored canoes gliding on the water. The breeze cooled our faces, the beauty and peace of the surrounding landscape calmed our recent misgivings, and we unanimously decided to stay.[30]

BECOMING SOMETHING SPECIAL

Nursing isn't something that you just find a book to read. Nursing is something you do very intimately with a person who's ill. You learn to know about people who are ill. I enjoyed that because it meant that we really did know the patient and we really did know what was going on. Hopkins was just so much more outstanding than anywhere else in the world as far as I knew. The Hopkins nurses had a very high standard. I was going to be a doctor but I just didn't have enough training so I thought, "Well, okay, I'll just go on and do the Hopkins training." The more I studied the happier I was I had decided to stay with Johns Hopkins. I really enjoyed being a nurse and I felt happy about it, too.

Frances Schlosser Scherer, 1944

Opposite: Instructors, like Cynthia Mallory, 1946, shown demonstrating how to give an injection to Margaret Grainger, 1930, c. 1948, had an enormous influence on their students and encouraged them to be aware of many aspects of the patient's disposition.

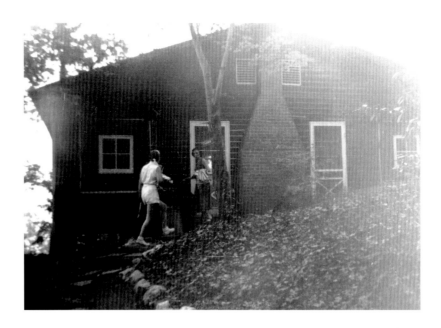

I was fortunate because I had access to a car and I was from Baltimore. My big brother convinced my father to get me a Buick convertible, which meant that two groups could go to Sherwood. One person could drive the station wagon from the alumni association and the others could go with me. The cottage in Sherwood Forest had bedrooms on the sides and then a big center room and a wonderful porch. Then you went down steps to the river. Eleanor Summers Kaschel had a little motorboat. We took that out. We would play cards. We would play games. We would dance. We would swim. We would relax. You could go down just for a day. Miss Wolf wanted you to go down even if it was just for a day, but we could stay overnight. Of course, we never got more than two days off.

Betty Borenstein Scher, 1950

Above: The cottage, which had been given to the nursing students by some hospital trustees and Dr. Hugh Young in 1917, was in a wooded setting, which made taking snapshots difficult. Mabel Gerhart, 1953, who took one of the few known photos of the cottage, noted in her scrapbook that "to recline in a cottage like this is heaven."

Right: Students in the summer of 1938 paddled their canoe on the Severn and probably went swimming or stretched out in the sun once they returned to the dock.

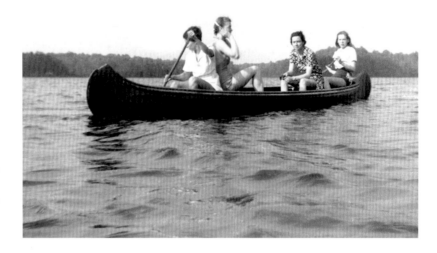

Our very favorite teacher during the first crucial six months, when we were all probies (probationers), was Miss Elizabeth Moser, who taught Nursing Arts. We sat in the tiered ranks of a small amphitheater that had originally been an operating room as she demonstrated with skill and grace the mysteries of bed making, bed baths, turning and positioning the patient, taking the temperature, pulse, and respiration, and later the deeper mysteries of enemas and catheterizations. To us she was blessed with a holy aura, and not once did we think of these tasks as menial.

Frances Schlosser Scherer, 1944

When the Gate House Shop Committee, an alumnae group that raised funds for the school and its activities, gave the station wagon to the students in 1947, their generosity meant that students could get to the cottage in forty-five minutes. Before that, they had to take two trains and a bus on a journey that took well over two hours.

Alumnae from the 1940s remember that everything changed constantly. In 1941 the student uniform was modified for the first time in many years. Gone were the black shoes and hose and the aprons, detachable collars, and cuffs that were too difficult to maintain and launder. Resources were in short supply, given the war preparedness restrictions on energy use and the availability of fabric. In their place, simple single-piece blue uniforms without aprons, tan shoes, and stockings were introduced. Members of the class of 1944 were the first to don rented tan lab coats and tan shoes and hose for their probationary period.

The other major change for the student uniform was the introduction of a student cap, which was made of washable muslin and could be laundered by the students. The upper-class students were told that if their old uniforms wore out, they would have to replace them with the new style, but they were not pleased with these changes, and many students wore rather shabby old-style uniforms rather than make the change.[31]

The student organization developed committees to address every aspect of student life. New social events were planned and opportunities to help others through a group called the Volunteers were added to student schedules. The social committee established monthly activities, which might be movies, dances, talent shows, or field trips—if transportation was possible. Student volunteers participated in Red Cross or community service activities to help veterans or the needy while other volunteers led Bible studies in the residence.

Students looked forward each year to the annual turtle derby held in May. This fun-filled social event raised money for special resources in the hospital, such as a house staff fund for new tennis courts adjacent to the Main Residence. The 1941 derby committee began publicizing early with the announcement of a new drug discovered at Hopkins as the result of the turtle derby. The drug, "Sulfaturtlene," came from the "sudor testudinous" excreted by turtles exercising for the derby, which would be coming up in three weeks. That year the turtles raced for the "Kolostomy Kup" and $50 in nickels. Hospital departments, students, house staff, and individuals could enter turtles for a fee. (The turtles were obtained from a nearby farm, where they were returned after the race.) The 1941 winner was Clanging Bell Out of Order by Marburg III. In 1946 the Johns Hopkins Turf and Turtle Club, Unincorporated, managed the first postwar derby. Patients who were able were wheeled to the "track" to watch the race. Bulletin boards announced favorites and refreshments were served to the tunes of an amateur band. The winner that year was Ulcers Out of Neurosis by Frustration, entered by nursing students Rose Pinneo, 1946, and Margaret Hawkins, 1946. They accepted the Kolostomy Kup filled with nickels.[32]

The work of a nurse in the 1940s was a little different from our work in the '80s. During the war materials were few and precious. We had to sterilize and reuse thermometers, syringes, needles, instruments, and gloves. To give a hypodermic injection we had to boil a few drops of water in a spoon over an alcohol lamp, then dissolve the correct dosage of medication in the water, and then draw up the solution in a boiled syringe. Often we had to sharpen the needles as well as boil them for reuse. Rubber gloves were mended like bicycle tires, with a dot of rubber and some cement. We mended, washed, dried, powdered, and sterilized them over and over again.

Frances Schlosser Scherer, 1944

Arriving members of the class of 1944 were the first to be called preclinical students instead of probationers. Like generations of students to follow, they wore tan lab coats over their civilian clothes while their uniforms were being custom-made. They also learned nutrition in a classroom instead of the old Main Residence's kitchen.

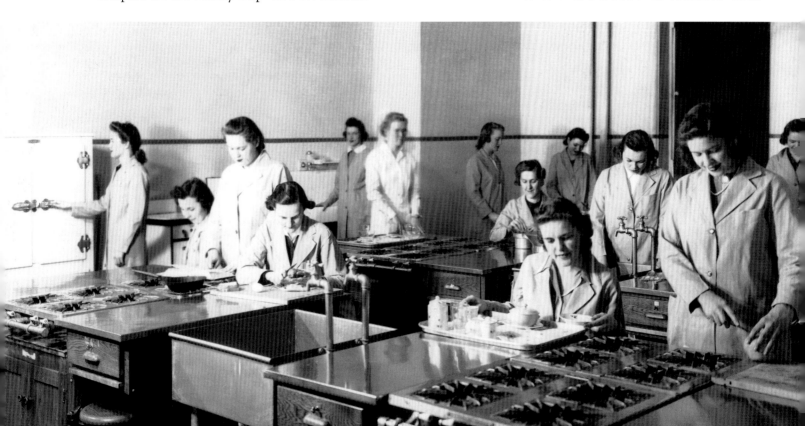

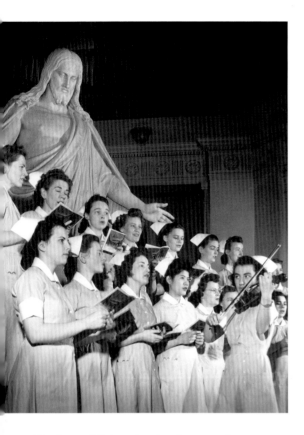

The figure of *Christus Consolator* has greeted everyone entering the Broadway entrance since 1896, when William Wallace Spence gave the copy of a statue created by Danish sculptor Bertel Thorvaldsen to the hospital. Nursing students in 1946 gathered at its base to sing, no doubt bringing holiday cheer to all.

Opposite, above: Increased enrollment during World War II provided enough performers in the class of 1945 to mount a production of *HMS Pinafore* on March 3, 1944.

Opposite, below: Even while serving in the military, Hopkins nurses and doctors in General Hospital No. 118 took time to lift their voices. On December 25, 1943, they started the day singing Christmas carols on the grounds of the hospital center at Herne Bay, twelve miles south of Sydney, Australia, where they maintained a thousand-bed unit.

We all had relatives and boyfriends who were in the service and were away. After some time I remember we had some German prisoners of war at the hospital. Hopkins used to have white brick walls in the corridors. I remember those prisoners of war washing those walls and washing floors.

Ethel Rainey Ward, 1947

A sense of foreboding filled students before and during World War II as hospital units were organized and the hospital prepared for war. There was concern that Baltimore's proximity to Washington, Baltimore's steel mills and shipping port, and nearby military installations made the city a target. Every strategic window was equipped with blackout curtains. Emergency supplies and facilities, including operating rooms, were established in the basement of the dispensary building in case of attack or emergency.[33]

Mary Agnes Gautier, 1942, in a letter to her family postmarked December 13, 1941, provided a vivid account of her thoughts and concerns during the week after the attack on Pearl Harbor:

I know how awful you all must feel and I'm certainly on edge but all we can do is hope for the best. . . . I just thought this was going to be the best Christmas I ever had in years, but no matter how much cash or otherwise I had to spend for my pleasure it couldn't be now. We seniors who graduate in February had a dinner with Miss Wolf (our sup't. of nurses) last night. Of course lots of the conversation was of the present situation. I asked her point blank several things about what they were doing here at the hospital in regards to evacuation of patients, instructions that we might be given in case of air raid, places of safety etc. . . . I've heard all kinds of rumors as to how the patients will be sent to outlying hospitals and all sent home that could be possibly discharged when Hopkins would be used as emergency hospital and evacuate injured to hospitals some miles from here. . . . There has been talk of other plans of action but nothing official. . . . The staggering thing about it all is how unprepared Baltimore apparently is for an air raid.[34]

Gautier described the recruitment of her class for the Hopkins hospital unit that was being formed. She expressed interest but had made no decision. Eventually, she joined and served with General Hospital 118. It must have been difficult for young nurses embarking on their careers to decide which direction to take as the world situation changed so dramatically.

Once the United States joined the war, worry for loved ones and friends added to the anxiety students felt. Constant messages about death and destruction overseas compounded the normal stress associated with working daily with people who were sick and dying from disease. Students had to cope with their own loss of personal freedom to do whatever they pleased after graduation, recognizing that deployment for war emergencies remained a possibility.

Even students arriving after the war faced tough times. Termination of funding for nursing education led to a decline in the enrollments, and staffing levels dropped. The severe shortage of nurses, which developed right after the war and continued throughout the rest of the decade, meant students learned quickly that there was always too much

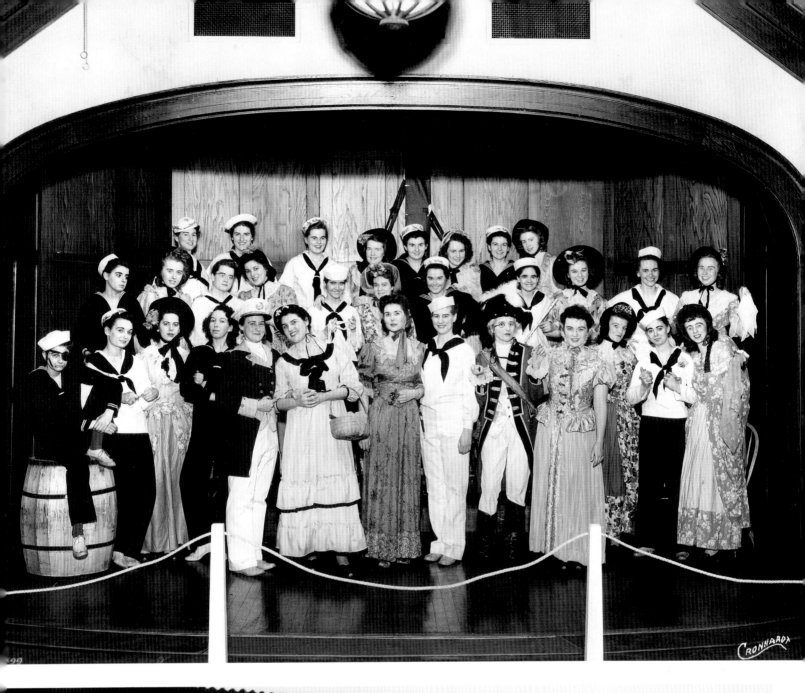

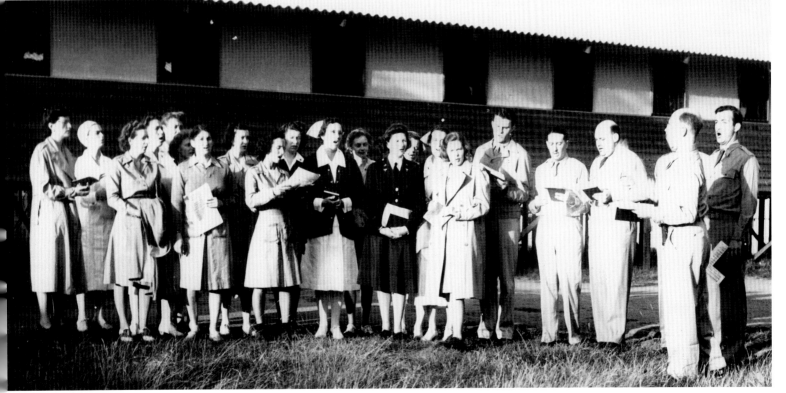

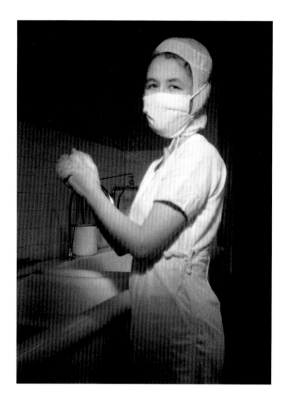

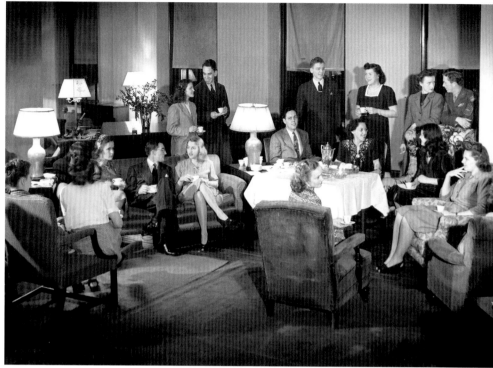

Like many a nursing student before and after her, Mary Agnes Hull, 1950, scrubbed vigorously as she prepared to work in the general operating room.

Above right: Students in the classes that graduated between 1947 and 1950, all of whom had bachelor's degrees, brought a mature ambiance to the nursing school. Medical students, young professionals, and servicemen who visited them in Hampton House found stimulating conversation as well as tea and coffee.

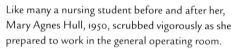

We worked 7 A.M. to 1 P.M. and then we would be back 5 A.M. to 7 P.M. In between those times we had classes. Then there were other days that we would work 7 to 9 A.M. and 1 to 7 P.M. Occasionally you would get 7 A.M. to 11 A.M. and 7 P.M. to 11 P.M. It was hard but it was interesting and you felt like you were learning and doing. In those days we had a lot of respect for our teachers. We were there to learn and we tried to be respectful and listen to them.

Constance Cole Heard Waxter, 1944

work for the hands available to do it. Illnesses that plagued the students throughout the decade also had an impact on the labor force. Quite often in her reports to the advisory board, Miss Wolf mentioned the loss of students through illness. Tuberculosis took a severe toll during this period, before the availability of effective medications.

Throughout this challenging time Hopkins students were grateful for the opportunity to learn in such a large and diverse clinical setting, and they wrote frequently in the alumnae magazine about how thankful they were for their education. Miss Wolf wanted more for these students, and yet they felt they had received an excellent education, and they went out into the nursing world and did great things with what they had learned. The idea that becoming a Hopkins nurse was something special did not diminish with the war years, in spite of the hard work, difficulties, and disappointments.

Close friendships that lasted a lifetime were forged in the crowded living quarters of the early 1940s, and each group seemed pleased to have been housed just where it was. Looking back, alumnae from these years treasured their clinical experiences in spite of the hard work and long hours. They saw Miss Wolf as a dignified, caring director who impressed upon them the need for the school to go forward. Nurses prepared in this turbulent period learned Miss Wolf's lessons well, including her message about the need to endow the School of Nursing for the future, which she repeated often and earnestly. These alumnae demonstrated Wolf's success in the years after their graduations, especially in their support of the school and its alumnae association.

A large group of graduates enlisted in the hospital unit that began organizing within the Johns Hopkins Hospital in 1940 in preparation for war. This unit was to be called General Base Hospital 18, as a similar group had been titled in World War I. This hospital was to have enough doctors, nurses, and support personnel to serve a 1,000-bed military hospital to be based overseas in time of need. In April 1942 the Office of the Surgeon General asked that the group, which had been recruited, screened, and enlisted, be divided into two hospitals, each with a 500-bed the capacity, so the 18th was split into the 18th and 118th units.

Originally Mildred Struve, 1926, a nursing supervisor at the hospital, was to lead the nurses in the 18th, but she was disqualified because of a vision problem, and Mary Sanders, 1934, was selected to replace her. When the units were split, Miss Sanders assumed direction of the 118th, and Jane Pierson, 1932, was selected as chief nurse for the 18th. Pierson was practicing in Tennessee when the call came; she reported to Baltimore within four days of her selection.

Once the units had been called up for service, there was a flurry of activity to prepare for their departure. Young nurses settled their personal affairs, said goodbye to families, and prepared to leave with their units.[35] On April 20, 1942, both units were scheduled to leave Baltimore for training. A few days earlier, the hospital's board of trustees and the women's auxiliary gave a farewell tea in the Hampton House lounge, where they presented the medical directors with $5,000 each for discretionary needs of the nursing staff in each unit. Then, they were on their way. The 118th went to Massachusetts and the 18th went to South Carolina for training prior to receiving their overseas orders.[36]

PROBING FOR SHRAPNEL, DRESSING RAW STUMPS

During World War II, two hospital units were composed primarily of Hopkins nurses and doctors. Mary Sanders, 1934, led General Hospital No. 118. Nurses of General Hospital No. 18 posed as a group before departing from San Francisco in 1942. Their travels took them to New Zealand, the Fiji Islands, and the Burma-India theater of operations.

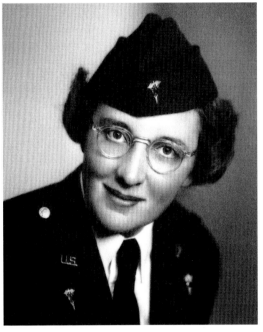

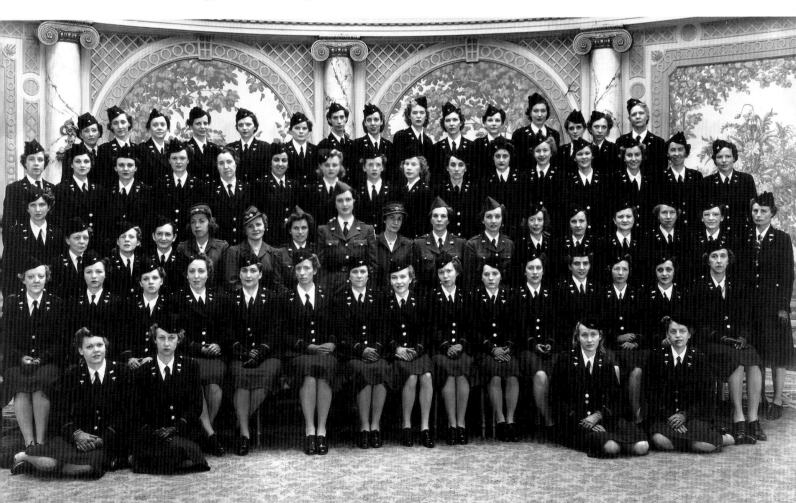

Both units spent a few days in San Francisco getting equipped and supplied before leaving the country. While they were there, Miss Lawler rode by bus from Santa Cruz, where she lived, and spent three days with her graduates. She wrote a lively article for the alumnae magazine about the experience. After spending time with both Miss Pierson and Miss Sanders, Miss Lawler wrote, "I have the consolation of thinking that even if I cannot go as an army nurse, I did have a glorious ride on the front seat of an army truck and lived with uniformed nurses for three days. I go with them in spirit and pray that things may not be too hard, but I know they will meet whatever comes and that Base Hospitals Nos. 18 and 118 will do good work and that we will be proud of them."[37]

The two units had very different experiences. The 18th moved often and had long periods of professional idleness, while the 118th moved less frequently and had fewer periods with low patient loads. Both groups did share common experiences, including the deprivations and struggles that go with practicing under primitive conditions and having to improvise in order to maintain care standards. Nurses experienced tropical monsoons and seas of mud in the midst of trying to provide sterile surgical care. The needs of local people who were not involved in the conflict were also a concern. All this was experienced against the backdrop of the uncertainties of war and being far from home and loved ones.

In spite of the stresses of war nursing, these veterans recalled many happy times. There were social occasions when staff would have parties or special dinners. Entertainments were arranged for staff, and free time between peaks in patient needs allowed for sightseeing and recreation. A nurse with the 18th remembered going horseback riding in Fiji. Elizabeth McLaughlin, 1915, wrote from the 18th that

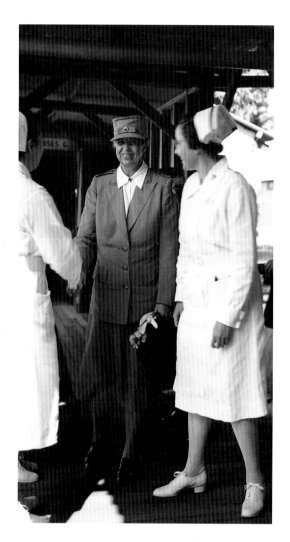

Mary Sanders escorted First Lady Eleanor Roosevelt as she visited the wounded and inspected working conditions. The visit was formal; Sanders and her colleagues rarely donned white uniforms once they left Australia and moved on to more difficult circumstances.

the limitations of an island outpost and the periodic enforced abundance of leisure have brought about the development of various hobbies. Lacking equipment is improvised. Photography has attracted a large group. Sergeant Julio, the painter, has made an enlarging machine out of an old lens and a few odds and ends. Corporal Marco, the electrician, furnished the enthusiasts with a printing box he makes out of some scraps of lumber, a beer bottle, and a bit of glass. From his machine even the rankest amateur can get good results. There is considerable and generous swapping of negatives, printing paper, solutions, and film.[38]

On February 17, 1944, Dr. H. Alvan Jones spoke to the alumnae association about some of his experiences with General Hospital 18. When they moved to the Fiji Islands in August 1943, the site for their hospital had not even been selected, but by late October they had taken over a school and were treating patients. "On the night before we received our patients they were pouring concrete and finishing up lighting fixtures and we—both men and nurses—were finishing up making the beds . . . until midnight. What a grand and glorious sight and feeling it was when

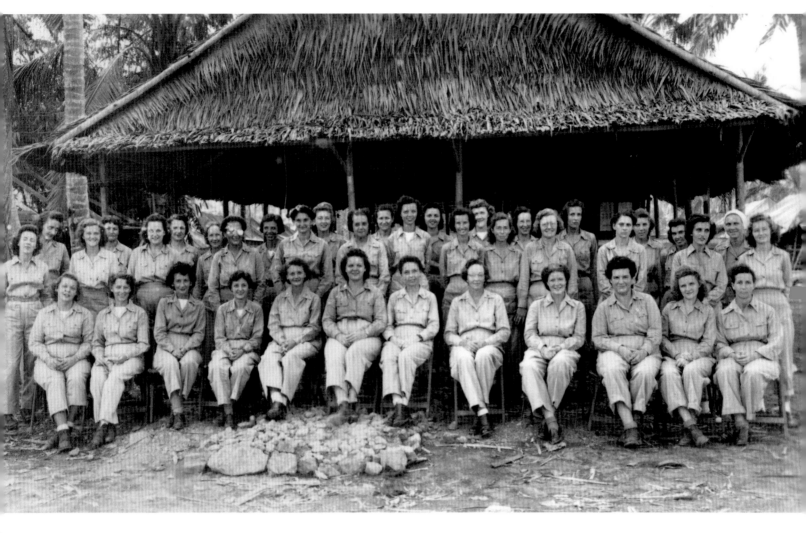

From 1942 through much of 1944, the 118th was ensconced in Australia, where they treated cases of malaria more often than battle wounds. They had plenty of time to sightsee and party on the beach and cruise in motor launches. Their work became less comfortable and more complex when they moved on to Leyte Island in the Philippines, where they posed in front of a building constructed for their unit.

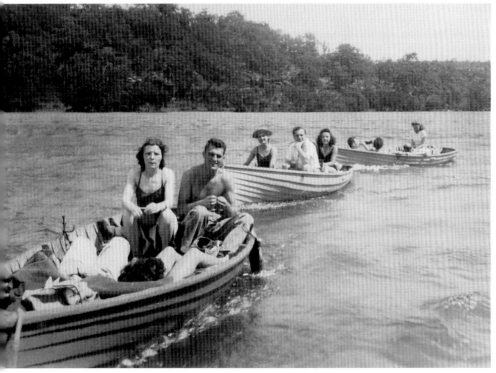

Really we could not have picked a more beautiful spot…. We are celebrating our year on this island by having a large party in the new Recreation Hall…. The nurses have nice quarters … in grass houses built by the natives….

Charlotte Fischer, 1928,
writing from General Hospital No. 18

Captain Mary Sanders married the Reverend Harry
Price, chaplain for General Hospital No. 118, on
September 25, 1945. In 1955 the couple would take up
residence in Hampton House.

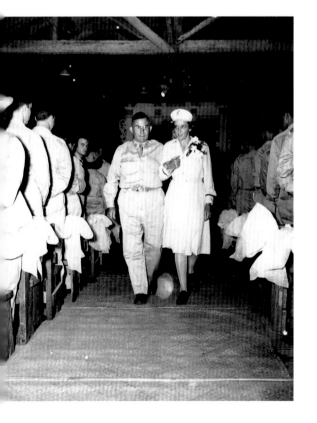

the ambulances began to roll into that hospital the following morning, and from then on many of us were kept busy."[39]

In November 1944, Captain Helen Weber, 1934, wrote home to describe conditions at General Hospital 118's new site in New Guinea, where, she reported, the temperature regularly reached 125 degrees. Frequent rains "turn everything into a sea of grimy mud." She observed that after their arrival,

for a few days we worked 6 hours, then 8, and finally, although posted 8, we worked 10 and 12 hours. As I write 23 of our nurses are on 12 hour night duty. Having had no time to accustom ourselves to the heat, we are becoming fatigued.

Nevertheless, we are getting valuable experience. Our people are probing for and removing shrapnel, dressing new, raw stumps, and doing many surgical procedures, which until now were done by our officers. One nurse not infrequently carries a ward of 40 bed patients. . . . Emergency major operations are done, frequently, on the wards and the ward nurse scrubs![40]

On one auspicious occasion, Edith A. Nunn, 1932, wrote to the alumnae magazine, exclaiming that she had experienced a high point in her tour of duty with the 118th by attending the marriage of the unit's leader, Captain Mary Sanders, to Chaplain Harry Price on September 25, 1945. She reported that the bride had been given away by Colonel Bordley and that she and Captain Virginia Thompson, 1940, had been attendants. She said that the bride was lovely and that both parties were held in the highest esteem by the entire staff.[41]

Other graduates served as rank-and-file nurses in various military campaigns, and some drew duty that had benefits as well as hardships. Mary Claire Cox, 1935, wrote from "somewhere in North Africa" that she and her colleagues had "a wonderful set-up here. It is a beautiful spot by the sea. We are lucky enough to live in houses and our hospital is also housed. The beach is just out our back door so, of course, we go swimming every day and are brown as berries."[42]

Mary Agnes Gautier wrote about her experiences with the 118th in a diary and in letters home. Her correspondence reflected the unpredictability of life in the service during the war. There were hectic times, but few weeks went by when she did not have time to write to her family. Her career took a significant turn when, having trained to give anesthesia in the operating room in the 118th, she grew to love this work. After the war she attended the Charity Hospital School of Anesthesia in New Orleans and served with the army in Georgia during the Korean Conflict. She then returned to her native Mississippi and practiced for more than thirty-five years as the director of the Department of Anesthesia at Singing River Hospital in Moss Point. She served as a leader in the Mississippi Nurses Association and among nurse anesthetists in her region. In 1998 she was inducted into the Mississippi Nurses Hall of

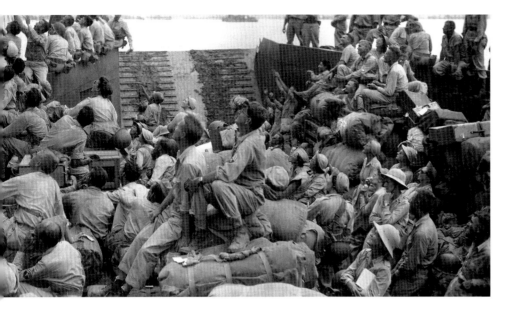

Between Australia and the Philippines, the 118th traveled through Hollandia, New Guinea. As they waited on a landing ship transport for a gangplank to be lowered into position, most seemed eager to move on.

Center: On June 4, 1944, not long before they left Australia, officers and nurses of the 118th commemorated their arrival there two years earlier by throwing a "landing party." Dr. W. B. VandeGrift, far right, whom Mary Farr, 1941, recalled as being in charge of organizing the alcohol for parties, was named "supreme admiral" for the occasion.

Below: Mary Farr remembered many good times at both work and play while she served with the 118th, especially in Australia. She and her surgical colleagues took time away from the operating rooms to pose for a group portrait. The caps they fashioned to cover their hair, she recalled, were made from diapers.

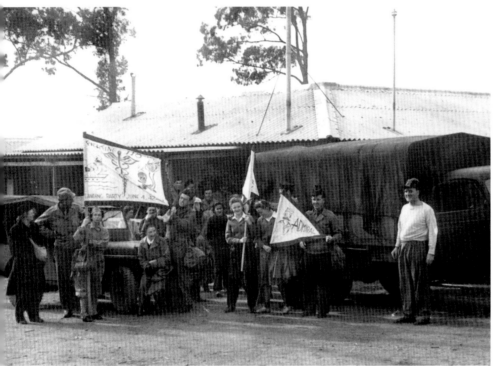

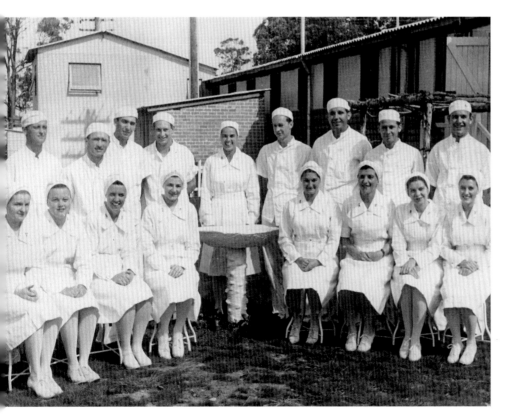

In Australia, we were not so busy surgically but we got the casualties as they were sent from hospital to hospital. We were improving on what had been done quickly up in the station hospitals. We did elective surgery in the operating room. In medicine, they had the tropical diseases. And we had psychiatric cases. We were not that busy in the operating room so we were farmed out and given the opportunity to be some other place and help out.

When we left Australia, we had no idea what we were going to do. The nurses left first and went up to New Guinea on this hospital ship. We were busy there. We were assigned to the hospital and were beginning to get patients from the Philippines. I was assigned to an orthopedic ward. In orthopedics, they had gas gangrene, oh my gosh, and they didn't have water to wash your hands. We had sterilizing solutions. I was scared. I really was.

Mary Farr Heeg, 1941

LINDA SABIN

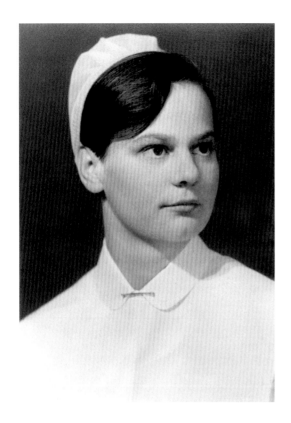

Esther Jacoby, 1930, who served with General Hospital No. 118 during the war, returned to her alma mater to become a favorite member of the faculty.

This was wartime and there was a cadet nurse program that Lucile Petry Leone was involved with. She's a Hopkins grad and she was in the surgeon general's office. Although I had graduated from college and I'd taught for three and a half years, I was interested in going into the nursing program. There was gas rationing then so I came on the train. I'd never been to Baltimore, so when I asked the conductor which station should I get off to be closest to the hospital, he told me Camden. When I got off the cab drivers were saying, "North Bawlimur, East Bawlimur, West Bawlimur." I couldn't tell what they were saying plus I had no idea which direction it was. I finally got in one for East Baltimore and they took me to Hampton House.

Ethel Rainey Ward, 1947

Fame. "A role model and nurturer of new graduates, colleagues and students, Gautier was highly respected by those who worked with her and the patients for whom she cared," the announcement declared.[43]

Several war veterans came back to their careers at Johns Hopkins or returned later to serve the school and the hospital. Mary Farr, 1941, was a beloved instructor in the school during the 1950s and '60s. Esther Jacoby, 1930, also became a popular staff member and nursing instructor, and Mary Sanders Price succeeded Miss Wolf as director of the school. Many physicians and other staff also returned to continue their service at the hospital.

In addition to the nurses who served with the Hopkins base hospitals, many graduates served in other capacities with the army, navy, and American Red Cross, and some assumed leadership positions in civilian and military capacities. In 1944 Virginia Dunbar, 1923, was appointed director of the nursing service of the American Red Cross. Dunbar had come to Johns Hopkins with a degree from Mount Holyoke College; after finishing at Hopkins, she earned a master's degree at Columbia.[44]

Lucile Petry Leone, 1927, had a distinguished career before the war and emerged afterward as a national nursing leader. She had served as the first woman administrator in the U.S. Public Health Service before the war. Then, in 1943, she had just been appointed dean at the Cornell University School of Nursing when Surgeon General Thomas Parran appointed her director of the new Division of Nursing Education of the Public Health Service. This division, established by the Bolton Act of 1943, provided for the establishment of the Cadet Nurse Corps. Leone was granted a leave of absence to take the directorship, and for more than three years she headed a national campaign to recruit more young women into nursing education—an effort that helped recruit more than 180,000 students into nursing.

After the war, Lucile Petry Leone served for more than two decades as the chief nurse officer and assistant surgeon general for the U.S. Public Health Service, in Washington, D.C. Mrs. Leone played a major role as a leader of nurses during the turbulent postwar years, serving as a teacher and mentor for young nurses late into her long life. She continued to support her alma mater through the alumnae association and was frustrated by the inability of the leaders at Hopkins to establish a baccalaureate program.

Elizabeth Lawrie Smellie, 1909, a Canadian who returned to her homeland after graduation, served in Europe during World War I. She went back to Canada after that war and led nurses as a director and superintendent in several key positions. On June 27, 1940, she became the matron-in-chief of the Royal Canadian Army Medical Corps Nursing Service and practiced in that capacity throughout World War II.[45]

The 1940s was an era of service and determination for the alumnae association. With many of its active members involved in the war effort and many others working at home, activities were pared down to the essentials. Alumnae continued their commitment to fundraising for the endowment and supporting activities for students. Each class that graduated in the 1940s presented gifts to the school and often to the alumnae association for the Endowment Fund. Membership in the association was considered a major step related to graduating from the hospital training program; wearing the alumnae pin along with the graduate cap (especially for those admitted after 1940) was part of the transition from undergraduate to graduate.

The association did an impressive job keeping track of graduates who were in service overseas and making sure the membership was updated on events at the school and changes at the hospital. With wartime shortages and limitations, it had to keep the alumnae magazine small, filled to the brim with only the most significant news. It followed developments in the profession, however, and members learned from detailed articles and reports about the challenges Miss Wolf and the school were facing. Alumnae struggled at times with necessary modifications, such as new uniforms, the elimination of morning prayers, and new requirements for admission and graduation.

This was also a period of loss for the group. Several of the early leaders died, including Christine Dick, 1899, who had managed the nursing residences for many years; longtime instructor Hester Frederick, 1912; and M. Adelaide Nutting, 1891. The sudden drop in nursing enrollments and the severe nursing shortage that occurred after the war stressed the entire system at Hopkins, and the alumnae became aware that even greater changes lay ahead. There was hope however, that the end of the war and the arrival of the mid-century mark would bring a new impetus for improvements that would benefit nurses instead of increasing their burdens.

Christine Dick was the housemother at Hampton House. She was kind of strait-laced. We were supposed to be in at ten-thirty, maybe eleven or twelve on the weekends. She expected the rooms to look pretty good. She did inspect them so she had keys to everything. It was wartime and we were to wear brown stockings. The graduate nurses could get white nylons. We would go to the five-and-ten and get Tintex and dye the stockings in our white enamel sinks. So we had brown sinks and Miss Dick had a problem with that. But we had no way of cleaning them and I don't think we were interested in cleaning them either.

Ethel Rainey Ward, 1947

Below left: Alumnae gathered in the dining room of the Main Residence for a Christmas luncheon and sale, c. 1940, probably an effort to raise money for the endowment fund. It was one of the last times they would be served by nursing students wearing uniforms like the ones they themselves had worn.

Christine Dick, 1899, here c. 1912, managed the nursing residences, as well as the cottage in Sherwood Forest, for more than twenty-five years. When she died in 1945, the cottage was named in her honor.

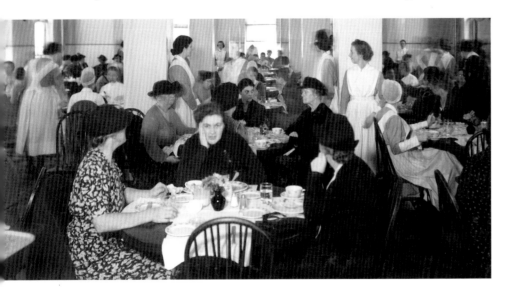

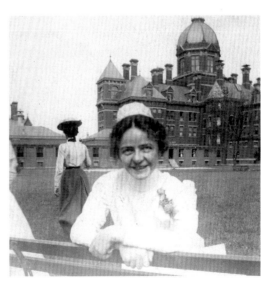

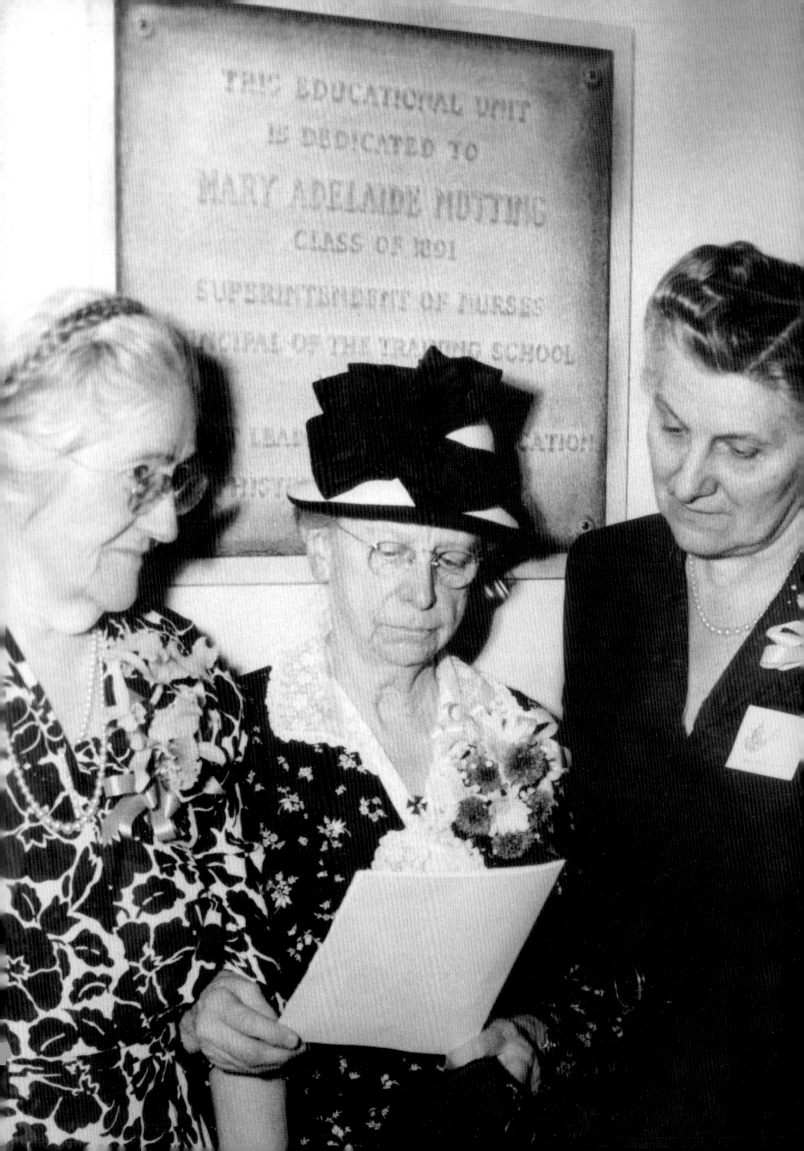

Nursing at the Crossroads, 1950–1960 · LINDA SABIN

3

On May 29, 1951, Elsie Lawler, 1899, Helen Wilmer
Athey, 1905, and Anna D. Wolf, 1915, joined fellow
alumnae to celebrate the dedication of a new
educational unit on the basement level of the old
Nurses' Home. The new facilities comprised fourteen
renovated rooms for class and lab work, ten offices
for faculty, and a new auditorium.

CHALLENGES confronted Anna Wolf on many fronts during her last five years at the Johns Hopkins Hospital. Relaxation of the short-lived degree requirement necessitated a return to lower admission standards; this, joined with a shortage of qualified students and the lack of movement on the nursing degree program at the university, increased Miss Wolf's frustration as she saw her goals slip away. By 1950 the nursing shortage in the United States had escalated, although some had feared there would be an oversupply when the war ended because of the Cadet Nursing Program. The opposite occurred because the number of potential candidates between the ages of fifteen and nineteen had fallen more than 20 percent since 1940, a legacy of hard times in the Great Depression. In addition, more than half the women between eighteen and twenty-four had married, which eliminated them from traditional nursing programs. The birth rate did not diminish in the early 1950s as expected, and the pattern of women dropping out of the workforce to raise children became the norm, which limited the duration of the professional careers of many graduate nurses.[1]

ADRIFT IN A CHANGING TIDE

The chronic turnover, recruitment woes, and staff shortages that plagued Miss Wolf and her colleagues were reflections of societal issues. That enrollments at the School of Nursing *did* climb modestly in the 1950s demonstrated the success of Hopkins' efforts, as well as the high quality of the program. There was also no discussion of closing units because of a lack of nursing staff during this period, when some other hospitals had turnover rates in excess of 60 percent and had to close units for years at a time owing to a lack of staff.[2]

By late 1950 nursing shortages had gotten the attention of the medical board of the hospital, causing it to send a strong recommendation to the board of trustees. The doctors on the medical board complained that nursing care had not been up to usual standards for some time because of inadequate recruiting of students and emphasis on college education as a qualification for nursing practice and advancement. They suggested that the number of students was directly related to the availability of nursing care and that graduates of the Hopkins program were not attracted to work at the hospital because of the emphasis on college preparation for advancement or promotion. Further, they reported that Hopkins nursing students were better trained than some degree-holding graduates from other programs who had been hired but did not meet expected standards of practice. The doctors had two specific recommendations for the board of trustees:

1. Wholehearted acceptance by all concerned that the minimal educational requirements for admission to the school of nursing is a high school education, with energetic recruitment efforts on that basis.

We were all awed at the hospital and how large it was. Our schedule was laid out for us as we all took the same classes. We were assigned to different clinical units in the hospital. There was no special order to it. You just did the six units during the time of your student days. We had to learn to not only talk to the patient but be observant while we were talking to the patient. There was a lot to learn. When we weren't doing clinical practice or clinical skills, of course, we had other classes, learning dosage and solutions, a lot of pharmacology. We had wonderful instructors. Usually an instructor would have about six students on an individual floor that they would be responsible for.

Betsy Mumaw McGeady, 1955

2. Wholehearted acceptance of the general principle that a college education is not essential for advancement in the field of hospital nursing.[3]

These sentiments indicate not only the problem of a chronic shortage in the hospital but also the opinion of many physicians regarding the education of nurses. In some ways the Hopkins medical staff had been spoiled over the years. Through the late 1930s and into the '40s, most of the students in the nursing program had college backgrounds and many were college graduates. Physicians had become accustomed to a mature, hard-working, and focused student population, yet they did not appreciate the significance of the college experience the nursing students possessed. The war, the shortage of students after the war, and Miss Wolf's attempt to admit only college graduates all led to the doctors' ill-conceived response. In addition, medical and hospital associations strongly opposed the postwar drive of nurses wanting baccalaureate preparation for practice. Fear of increased labor costs, concern about the demands of college-prepared nurses, and an ongoing satisfaction with diploma-prepared nurses fueled this opposition. Physicians at

The corridors of Johns Hopkins Hospital were usually busy, with doctors, nurses, and visitors bustling or conversing, sometimes both. Marlene Lowder, 1960, took a few minutes to chat with an alumna instructor at the entrance to the Osler Medical Clinic in 1959.

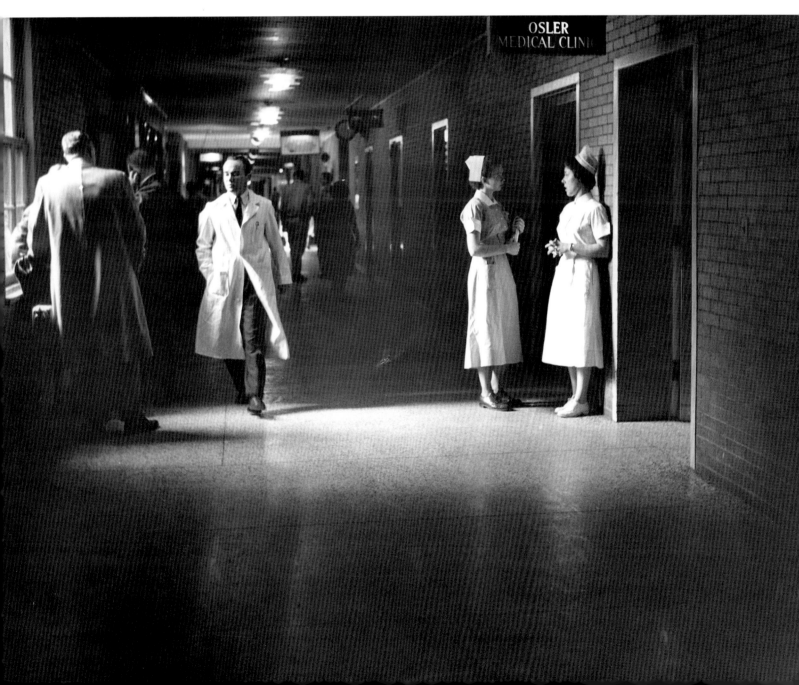

*I came to Baltimore in 1959 right smack
out of high school. I chose to come to Baltimore
rather than to pursue the degree channel.
It was the shortest route to a career given the era.
It wasn't as important for me to think in terms
of degrees. I wanted to be a bedside nurse.
In today's nursing, you really can't do that.
Once you have your degrees, you're really kind of
forced up the chain and that's not what I wanted.
In the early '60s, you didn't need degrees if
you wanted to be head nurses and supervisors.*

Lois Grayshan Hoffer, 1962

*Miss Wolf allowed married students but you
couldn't be pregnant. At our graduation
Mary Agnes Hull Stewart was married and she
held up the diploma and whispered, "Is it mine?"
We said, "Yes." "Can they take it away from me?"
"No." "Are you sure?" "Of course." She unbuttoned
her waist and she said, "I'm pregnant."*

Betty Borenstein Scher, 1950

The class of 1950 was the last in which all members
arrived at the School of Nursing having already earned
a bachelor's degree. In less than a year, Betty Borenstein
(front row, center, holding her diploma in her right
hand) was a head nurse in the Wilmer Institute. She
recalled that "Miss Wolf had told us that we were
graduating as excellent bedside nurses, but we were not
equipped for anything more until we had more
experience and more education."

Hopkins felt frustrated and inconvenienced by Miss Wolf's attempt to modify a program that had met their needs throughout the history of the institution. But the change Miss Wolf wanted was only partially the issue; social dimensions of the postwar era were also driving the shortage of students and practicing nurses. The doctors' recommendations and wishes were late and missed the target altogether.

The hospital board of trustees sent the recommendations to the Advisory Board of the School of Nursing. Miss Wolf responded by pointing out that enrollment of only bachelor's-prepared students had ended in 1947. She reported that there were efforts under way with McCoy College to set up a bachelor's degree program for Hopkins nursing students with two years of college. She also cited the decision, then more than two years old, to make a high school diploma and an age of eighteen years the minimum requirements for admission into the School of Nursing.[4]

The shift to high school graduates became pronounced in the transition from the 1940s to the '50s. Admission profiles for the classes of 1951 and 1954 demonstrate how dramatically the change occurred:

	% of class of 1951, admitted 1948	% of class of 1954, admitted 1951
High school only	6	29
1 year college	3	7
2 or 3 years college	58	53
4 years college	33	11

The class of 1956, admitted in 1953, comprised ninety-six students, exactly half of whom were admitted directly from high school.[5]

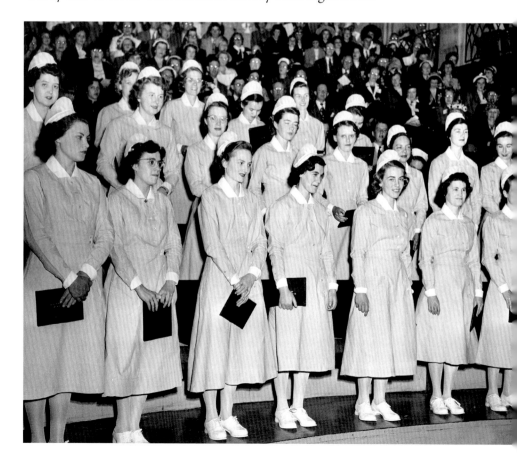

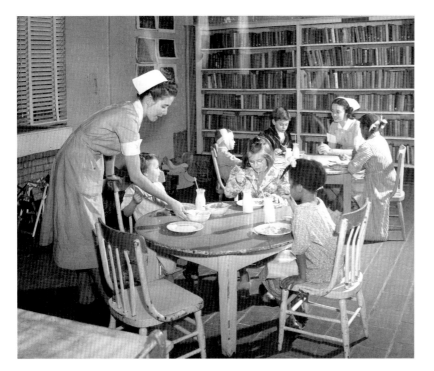

Black children from the nearby East Baltimore neighborhood mingled with white children, some of whom had traveled great distances to be treated in the Harriet Lane Home—an unusual occurrence in a Southern city that cherished traditions. For many years, most nursing students and their instructors were white; the School of Nursing accepted and graduated its first black students in the 1950s, almost a decade ahead of the School of Medicine.

The advisory board took no formal position on the recommendations from the medical board, but Dr. Francis Horn, dean of McCoy College, wrote a response in opposition to the recommendations citing recent research on the nursing shortages nationally and pointing out that current and future shortages would not be affected by intensified recruitment of students. Dr. Horn also presented the argument that lowering the admission standards would diminish the school's ability to attract top students. He emphasized the history of the school as an incubator for nursing leaders and asserted that national trends in the profession pointed toward more advanced education. He warned that approval of the board's recommendations would end the school's national leadership in the profession.[6] One can only wonder if Dr. Horn realized just how prophetic his words were.

The Hopkins community's inaction in addressing issues in the School of Nursing was compounded by dramatic changes taking place in the nursing profession throughout the United States in the early 1950s. Organized nursing, led by the American Nurses Association, voted in 1950 to merge with the National Association of Colored Graduate Nurses; following this move the National League of Nursing Education, the National Organization of Public Health Nurses, and the Association of Collegiate Schools of Nursing merged into the National League for Nursing. These new associations would redirect the goals of the profession over the next thirty years. The positions of these two groups regarding nursing education and nursing practice would remain in conflict with the views of the American Medical Association and the American Hospital Association throughout this

Across the city was the University of Maryland, which was a hospital diploma school too. But in the '50s, they made that transition to a baccalaureate program very easily. They were recruiting and graduating young women with academic credentials and Hopkins was not. It was totally unfair because the Hopkins graduate found himself or herself at a real disadvantage in the workforce. They still were faced with a long haul in order to get their bachelor's. It really was an ethical dilemma to recruit the best into a system that was archaic. It was no longer the way the profession was moving. If you were academically talented you certainly belonged in a university with the appropriate credentials when you graduated.

I went back into the archives and I read the notes of meetings. There was a task force put together to look at baccalaureate education for nurses. There were people, according to the minutes, who felt that putting females in any of the classes with the males would just be so distracting that the seriousness of study for the males would be totally disrupted. Yale, Vanderbilt, and University of Maryland, some of our peer elite institutions were able to move from diploma education models to academic collegiate models for nursing, and it took Hopkins more than fifty years longer than these other institutions to do it.

Stella Shiber

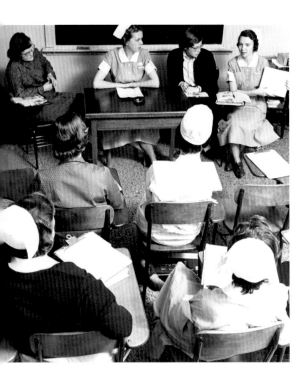

Students were expected to be able to lead class discussions, explaining how their clinical experiences corresponded with or differed from textbook cases. Many graduates would go on to become nurse educators, following the example set by their teachers.

Our teachers expected us to really think about what we were doing—the ramifications of what you would do, a treatment or medication—and we learned to see and care for the whole patient. The patient was not the heart attack or the appendectomy or the depression. You were taught to care for the whole patient, and that was the thread that went through all of the different clinics. It really helped to make us more observant, more aware of signs and symptoms. That was one of the things that has stuck with me over the years in every place that I worked.

Everybody was supposed to do their best and that was all that was acceptable. This is what you're expected to do. It may not be easy and you may not like it, but this is what you do and this is how you do it and you don't do it any other way.

Betsy Mumaw McGeady, 1955

period. Tensions between nursing as a hospital service and the need for students to learn within care facilities would dramatically shift nursing educational philosophy. The era of training a nurse by means of lengthy periods of repetitive practice with limited theoretical education was coming to an end.

Both of the newly reconstituted professional organizations addressed nursing education standards and working conditions as critical issues in the ongoing nursing shortage. Neither group, however, looked to lowering requirements or decreasing educational expectations as methods for addressing the problems. The efforts of the '50s reveal a constant drive to raise educational and practice standards to keep pace with rapidly changing medical technology and community health programs. The world was moving on while the School of Nursing was drifting within the Hopkins community and little was being done to respond to the external developments in nursing and health care.

During the late 1940s and early '50s development of the State Pool Licensing examinations was completed. The results of these standardized exams, which were administered throughout the United States by 1950, were reported faithfully each year to the advisory board. In spite of Miss Wolf's and the board's concerns, the performance of Hopkins graduates consistently exceeded all state and national norms for the exams. Students performed exceedingly well, especially when compared to bachelor's degree graduates within Maryland and nationally. The exam was designed as a test of safety and competence for the beginning nurse, and the test results were interpreted as a sign of excellence in the school, which contributed fodder for the physicians' arguments.

The other problem plaguing national nursing leaders during this period was that standards within some of the fledgling degree programs were lower than those at hospital schools. Some of the early baccalaureate programs had so few physical and social science courses and such traditional clinical formats that it was hard to tell the difference between the collegiate programs and strong hospital-based programs. The Hopkins nursing faculty continued to do an excellent job regardless of the age or experience of the students, so it was difficult for the doctors to understand how a college degree could be an improvement. Physicians and university leaders viewed nursing as a dependent vocation that had evolved in response to medicine. Nurses in the hospital system developed an ascribed status based on their relationship with a hospital and school. What nursing leaders and Miss Wolf were advocating was status based on the same discipline and research focus as all other professions on American college and university campuses. This goal seemed superfluous and unnecessary to Hopkins leaders of the time. It was a case of looking at a long-range problem from a here-and-now perspective.[7]

One bright spot in the early 1950s was the opening of the new educational unit on the ground floor of the old Main Residence. Fourteen rooms had been renovated for class and lab work, and there were ten offices for faculty. A new educational auditorium was constructed from the World War II–era east dining room, and twenty-three patient units and a utility room were designated for lab practice. The unit was dedicated on May 29, 1951, and many of the school's past and present dignitaries attended the event.[8]

Miss Wolf's leadership team continued to undergo modification. Faculty and supervisors left as they chose marriage, new professional opportunities, or continuing education. Some of her contemporaries recalled that Anna Wolf struggled with those adjustments. Often she was dismayed by the decisions of long-term employees, taking these decisions personally, as hurtful to the cause of better nursing at Hopkins.[9]

The perception of nursing in this period was determined by a view of women that limited nurses' potential in ways no longer at issue today. At a convocation speech given by Dr. Richard W. TeLinde in 1952, one can glimpse how a Hopkins physician who obviously cared deeply about the welfare of the students viewed the nursing profession:

Although bedside nursing still remains the foundation of all nursing the scope of nursing has enlarged tremendously and you may select a special field compatible with your talents, taste and personality.... I could talk indefinitely about the opportunities in nursing, but I believe I have said enough to indicate that the demand for nurses in all fields is far greater than the supply, and you are limited in attainment only by your ambition and ability ... let us consider for a moment, nurses training as a preparation for marriage. There is no college in the land that can give you comparable experience and knowledge that will be as useful to you

The dedication of the Mary Adelaide Nutting Educational Unit occasioned great celebration among alumnae. Representatives of many classes attended, including (left to right) A. Ethel Northam, 1921, Loula E. Kennedy, 1903, Elsie M. Lawler, 1899, Helen Wilmer Athey, 1905, Helen French, 1937, Blanche Pfefferkorn, 1911, and Anna D. Wolf, 1915; each wore a corsage.

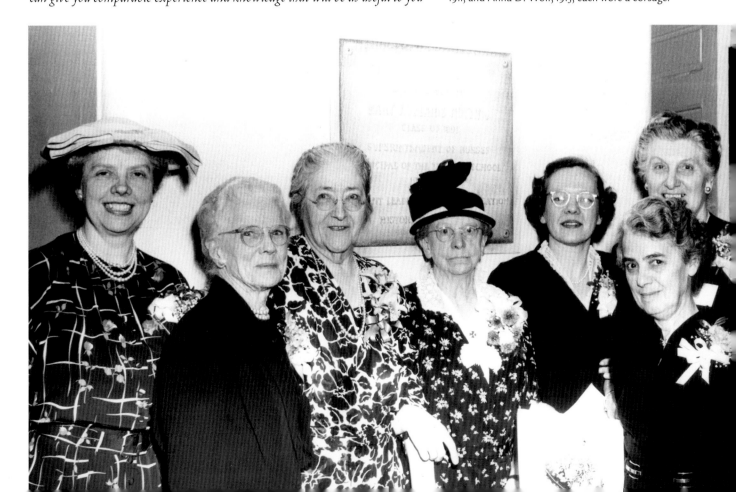

The doctors always stopped at the head nurse's desk to say, "I'm here for rounds. Can you come with me?" I remember going to Dr. Blalock's floor in Halsted when Louise Thomas, who later married Denton Cooley, was doing something and she said, "Can you give me a few minutes, Dr. Blalock, or I can get one of the other nurses to go with you." He said that he would wait.

Betty Borenstein Scher, 1950

Hampton House was the setting for many wedding receptions after restrictions on married students were lifted. When Joan Lucy married Paul Hurlock on January 1, 1953, the portrait of Adelaide Nutting kept watch over the party.

as a wife or mother. Your psychiatric training will help you to understand a temperamental husband or child. Your pediatric training fits you for the care of your children. Your general medical and surgical knowledge should enable you to more intelligently combat the inevitable vicissitudes of family life. . . . You have decided to study nursing at The Johns Hopkins Hospital. You, who are finishing your training will understand what I mean better than the incoming class when I tell you that Hopkins has something to give you that is not found in many training schools. I mean a fine tradition based on years of accomplishment.[10]

Dr. TeLinde's remarks included data about his view of nursing and its possibilities, the significance of nursing as preparation for marriage, and the role of Hopkins as an extraordinary institution. He also mentioned the outstanding nursing leaders who had established the program but said little of the program itself or of its future. He seemed truly to believe that simply by being part of the Hopkins institution the school would remain viable. But standards or prestige by association were not the goal of Miss Wolf and her colleagues. They wanted a school that could stand on its own as a university division that would be autonomous and would contribute to the expansion of nursing knowledge.

One event in 1952 that would prove beneficial to the school was the appointment of Dr. Russell Nelson as head of the hospital. Dr. Crosby, who had succeeded Dr. Smith, maintained an interest in the school, and Miss Wolf reported a cordial working relationship with him.[11] During his relatively short tenure as hospital director, he played a significant role

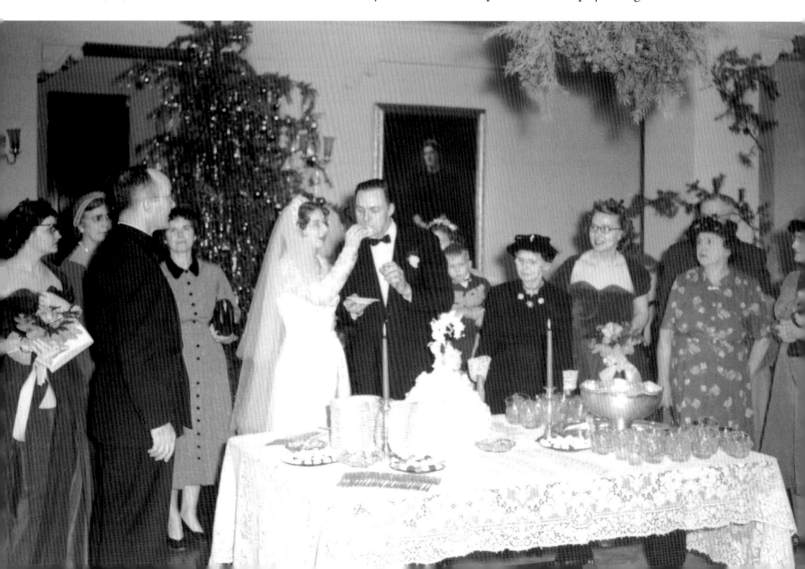

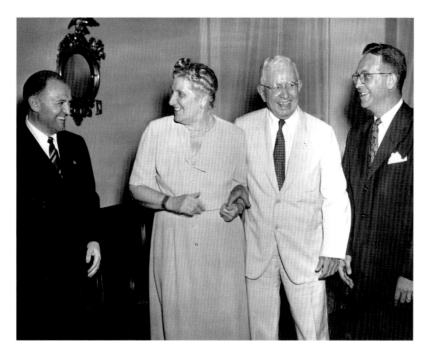

Maintaining good relations with hospital presidents who wanted to preserve the status quo was a challenge for Anna Wolf. Winford Smith, standing with Wolf, was president when she arrived, and together they guided the hospital and the school through the turbulent war years. Edwin Crosby (left) became president in 1946 but stayed only six years and had little impact on the school. Russell Nelson (right) took over in 1952; of the three, he was the best advocate for change.

in moving the hospital from the Smith era into the 1950s, but radical advancement for the School of Nursing was not his priority. He left Johns Hopkins to become the first executive director of the Joint Commission for the Accreditation of Hospitals. In contrast, Dr. Nelson had a strong interest in the welfare of the school and became a staunch supporter of advancement for the program. He was married to a Hopkins graduate, Ruth Jeffcoat, 1937, and had been at the hospital many years before becoming its president. Nelson understood Miss Wolf's dream and was willing to work within the system toward the goals she envisioned. He guided the hospital and the School of Nursing through twenty years of turbulence and change.

Although the 1950s were hard on Miss Wolf, she never lost hope but continued to tell her students bluntly that they needed more education. She redirected resources and used the power of her position to send nurses to graduate programs in order to benefit the School of Nursing and the hospital. She reported regularly in advisory board meetings about the immaturity and lack of preparation of the newer students compared to previous admissions. Although she still gave preference in admissions to applicants with degrees, the numbers of college-prepared applicants continued to drop. With the admission of the class of 1955, a double track for students was announced: college-prepared (at least two years) matriculants would complete 129 weeks including orientation, whereas high school graduates would complete a full thirty-six month program. This lengthened the preclinical period by eleven weeks, providing more background for the clinical rotations that followed.[12]

One of the hardest years in Miss Wolf's tenure was 1953, when the Russell Sage Foundation published a study titled *Collegiate Education for*

When we were seniors, Miss Wolf was teaching two classes. One was the history of nursing and one was the ethics of nursing. The rule was that you waited fifteen minutes. If the instructor didn't come, you could leave. But what do you do with Miss Wolf? When she finally came in, she was as gray as her uniform. I later asked a fascinating alumna, Annabelle Gleason Brack, about that day. Mrs. Brack said that was the day that Ed Crosby, who was head of the hospital, told Miss Wolf that wasn't it a shame, she was due to retire in a few years. Now wouldn't it be terrible if she lost her pension? In other words, "Shut up about the collegiate school of nursing." One time I had Miss Wolf over to my house for lunch and I asked her if that was true and she said, yes. So they did make that threat and yes, she did shut up because she was a single lady. I hold no grudge about that.

Betty Borenstein Scher, 1950

Mary Farr, 1941, Mary Jane Donough, and Gerry Jordan, 1945, taught clinical medicine on the Osler medical service and they seem to have left lasting impressions on generations of their former students. Alumnae thought so much of Donough that in 1968, they made her an honorary member of the alumnae association. Paula Einaudi, former director of development, explained that "these were women who had been brought up by these very hard-driving, high standard–bearing women who wanted the School of Nursing to maintain that standard, so they were very hard on their students."

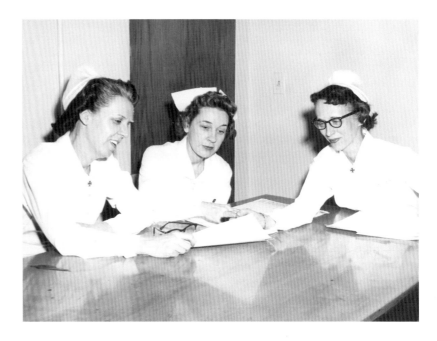

We had classmates from all over the United States. At that time they limited the number of students from Maryland so that other students in the country had an opportunity to come. We had students from the West Coast, and Pennsylvania, Delaware, Ohio, Georgia, Florida—a wide variety of the states. One of my college classmate's uncles was a practicing physician in Baltimore and he said to her, "Under no circumstances are you to go to any other nursing school except Hopkins."

Betsy Mumaw McGeady, 1955

Nursing, written by Margaret Bridgeman. Known as the Bridgeman Report, this document was designed to analyze the current state of collegiate programs in nursing. It called on colleges and universities to address nursing as they would any other academic discipline and to meet their responsibilities to nursing as they did to all other fields in an institution for higher learning. Bridgeman was critical of many of the programs in existence at the time, and she singled out the collegiate arrangement between the Johns Hopkins Hospital School of Nursing and the Johns Hopkins University (at its McCoy College).[13]

When Bridgeman visited Johns Hopkins, she found students with two years of college credit receiving a bachelor's degree at the completion of their diploma program without ever having entered a classroom at the university. She labeled the blanket credit arrangement educationally unsound and criticized both institutions in her study. Not only was the school having difficulty getting students with college backgrounds, suddenly the program that might have attracted them was cited as educationally inferior.

Miss Wolf had to respond, which she did at a subsequent advisory board meeting—but in her heart she had to agree with some of what Bridgeman had written.[14] Some of the extracts from the study are similar to things she herself had said in the drive to improve standards. When Miss Wolf first learned of the report she firmly believed that Bridgeman was criticizing the university and how it related to the school rather than the educational program itself.[15] She addressed the report in a written response to the board, identifying each negative point in the study and addressing the Hopkins position on the issue. She pointed out that members of the university faculty had participated in the development of the current curriculum at the school, so the charge that the university had no control over the program was not totally accurate. Bridgeman had charged that a university would not establish a degree program in engineering and then send its students off campus for their major; Wolf pointed out that the university was also granting degrees to students in music and art who did their major work at the Peabody Conservatory and the Maryland Institute of Art.

One of the most interesting aspects of Miss Wolf's reply to the study was her ability to provide detailed information about all that was wrong with the Hopkins arrangement and the limitations of diploma education in the midst of her defense against Bridgeman's charges. She used her reply to lay out for the advisory board the entire landscape of problems, from the financial needs of an education program in a service institution to the reality that the preclinical program had become too heavy for students entering without college preparation. Miss Wolf defended the quality of the theoretical and clinical education offered at Johns Hopkins as worthy of sixty credits while recognizing that few college-prepared students were still entering the program. In later years, Wolf reflected on her resentment of Margaret Bridgeman, who painted the darkest picture possible of what she had tried to do in a tough situation, but this report to the board truly summed up her frustrations and despair over the situation as it existed in 1953.[16]

Reaction to the Bridgeman Report separated Miss Wolf from those of her nursing colleagues who supported Bridgeman's position about the placement of nursing programs in the university setting with university control. Miss Wolf deeply resented Hopkins having been singled out and used as an example in the study. She believed that many other programs were having problems at this time and that Bridgeman had cited

Hopkins has gone through a lot of changes in nursing education. For a while they only took people with baccalaureate degrees. The thirty-six-month program was for students who came out of high school. The difference between thirty-two months and thirty-six months, you know, is not worth two years of college. Our preclinical was six months and the high school's was nine months. They maxed it up so that at the end of the first year, we were all the same. Preclin was the only time we had separate classes because when you went into the clinics—major clinics like surgery, medicine, obstetrics, pediatrics, and psych— it was all the same.

I graduated from the School of Nursing and a month later I went out to the university and picked up my baccalaureate degree there. If you had at least two years of college you could transfer those credits to the university, couple that with your three years of nursing school, and get your baccalaureate at the end, which is what I did.

Trudy Jones Hodges, 1959

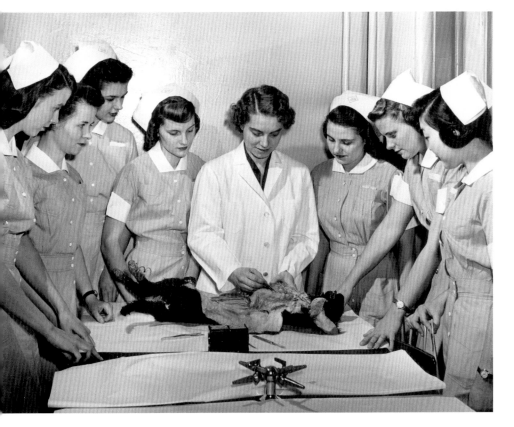

Members of the class of 1953 watched intently as their lab instructor dissected a dog, preparation for later experiences they would have in the operating room. Once the educational unit opened in the Main Residence, attending lectures and labs was much easier for everyone, since they were held in close proximity, and faculty offices were nearby.

LINDA SABIN

Hopkins because of its reputation as a first-rate program. In addition, she believed that Bridgeman had overlooked the fact that the school had been the first to receive accreditation under the new system introduced by the National League for Nursing in the late 1940s and that she had focused only on the school's relationship with the university. Wolf found the entire issue quite ironic, since fewer and fewer students eligible for university credits were even applying to the program. Her report to the advisory board was her last attempt to make plain how the world was changing around the school and how, without conversion to a university-based system, the program would be left behind.

During this time dramatic innovations related to medical discoveries such as the development of antibiotics and psychotropic medications were rapidly altering care within and outside the hospital, but there was little impact on the School of Nursing's organization. Hospital administrators, physicians, and university liaisons were blind to the future potential of university-educated nurses. The view persisted that nursing was nursing and all that faculty and students had to do was continue their supportive work, which would help patients and doctors as new treatments were developed. The faculty had to continue to plan for diverse

Body mechanics classes were held in the gymnasium in the basement of Hampton House. Students not only mastered exercise and stretching techniques but also learned how to move patients and heavy equipment safely, so that they would not injure themselves.

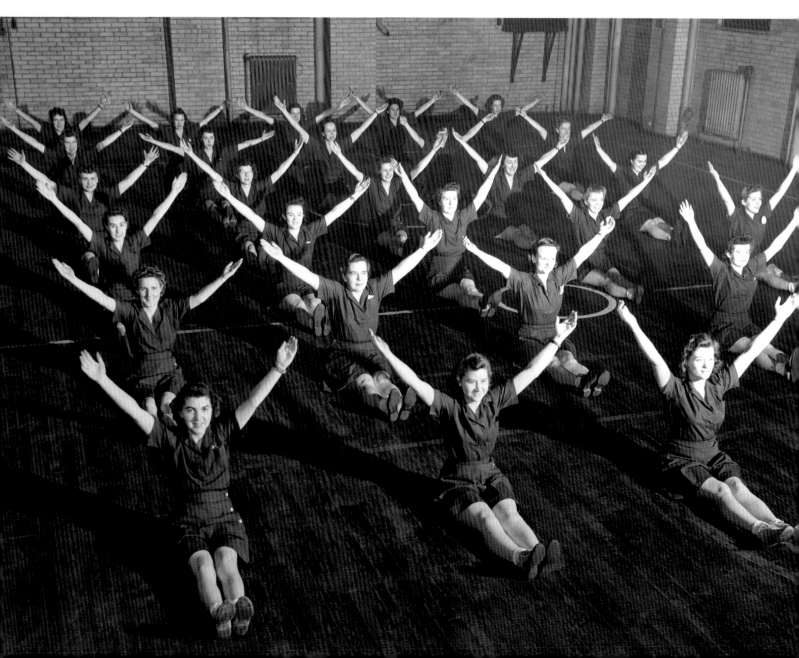

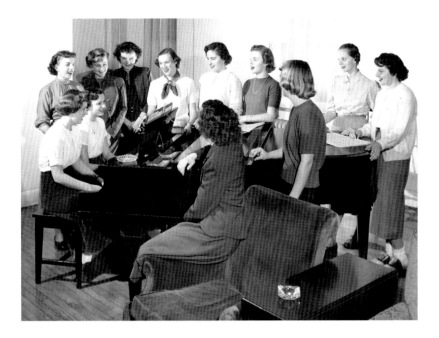

Members of the class of 1952 were a mixture of young women with some college experience and many who came straight from high school. Scenes like this gathering around the piano in Hampton House were staged for a recruitment brochure, an attempt to lure prospective students who were beginning to realize that a baccalaureate degree might be more valuable than the superior clinical experiences Hopkins offered.

student populations consisting of college graduates, students who had completed some college, and high school graduates. Some of the medical members of the advisory board could not see a problem when faculty expressed dismay about curriculum planning in this situation. This attitude was hard to take when the faculty already had dual roles of teaching and supervising. (Each faculty member served as a unit supervisor and taught students, who provided much of the care.)[17] With the shortage of nurses so severe, the difficulties for faculty increased. Monthly reports of the director of the school are filled with faculty resignations and transfers. In just one monthly report at the end of 1953, almost half of the staff nursing positions (109 of 244) were open and a third of the assistant head nurse positions (19 of 58) needed staffing.[18]

In spite of the challenges faced by the faculty, the school was able to keep pace and produce practitioners who had mastered the latest theory available. In late 1953 the preclinical curriculum and clinical rotations were modified to meet the needs of the high school and college-prepared students in a more efficient manner. The advisory board minutes from the first half of the 1950s are peppered with alterations and adjustments in courses as the faculty attempted to meet the needs of both students and patients.

On September 15, 1952, the hospital discontinued the Dispensary Visiting Nurse Service, which had begun in 1934 with financial help from the Adelaide Nutting Endowment. Miriam Ames developed the service and served as its director until 1949, when she retired. Between 1949 and 1952, half the students worked in the Eastern Health District for their public-health nursing experience and the other half stayed in the Dispensary Service (the hospital's outpatient department). After 1952 all nursing students completed their public-health experience in

We were from all over. The majority of us were right out of high school, but we did have some college graduates and more that were just two years into college. The oldest was probably about thirty-three. Probably 95 percent of us were in the eighteen-to-twenty-year-old range. Kathy Hopkins came from California. Her parents scraped together the money to get her here and she was not going to go home for three years. We weren't all really interested in nursing. Some knew they'd wanted to be nurses from little, bitty girls. Others were there looking for a husband. Some people had never been away from home and it was difficult. Several left within the first week or ten days.

Lois Grayshan Hoffer, 1962

The School of Nursing always attracted international students, some of whom stayed on to work and teach at the hospital. Mary Farr Heeg recalled that after World War II, several students of Japanese descent came from Hawaii.

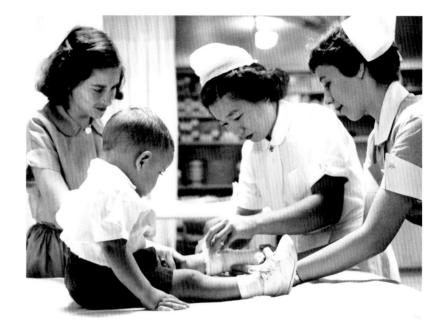

There was always this battle between education and service, but when you realize you're the only staff on the floor, you know you're being used for service. We had a forty-four-hour week. That included work and formal class time. We got down to forty hours before I graduated. Those are long days especially if you're working on the weekend, you do an eight to six. That means you've got breakfast, lunch, and dinner, so those were some long, hard days. We have to realize, when we look at the difference in the tuition between the diploma school of fifty years ago and what it is at Hopkins University today, we were literally providing service.

Trudy Jones Hodges, 1959

the Eastern Health District, which was located just east of Johns Hopkins Hospital.[19] The program never achieved accreditation, however, because there was no sanction by a university.

The agitation caused by the efforts of organized nursing and the Bridgeman Report stimulated a broad wave of antibaccalaureate feeling, especially among hospitals with training programs.[20] Nurses graduating from diploma schools felt pressure to demonstrate their excellence and superiority to bachelor's graduates, who were viewed as less experienced. Scholarships to the top three outstanding graduates from the school in the years since World War II had gone unused. This was a dramatic change from the pre–World War I era, when Miss Wolf had graduated and scholarship recipients were simply expected to continue their education to prepare for leadership.[21] As a result, in 1953 the advisory board voted to discontinue awarding Trustees Scholarships at the time of graduation. Instead, they decided to grant up to $2,400 to one or more graduates to continue their education in nursing. Hopkins employees received priority for these scholarships, although recipients were not required to return to the hospital after receiving their degrees.[22]

In early 1954 recruitment efforts escalated, with over thirteen hundred school bulletins and posters sent to colleges and more than forty-eight hundred aimed at high schools throughout the country. The Women's Auxiliary to the Baltimore City Medical Chirurgical Faculty planned special programs for nurse recruitment in an effort to help the programs in Baltimore.[23] This same year the first class to graduate with predominantly high school prepared students began a new era in the program; even though there was still a significant number of students with some college courses entering the program, two distinct student groups remained.

By the time Anna Wolf announced her retirement she was drained from the battle she had failed to win. Her efforts had led her to the end of a professional career in which much had been accomplished, but her dream remained unfulfilled. In later years she reflected on this disappointing aspect of her administration:

National emphasis and impetus upon university and college education for all professional nurses was greatly stimulated and accelerated postwar. It was obvious that historic prestige of the JHH School of Nursing (et al.) could not survive without full university control and administration. The handwriting was on the wall. It was also obvious the writer had utterly failed to convince authorities of the hospital and university: 1) that professional nursing was worthy of university inclusion, 2) that adequate funds were necessary to establish a school, 3) that a strong, qualified faculty was necessary, 4) that with the long prestige of JHH School of Nursing and the University there would be no doubt of highly qualified students, 5) that the future should include undergraduate and graduate programs with research as a productive feature.[24]

Miss Wolf may not have swayed the medical and academic leadership at Johns Hopkins, but she convinced hundreds of nurses who graduated from the program during her tenure. These nurses believed in her goal and supported its fulfillment when they finally had the opportunity to do so years later. Many of the students she taught went on to school after completing their education at the hospital and moved into leadership positions across the globe. She sowed seeds she never got to harvest. In an unpublished biography of Anna Dryden Wolf, Sarah Allison succinctly summarized: "While educated, committed professional women like Wolf personally did not achieve all of their goals, they serve as role models for others to follow. More importantly, they conveyed their value systems—their visions and beliefs—for others to emulate and develop."[25]

In her zeal to achieve the dream, Anna Wolf had polarized medical opinion about the program, and the nursing community had tired of the constant committee activities that produced no results. Miss Wolf's

We were Anna Wolf's last class. I remember her being a striking figure. She had a presence when she walked into the room. She gave classes during senior year about the history of Hopkins nursing. It was wonderful to see her stand at the podium. She didn't need notes. She knew. She knew the whole history of Hopkins nursing and the importance of Hopkins nursing and the difference that it had made in other parts of the world. Her classes were outstanding.

Betsy Mumaw McGeady, 1955

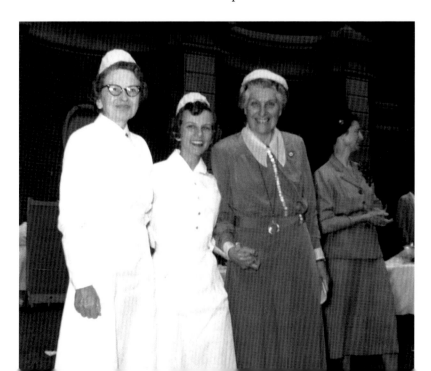

K. Virginia Betzold (left), 1933, associate director of the School of Nursing for twenty-two years, and Anna D. Wolf (pictured here with Mary MacSherry, 1954) were united in their determination to see the school become a degree-granting division of the university. As a result, Betzold was passed over when the time came for the hospital trustees to choose Wolf's successor.

LINDA SABIN

loyal supporters knew that she was right about the need for a collegiate program in nursing, but issues regarding funding, concern about the presence of female undergraduate students at the Johns Hopkins University, and medical disregard of nursing as a profession blocked progress toward her cherished goal. She was tired, and the Hopkins institutions were vested in maintaining the status quo in nursing. It was time for a new approach, a fresh start.

Miss Wolf was feted at several farewell events and recognized for her unfailing service to her hospital and school. The sum of her accomplishments in the fifteen years she served as director was awe-inspiring. During the war she led the school and nursing service through the dramatic transformations dictated by the Cadet Nursing Program and maintained service without many of her experienced leaders, who were serving in the war effort. She learned how to use non-nurses in administrative positions and began team nursing with Red Cross–trained nursing aides. Although the postwar period did not bring the major change Miss Wolf desired, there were dramatic alterations in both the school and the hospital. Separation of nursing service and nursing education under individual assistant directors strengthened the school's control over student practice. The assistant director in charge of the school had the duty of assigning all student hours. The process of separating the school's budget from nursing service was begun. The curriculum was revised frequently, and significant changes were made to the

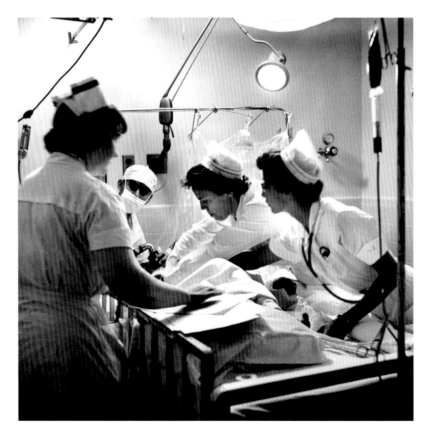

A new generation of nursing leaders emerged from the classes graduated in the 1950s. Sarah Allison (in long sleeves), 1953, was one of several alumnae able to continue their education because of funds offered by the nursing school's advisory board. Allie Sanborn, 1955, worked at Allison's side in the recovery room in 1959.

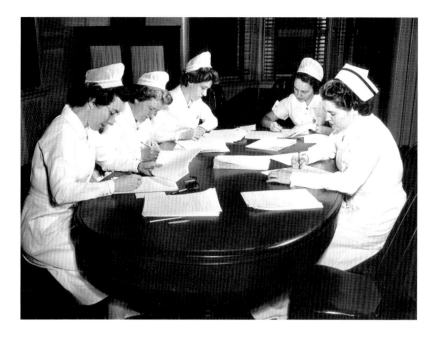

Alumnae, easily recognized by their distinctive organdy caps, dominated the faculty throughout the life of the hospital school. In 1955, when this group of instructors reviewed examination papers, they utilized a new grading system that acknowledged the new realities of the less well-prepared incoming students.

educational process, bringing theory and practice into greater alignment to facilitate student learning. The preclinical program was dramatically altered in the 1950s to meet the needs of students lacking college preparation and a shift was made to include more psychological, social, and health-promotion content to nursing practice. Hours of practice and education were adjusted and time allocated to night duty limited. A major renovation of the Main Residence into modern classrooms, an auditorium, and a modern library brought new assets to the school.[26]

In 1954 the grading system in the school was altered to reflect more closely the new realities of younger, less well prepared students and evolving collegiate grading systems. The grades Low Satisfactory and Highly Satisfactory were added to Honors, Satisfactory, and Unsatisfactory.[27] Upgrading the curriculum was combined with improved house rules and opportunities for employment for students.

In the hospital, nurses continued to work in teams after the war. The assistant director of nursing service was able to develop staffing patterns that included increasing numbers of graduate nurses and unlicensed assistants. She introduced new approaches to staffing and care delivery. Miss Wolf encouraged the consideration of employment of African-American staff and the acceptance of African Americans in a variety of roles, including pediatric nursing aides, staff nurses, and students.

Anna Wolf personified the strengths of her generation of nurses and attempted to achieve her vision for higher education for Hopkins nurses. Her philosophy of nursing never wavered: "[Nursing] must . . . be family and patient centered. It can't and it mustn't lose [sight of] the patient's needs. The minute we lose that we are going to lose something else: we are going to lose really a spirit of helpfulness. I think it is because a person needs help that the person responds to give help."[28]

The first African-American student did not graduate. She was engaged to a fellow who was in the army or the air force. He was transferred to England and she elected to leave. It seemed very different, I think, to most of us; very different to those from farther south. I did not mention it to my grandmother because she would have been upset. I think she was a good student. I never felt that there was a problem. She was accepted by the other students.
Betsy Mumaw McGeady, 1955

I had planned to go to Bellevue Hospital because I had gone to NYU for two years, from 1953 to 1955. You went two years to NYU, took a prenursing course, and then you transferred to Bellevue Training School for Nurses. During the summertime I went to work in the Catskill Mountains as a short-order cook. The gentleman who hired me had a brother who was an orthopedic surgeon who had a son who was premed and they talked about going to Johns Hopkins. I sat down and took pen and paper and wrote to Johns Hopkins. I said, "Now, I know if they have a medical school they must have a nursing school." I wrote to New York because I thought everything was in New York City. Lo and behold, they got the letter.

Trudy Jones Hodges, 1959

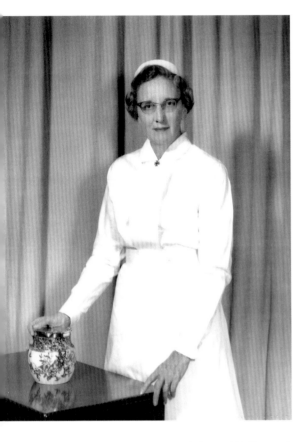

Mary Sanders Price, 1934, succeeded Anna Wolf as director in 1956. Mary Farr Heeg, 1941, who had served under her with General Hospital No. 118 during World War II, recalled that "Mary Sanders commanded respect and you would not do anything to displease her. She was fair. Things went very smoothly with her in charge of the School of Nursing."

Mrs. Price was a very prim and proper lady at all times. She was certainly the epitome of a Hopkins nurse, with her long-sleeved uniforms and cuffs and impeccably put together. She was a small lady. I think the key word probably was lady. *She was very much a lady.*

Stella Shiber

Johns Hopkins Hospital Board of Trustees and Dr. Russell Nelson turned to Mary Sanders Price, 1934, to succeed Anna Wolf as director. Mrs. Price was living in Pennsylvania with her husband, Harry Price, a Methodist district superintendent. Reverend Price was also invited to come to the Johns Hopkins Hospital—as chaplain—so both the Prices began new positions in 1956. Dr. Nelson recalled in later years that Mrs. Price was chosen because she was well known in the medical community for her leadership with Base Hospital 118 and her postwar service in Marburg. Her quiet dignity and nonconfrontational style would be welcome after what the doctors perceived as years of turmoil with Miss Wolf.[29] The board avoided K. Virginia Betzold as Miss Wolf's successor because of her known support for a baccalaureate program at the school.

Mary Sanders Price was a different kind of leader from Anna Wolf. Not as tall or impressive in appearance as Miss Wolf, she nonetheless had a quiet confidence. Esther Jacoby, 1930, who had served with her in the war, described Mary Sanders Price as a "regal person, reserved, well thought of by her nurses [and] impassioned about her students."[30] Her war years had taught Price how to work for change from within an organization. She was used to being in charge and understood the art of collaboration and delegation. Margaret Courtney, 1940, who was an associate of both women, commented that she felt as if she worked *with* Mrs. Price as a colleague, while she worked *for* Miss Wolf—as a subordinate.[31] Mrs. Price came from the generation of graduates who studied under Miss Lawler, Miss Kennedy, and Miss Struve. As Mrs. Harry Price, she adapted to the role of a minister's wife and worked part time at Johns Hopkins, which gave her insight into the issues of nursing service in the hospital.

Mrs. Price brought a new approach to managing the school and the needs of working nurses. Miss Wolf's devotion to the ideal of excellence through higher education for nurses had created conflict with physicians who believed, just as strongly, that nurses did not need such preparation, especially if they were trained at Hopkins. As the setbacks from the Brown Report,[32] the Bridgeman Report, and the decline of college-prepared students mounted, Miss Wolf had become more strident in her pleas for change. She wanted the school to be a leader in the process of change to university-based education, which she believed to be inevitable. In contrast, Mrs. Price approached the medical community very differently. She presented the advisory board and the hospital board of trustees with the facts and worked for modest changes that she hoped would bring about a transition in keeping with trends in the profession of nursing. Mrs. Price's views were similar to Miss Wolf's but she expressed them differently, and she was perceived as a peacemaker within the hospital community.

The problems Mrs. Price faced in her early years as director were significant. Like Miss Wolf, she had to address serious staffing shortages in the hospital and chronic turnover of instructors in the school of nursing. Faculty members were still fulfilling dual roles as clinical teachers and unit supervisors, which led to routine absences from the units and limited clinical instruction time for students. A forty-four-hour week for students was still the norm. Some students were spending too much time on the evening and night shifts in order to cover patient needs, or they were being sent onto night duty before they were properly prepared. Mrs. Price also found students spread out on so many units that appropriate supervision was impossible. In addition, staffing was so reduced that only minimal time was available for the most critical of patient needs, with no coverage left for patient education or discharge planning.[33]

The Eighty-fourth Congress passed legislation to provide traineeships for graduate nurses seeking bachelor's and higher degrees in an attempt to improve the supply of well-prepared nurse faculty. None of the Hopkins faculty could take advantage of this new opportunity because there was such a severe shortage of teachers.[34] The faculty and its leadership maintained a commitment to student learning and constantly sought new experiences to strengthen the theoretical and clinical performance of their students. They were able to accomplish this by attending national meetings, training events, and short-term courses to update their skills in education. For example, in 1954 Margaret Courtney, at the time the assistant director for nursing arts in the School of Nursing, attended a conference on nursing care of polio victims, and Mary Farr, instructor and supervisor of medical nursing, attended conferences on tuberculosis in Washington and at Baltimore City Hospitals.[35] In spite of the shortage of faculty, the demands of caring for patients, and the need to educate two levels of student, two strong curricula were in place, for thirty-two or thirty-six months, depending on the student's preparation. Most of the faculty was highly experienced in the fields they were teaching, but many lacked degrees in nursing. Mrs. Price quickly learned to value Miss K. Virginia Betzold for her skill at leading the faculty in designing a curriculum that was obviously working well in spite of other problems.

Mrs. Price spoke at commencement in May 1956, during the first year of her tenure. She began by speaking of the past:

I cannot move away from this part of my brief account of school activities without paying a heartfelt tribute to one who had more to do with inculcating in me a love for and pride in profession than any other living person—one who lives in our midst as a patient in Marburg and whose presence graces this occasion today—Miss Elsie M. Lawler.[36]

I was fortunate enough to have almost four weeks of night duty (12–8 A.M.) and much evening duty in Osler. This experience taught me better than any other how to plan and give total care to a large number of patients even with limited means. The work in Osler was difficult physically, and sometimes one feels almost nothing was accomplished. But still, at the close of a day, with tired feet and aching muscles, we remember the quieted faces of those we nursed. To know they are comfortable gives us restful sleep. Osler is the heart of what is called "bedside nursing." Its many varied experiences present a true challenge to each one of us.

Mabel Gerhart, 1953, writing in her scrapbook in 1953

Neonatology was a new field in the 1950s. At Johns Hopkins, healthy babies usually stayed near their mothers in obstetrics, but those with complications were taken to the premature nursery in the Harriet Lane Home. Working with newborns brought extraordinary responsibilities, and nursing students worked attentively with their instructors to learn what to do.

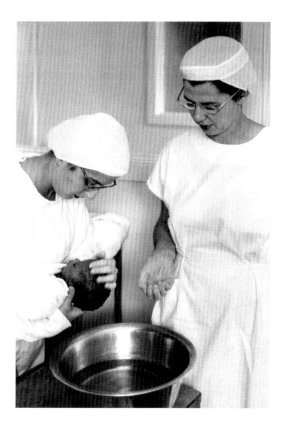

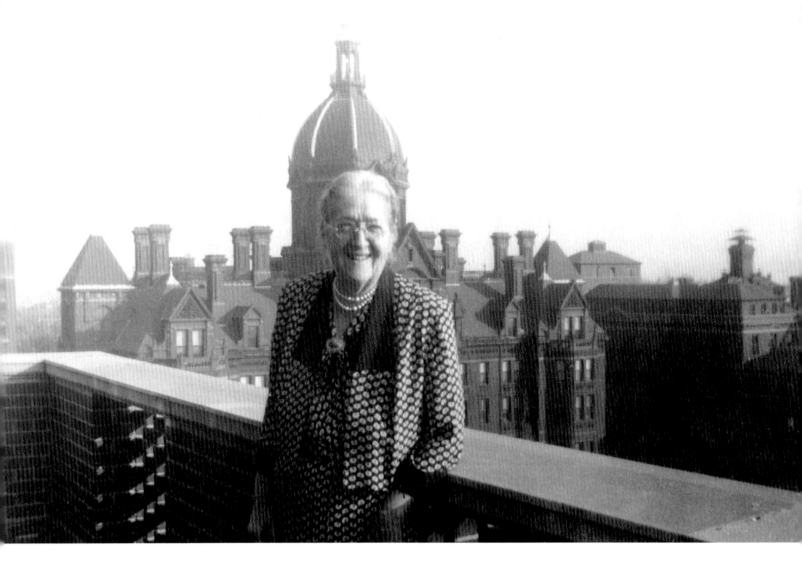

Elsie Lawler was a presence at Johns Hopkins through-out the 1950s. After her retirement in 1940, Lawler lived in California for a while and traveled, but after she had a stroke, Anna Wolf arranged for her to be transported back to Baltimore. There Lawler took up residence in the Marburg Pavilion, where Agnes J. Doetsch, 1931, cared for her. She remained there until her death, in 1962.

To have known Miss Lawler and Miss Wolf and to follow in their train pro-duces a feeling of thrilling pride, tempered with genuine humility.

She finished by turning her attention to the students and their future:

Since you entered this school 32 months ago you have worked hard, undergone anxieties, pleasures and at this moment can fully appreciate the hour and the honor with its privileges and concomitant responsibilities. Many have invested in you—your instructors who may feel that they worked harder and worried more than you, the patients from whom you have learned and gained inspiration, the doctors who have given generously of their abilities and time in both formal and informal instruction. . . .

To you graduates, we covet for the road that opens before you substantial sat-isfaction, a measure of success and happiness.[37]

At the end of her first ten months, Mrs. Price presented a report to the advisory board on the School of Nursing that included many famil-iar themes: hospital service was weakening the student program because the demands on student and faculty time limited educational activities; graduates of the program were performing on licensing exams above the average when compared to hospital and collegiate schools. Mrs. Price pointed out that the faculty lacked preparation to continue to produce outstanding graduates. She believed that the school was caught in a rapidly changing environment and she called for the establishment of a special committee to study present trends in nursing education, noting that "there is a widening gap between expected outcomes of collegiate and hospital schools which will before long affect the graduates of our school."[38]

Dr. Russell Nelson chaired the committee requested by Mrs. Price. There is no evidence that the committee ever became active, but Dr. Nelson did meet with Milton Eisenhower, the new president of the university, in 1957, and he requested that the faculty send the four-year curriculum it had developed to Dr. Eisenhower for review. Nothing would come of this effort until 1960.

By the end of Mrs. Price's first year the curriculum was again under scrutiny. The elimination of cookery classes, which required twenty hours, marked a transition. Isabel Hampton Robb had introduced cookery classes in the earliest days of the school. Food preparation had begun to fade from the curriculum in the 1940s, when students who could pass a pretest were permitted to go directly to the nutrition course. The faculty of the 1950s eliminated cookery altogether and replaced it with twenty additional hours of nutrition. They also extended the number of hours in the preclinical period devoted to social science.[39]

The thirty-two-month accelerated curriculum was discontinued in 1958 because of the decreasing number of applications from students with college backgrounds. The primary reason was believed to be unfavorable publicity from the Bridgeman Report, which had influenced high school counselors to send students to four-year university schools. It was also thought that a new trend of two-year nursing programs, which had started in Florida and California during the previous three years, was likely to spread. Under the new plan all students would matriculate into the thirty-six-month program for the diploma in nursing.[40]

During this same period severe staff shortages continued, and more than ninety beds in the hospital had to be closed owing to the lack of head nurses, assistant head nurses, and general staff nurses. Falling enrollment in the program and increasing pressure to limit practice hours for students complicated the staffing picture.[41] In an attempt to spur recruitment, Mrs. Price hired Dr. Leila Skinner, an experienced educator with advanced degrees in the behavioral sciences, as a full-time recruiter.

By 1959 the National League for Nursing warned the faculty and the advisory board in a routine accreditation visit about incipient problems that had to be addressed. The NLN was concerned about the faculty's limited education and experience, and about job descriptions of faculty who were also involved in nursing service, which was disruptive to their work as educators. The curriculum was cited for its placement of evening and night experiences for the students, which was not reflected in written plans. Warning signs that all was not well were increasingly evident.[42]

We had to take cooking class. The nutrition department wasn't as well organized then as it is now. We were supposed to know what the diabetic diet was for that patient. The cooking class was to make sure that we knew how to prepare those foods. After we prepared the food in this cooking class we had to eat it. The idea was that we would see if that was the right preparation. Eggs— soft-boiled, scrambled—and gruel, those are the things I remember fixing. They were so distasteful. There was a girl in my group and she would eat everybody's. She just had an insatiable appetite and we were so happy that we didn't have to eat it.

Ethel Rainey Ward, 1947

We had to work hard, not only the physical work but also the study. We had forty-eight hours a week clinical plus class. If you had an off day in the middle of the week, that didn't mean you didn't have to go to class. Sometimes you could go for several weeks without having a real day off because you may have had clinical on the weekends and then maybe you were off on Monday, but you had two classes on Monday. That was how the program was set up and everybody did it.

Betsy Mumaw McGeady, 1955

*The first day it was chaos because you had
to find your room and lug all your stuff.
That was the only time that fathers could go
up onto the floor. Other than that, men were
not allowed above the first floor.*

Betsy Mumaw McGeady, 1955

*Once I got through my first clinical, I could
work ten hours a week for a dollar an hour;
that's $10. It did give me some money that
I sorely needed but it also gave me extra practice
in things that I was doing, so for me it was
a plus-plus to work. That was a good thing.*

Trudy Jones Hodges, 1959

Below left: Patients accepted care from nursing
students, but those who were alert soon realized that
those wearing faded uniforms had more experience
than those in fresher, bluer attire.

Below right: Students discovered a wealth of both
current and historical information relevant to nursing
in their library in the basement of the Main Residence.
The collections were dedicated to Loula Kennedy in
1949, when her portrait was hung on the wall.

Students in the school during the 1950s had many advantages over the previous generation as work hours gradually declined and the pressure to achieve a BSN shifted under the arrangements made in the late 1940s. Yet student and staff shortages created heavy workloads on all units and at times interfered with learning activities.[43] Graduates from the '50s remember strict adherence to nursing practice. Betty Borenstein Scher, 1950, recalled being assigned to a patient with a bedsore and being told by the head nurse that, although the patient had come in with a bedsore, he would not leave with one—and he didn't. It took much of Scher's clinical time for many days to accomplish the assignment.[44]

The clinical experiences of the students in this period were as rich and varied as those of previous generations. Dr. Alfred Blalock frequently performed "Blue Baby" procedures for pediatric tetralogy of Fallot malformations, some of the earliest heart surgery attempted anywhere in the world. Students became adept at handling polio victims in iron lungs. When students worked overtime on the units they earned the princely sum of 50¢ per hour, a fee that rose to $1 by the end of the decade.[45] (The cost of attending the school had gone up to just over $600 by 1950.) Students were able to integrate their theory, read about advances in health care practice, and then actually participate in modern innovations during clinical experiences within weeks of having learned about them in class. They felt that they were part of a large team doing excellent work, and they were stimulated by a fresh environment in parts of the hospital that were being renovated or replaced with new facilities. Students also felt like a team within their own community. Studying together, weathering social events, and keeping up with clinical demands provided a sense of family that was appreciated by those far from home.[46]

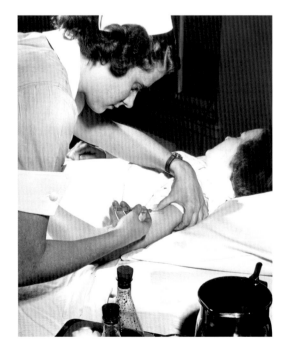

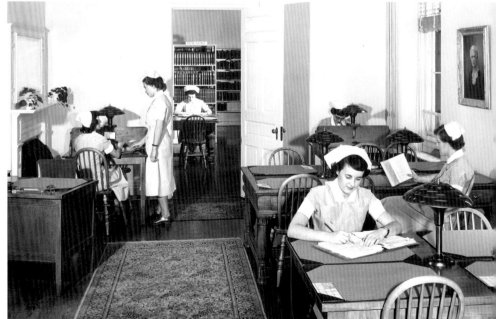

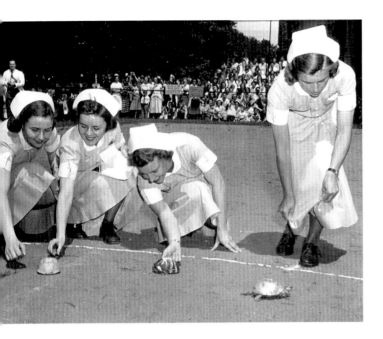
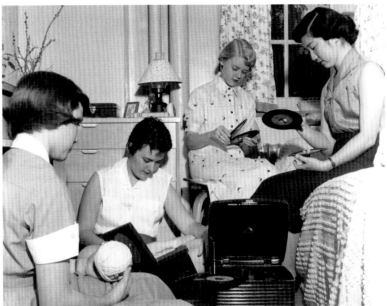

There was still plenty of heavy physical labor for nurses and nursing students on the units. Few materials were disposable yet, so cleaning, sterilizing, scrubbing, and managing reusable equipment still played a big part in daily activities. Patients received considerable bedside attention because of the nature of surgical wound management, treatments for chronic illnesses, and the necessity to provide both physical and respiratory therapies since those specialties of professionally trained workers had not yet evolved. Administering medications and intravenous drips often involved mixing and measuring by the nurse on the floor, and preparing injections required coping with reusable syringes.

Without the gas rationing of the war years, students had greater access to the cottage in Sherwood Forest, which had been named Dick Cottage in 1945 as a memorial to Christine Dick, who had been the keeper of its keys until her death.[47] Students piled into the school station wagon and drove down frequently in the summer months. Many fondly remember group outings to this peaceful setting and the friendships that grew during these brief periods of relaxation away from the hospital—despite the myriad daunting rules and guidelines to follow when using the cottage that were printed in the student handbook.[48]

Organizations established in the 1940s flowered in the '50s with a full calendar of student-planned and student-led activities. Participation in the resurrected turtle derby and annual dances added to the social calendar. Nursing students became popular guests at parties held at university fraternities and at tea dances at the Naval Academy, in Annapolis. Alumnae from the 1950s also admitted to watching events and performances at the medical school's Pithotomy Club through open windows and doors; the Pithotomy Club then was an all-male bastion where medical students and medical faculty came

Although students enjoyed private rooms in Hampton House during the 1950s, they often clustered in each other's rooms to talk and relax. In 1956 the student on the left seemed to be considering a possible knitting project as her friends decided which of the latest 45-rpm records to spin on the portable player.

Above left: The first turtle derby was run in 1931. Doctors and nurses in each hospital department sponsored a contestant and contributed to the purse, with all proceeds contributed to charities. Like many other lighthearted activities, the derby was suspended during the war, but it came back afterward, bigger than ever. In 1951, their senior year, Peggie-Louise Lee, Matilda Snelling, Katie Kennedy, and Geraldine Waybright posed with their contenders.

*You worked as a nurse with all the responsibilities and you worked mostly evenings and nights.
I worked on Osler 8, which at that time was the only communicable disease floor, with an aide and an orderly. I didn't realize at that time what trust the school put into the people who had educated us, that they would put us on a floor. You had a supervisor that you could call if you had a problem. I don't know anyone who did not live up to expectations. It was done that way for us to really accept responsibility and then to challenge us to put our education into practice. And we did.*
Betsy Mumaw McGeady, 1955

It was early spring of 1956. I wasn't really a person who read a lot of news. I knew there was something about desegregation and I didn't know it didn't apply to private schools. I wrote a letter to say "I'm interested in coming there and I don't know if you'll accept me because I am colored" and "Do you have any other colored people there?" The answer I got back was, "Yes, pending passing the application, we would accept you." I then got a letter saying, "We would like you to come for an interview." The appointment went smoothly. I came home and I said to my mother, "I'm going to Hopkins."

My brother brought me down with my mother. There's a tunnel underneath Broadway so my brother said, "Let's go through the tunnel and see what that's like." As we came up we came through the door, on the left were two bathrooms and on the right were two bathrooms. They were labeled White Women, Colored Women *and the same for men on the other side. My brother looked at me and I looked at him. Now you have to remember, I'm not from the South and I've never seen any of this before. We got upstairs to my room and he said, "You know, you don't have to stay here." I said, "No. I put my money down. I'm here now. I'm going to stay." So I got myself settled in and my brother and my mother went back home.*

I have very fond memories of Hopkins although the reality is, it was there, the prejudices, and it did show at particular times. While I didn't go out socially with any of them, the camaraderie in the rooms was fine. It was a good time for me. I just found it fascinating. There was just so much to learn. It gave me a good foundation for what I was able to do the rest of my life.

Trudy Jones Hodges, 1959

together to socialize and enjoy shared—and often bawdy—humor. Holidays were still a highlight in this period, with the disappointment of having to work tempered by special events in the hospital and at Hampton House. Christmas caroling remained a strong fixture of each holiday season, and the students organized to sing for patients on every unit on Christmas day.

With changes in the workload for students, especially late in the decade, there was more free time to participate in outside social functions than ever before. "All those talk sessions with our backs up against the wall in the hall—we were trying to solve all the problems of our lives. How innocent we were," Doris Higgins Thompson, 1951, recalled.[49] Her classmate Adele Sparks Birx remembered awakening in the night when the ceiling of her fifth floor room fell down around her bed.[50] Denizens of Hampton House had to get used to the tunnel that connected the residence to the hospital; some found this unnerving at times.

Students had to put up with air pollution from the Patapsco River and nearby steel mills and with the aging infrastructure of postwar Baltimore. But "Hoptown," with a healthy supply of shops, movies, and restaurants, was just a few blocks away. New arrivals' sense of fashion was increasingly affronted by the ugly brown duty booties and lab coats mandatory in the world of nursing in the preclinical phase. War emergencies were long over and the outfits seemed unusually disreputable.

In 1956 the first African-American student who would finish the program was admitted to the nursing school. Trudy Jones came to Baltimore from New York State and settled into Hampton House. Classmates welcomed her but she soon learned that she was living in a Southern city and could not participate in all social activities. Restaurants and other settings were not open to African Americans at that time. She also had to deal with segregated units in the hospital and with the insensitivity of some patients and of others who could not believe she was truly a nursing student. She completed the program successfully and developed strong friendships with many she met along the way. After graduation she continued her education, practiced nursing, and became a nurse educator and a leader in the Baltimore community.[51]

Adjustments during the 1950s did little to alter the basic demands of the nursing program or the expectations of student behaviors under the honor code. Strict adherence to dress regulations, house rules, and classroom requirements continued unchanged. The workload was still demanding because of chronic shortages of staff throughout the hospital, yet students were expected to aim for excellence in all they did. They understood authority, and although they were not above a bit of high jinks once in a while, they attended to business—and they developed strong bonds and lifelong friendships that endure to this day.

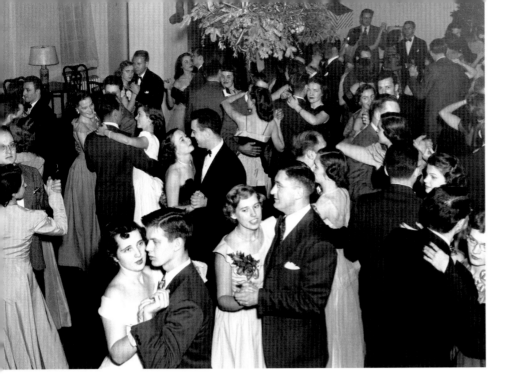

Christmas dances in Hampton House were formal occasions. Students often invited medical students as their escorts. Beginning with the class of 1951, however, when the age of nursing students began to drop, some preferred dates who were closer to their own age and turned to undergraduates from the Homewood campus of the Johns Hopkins University or from other nearby schools.

Center: Hospital president Russell Nelson, whose wife was an alumna, was a major booster of the nursing school. He enjoyed participating in school events, including raising a toast with students at a formal dance in 1954.

Below: As in years past, students in 1958 took pleasure in singing Christmas carols in the hospital on Christmas Day. One student found the indoor atmosphere chilly enough to don a sweater.

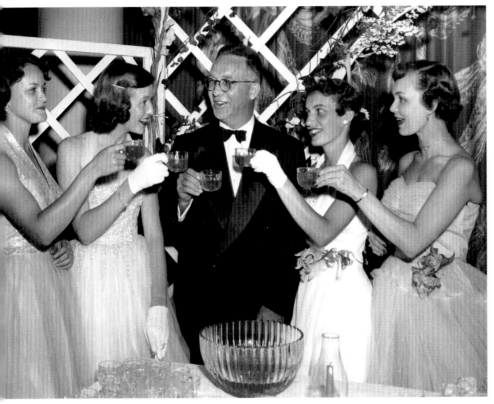

We were awakened at 5:45 on Christmas morning. First we all had coffee, then prayers led by Miss Wolf in Hampton House lounge. We were all happy and cheerful on this happy morning. The weather was cold and brisk but our hearts were warm with merriment. We rotated through the hospital, singing carols early Christmas morning for our patients. The quality of the music was marvelous, each putting her heart into the singing. We nurses experienced a great thrill being able to spread joy in what little way we could, and I'm sure the patients appreciated the carols. That day I worked on Halsted 7, the neurosurgical floor. By the time evening came, I was a very tired little nurse. But the wonderful experience of this Christmas 1951 will always remain a joy to my memory and a thing most dear to my heart.

Mabel Gerhart Hollowell, 1953, writing in her scrapbook in 1951

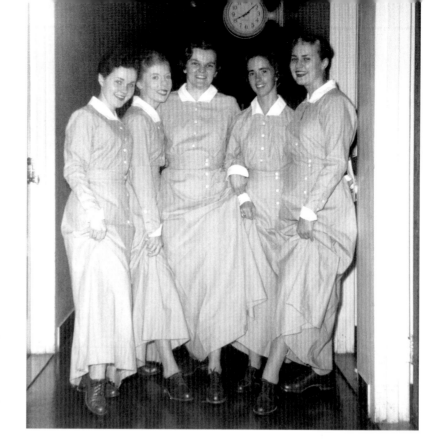

We were measured for our uniforms as part of that first week. When we came back after Thanksgiving, we had a candle-lighting ceremony and wore our uniforms to that. There was a feeling of belonging after that. You were accepted at that point. You'd at least done enough to earn a uniform. We had reached the point where we could go and work with a patient and they would see us in a uniform instead of this pinkish, tannish lab coat and wonder "What is this person?" Even though our uniforms were a little bit bluer than the ones that had been washed many times, they would be more accepted by the patients and that gave you the confidence to do things.

Lois Grayshan Hoffer, 1962

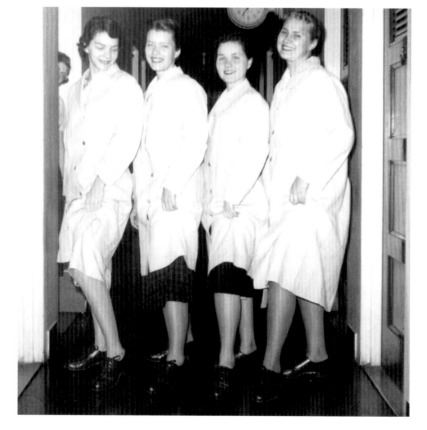

Above and center: Although significant changes occurred during the 1950s for students, the decade ended much as it began. New arrivals were fitted for their short-sleeved everyday uniforms as well as one long-sleeved dress uniform. Until their blue uniforms were ready, preclinical students wore tan lab coats over their civilian clothes. What remained constant in their attire were the dark brown oxford shoes they were told to bring with them, which they soon learned were known as duty booties.

On June 3, 1959, preclinical students donned professional attire and put on a skit spoofing the personality quirks of their instructors. In the 1960 yearbook, the *Dome*, this photo was captioned, "They entertain us . . . we entertain them."

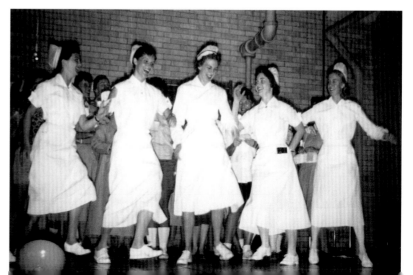

The alumnae magazine overflowed in the 1950s with contributions and awards garnered by the graduates of the Johns Hopkins Hospital School of Nursing for the marks they made on the profession. Effie Taylor was in her later years in this period, having retired as the dean of the School of Nursing at Yale in 1944. She remained active by serving in the American Red Cross in New Haven, Connecticut. After graduation in 1907 she had practiced at Johns Hopkins and then completed her bachelor's of science in nursing degree at Teachers College, Columbia University. Returning to Hopkins, she established the nursing service in the new Phipps Psychiatric Clinic just before World War I. In 1918 she went to Fort Meade, located between Baltimore and Washington, as director of the nursing education program that was part of the Army Training School for Nurses. There she served under the leadership of Annie Goodrich, and the two became close friends. In 1923 Miss Taylor joined the faculty at Yale, and she was named its second dean for nursing in 1934 upon Annie Goodrich's retirement. In 1937 Taylor became the first American nurse to be elected president of the International Council of Nurses, a position she held throughout World War II. She contributed regularly to alumnae activities and provided moral support to nurses advocating a degree program at Johns Hopkins. On May 21, 1955, when the new chemistry laboratory at the school was dedicated to the memory of Lavinia L. Dock, the first instructor appointed by Isabel Hampton to the Johns Hopkins Hospital School of Nursing, Effie Taylor was the featured speaker. She declared that

Johns Hopkins Hospital graduates are now occupying positions of trust and responsibility, not only in hospital, but in university schools of nursing, and other institutions of higher education. They are also sought after for supervision in the education of children. They are filling with great success, important posts in government and in the broad fields of public health, industry and business. This record can be attributed to the quality of young women admitted into this Nursing School; to the character and caliber of the women who created the School and formulated its policies; and to those who have since directed its activities, upheld its traditions and enlarged its scope of usefulness through maintaining one of the most comprehensive and broad courses of study in nursing education. Unquestionably it is due in large measure to the fact that this School is part of the great Johns Hopkins institution.[52]

Articles written about Miss Taylor portray a woman who gave her energy to encouraging others and reveal how much her peers respected her. In 1959 three nurses received the Florence Nightingale Medal, the highest award given to a nurse by the International Red Cross, and two of the recipients were Johns Hopkins alumnae: Effie Taylor and Lucile Petry Leone, 1927.[53]

Virginia Dunbar, 1923, had completed twelve years as dean at Cornell University–New York Hospital School of Nursing when she

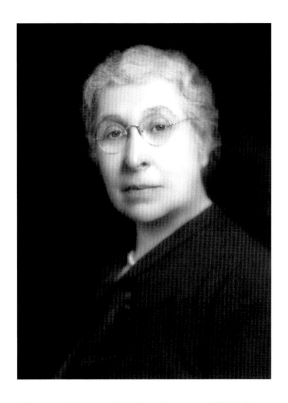

After pursuing a particularly active career, Effie Taylor, 1907, spent much of the 1950s working with the American Red Cross in New Haven, Connecticut, where she had served as dean of the Yale University School of Nursing for ten years. Taylor was a force in alumnae activities at Johns Hopkins throughout her life and a vocal champion of bringing the nursing school under the auspices of the university. In 1959 the International Red Cross awarded her its highest honor, the Florence Nightingale Medal.

retired in 1959. A pioneer nursing scholar, educated at Mount Holyoke, Johns Hopkins, and Teachers College, Columbia, she set out to improve schools in several states through innovation and support of nursing research. Her studies took her to the Florence Nightingale International Foundation in England, and she served as the director of Red Cross nursing during World War II. She was an avid supporter of the degree proposals for Johns Hopkins and served on numerous committees in the alumnae association. Miss Wolf wrote that Miss Dunbar's "steadfast faith in university education of nurses for nursing services to the public and also her conviction of the need for substantial endowment to further such a program are outstanding characteristics of her professional philosophy."[54]

Frances Reiter, 1931, was a distinguished graduate of the program who reached the pinnacle of her career as teacher and administrator in this era. She completed bachelor's and master's degrees at Teachers College, Columbia. A strong advocate of advanced clinical education for nurses, she introduced the term "nurse clinician" in 1943. Reiter achieved the rank of full professor at Columbia in the 1950s and then became the founding dean of the New York Medical College Graduate School of Nursing, which later became the Lienhard School of Nursing at Pace University. In 1965 she chaired the American Nurses Association's committee on education, which issued the historic position paper stating that all persons licensed to practice nursing should be educated in degree-granting universities. It took courage to produce this paper in a system that was still overwhelmingly dominated by hospital-owned schools of nursing. Two years later she wrote in the *Johns Hopkins Nurses Alumnae Magazine*:

In 1901 Dr. Richard Cabot publicly affirmed that he considered the practice of nursing so valuable to society that the preparation for this service should incorporate a broad and solid basis of general and liberal education. . . .

Had our professional progenitors stood with Dr. Cabot in 1901 or kept in step with the progress in education of medicine and social work following the Flexner Report in 1910, or taken the position of the Goldmark Report in 1923, or the Brown Report even as late as 1948, we would not in this generation, be facing a task that is more monumental and a transition more complex because of prolonged delay.[55]

"Clinical practice in hospitals is essential in the preparation of students," Reiter continued, "but learning only hospital nursing is not sufficient preparation for professional nursing practice." Reiter also received the Florence Nightingale Medal from the International Red Cross and many other national and international honors. She established herself as one of nursing's older, wiser visionaries and played a significant role in new developments over the next decade.

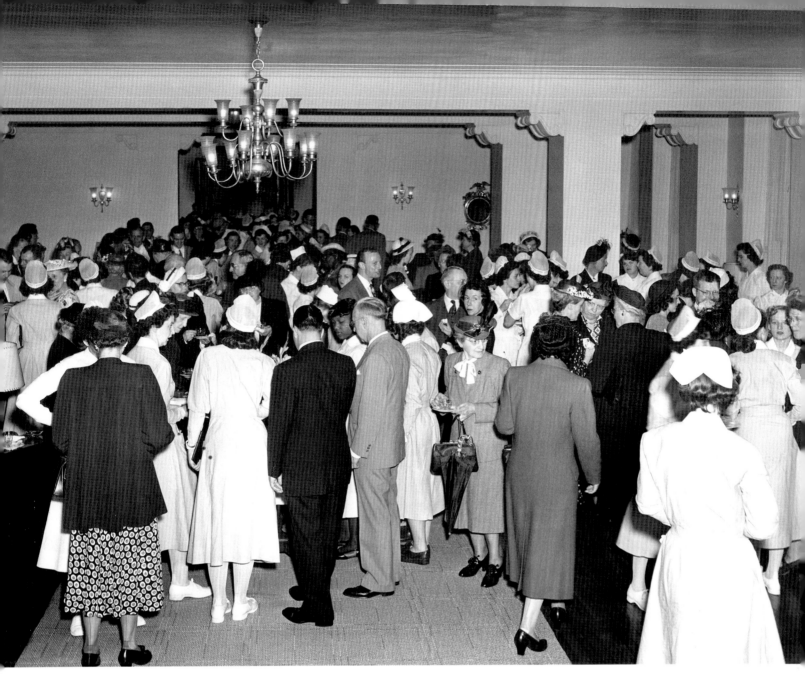

Many of the nurses who began their careers in the 1950s and are now reaching the end of their professional journeys characterize their achievements according to the values ingrained in them at the School of Nursing. Barbara Russell Donaho, 1956, the first nurse to serve as president and CEO of an American hospital, who became a trustee of the Johns Hopkins University in 1992, summed up the achievements of her contemporaries when she gave the keynote address at homecoming in 1996:

I doubt we really know the heights to which many of the Hopkins graduates have risen—the influence they have had in nursing, on patient care, on health care policy and standard setting for nursing in this country. As I have traveled this country, I have had the opportunity to meet and work with many, in a wide variety of positions—from directors, vice presidents, members of state boards of nursing, faculty, members of hospital boards, officers in nursing organizations (at both state and national levels), clinical specialists, researchers, and staff nurses. It always has created a strong esprit de corps when the connection with Hopkins is identified.[56]

Graduation receptions were always an opportunity for alumnae to mingle with faculty and students, as well as to welcome new graduates and family members. Signs of change were apparent in this scene, c. 1950: a young black woman stands almost at the center of the photograph.

Miss Pfefferkorn lived on the second floor of Hampton House in one of the student rooms. She did a lot of her research and writing in the library, which at that time was called the fishbowl. It was off of the corridor between the main hospital building and Wilmer. It was all glass on all sides so that's why they called it the fishbowl. You'd go in and she would be there writing away. We all knew who she was and what she was doing. We knew that this was very, very important, but none of us realized how really important it was until much later.

Betsy Mumaw McGeady, 1955

The alumnae association voted unanimously in 1952 to approve guidelines to replace the regimented code of ethics adopted in 1896. The new approach eliminated the subservient attitudes espoused earlier and instead took a new stance, in which nurses and doctors would act together as colleagues with separate but equally important responsibilities.

SOME ETHICAL CONCEPTS FOR NURSES

WE, who have chosen nursing, an essential and universal service to mankind, as our profession, have obligated ourselves to accept large responsibilities inherent in a great social service. Implicit in our decision to practice nursing is an acceptance of ethical concepts by which we carry on our work for and with others. In the consideration of these ethical principles which may guide our judgments, it seems appropriate to discuss them as especially applicable to patients, co-workers and others with whom we as nurses have close professional relationships and for whom we bear great responsibility. In many instances the specific guiding principle for ethical practice applies to all groups but has not been repeated, hence its application should be made as may be found significant. All practice, and all relationships in that practice, have a direct bearing upon the welfare of the patient or the community.

Basic to all nursing practice are respect for and understanding of human needs. With this fundamental concept in mind, may we practice

8

During the 1950s the alumnae association tried to keep up with the rapid changes in the profession while providing support for the students, school, and graduates. *The Johns Hopkins Nurses Alumnae Magazine* continued to report events at the School of Nursing as well as news about graduates and developments in the profession. In 1952 the alumnae underwrote the $750 cost of producing Anna Dryden Wolf's portrait, which was presented to Miss Wolf on May 27, 1952, at Hurd Hall. In later years, Miss Wolf spoke of the portrait and of the artist, Ann Schuler, who had painted it.[57] She described Mrs. Schuler as a "grand little person," who had a good rapport with her subject and who worked hard to get a good portrait. But Miss Wolf was afraid she looked "pompous" and "dictatorial" and wondered if she had been so severe in her manner.[58] Yet the alumnae recollections tell a different story—of a lady who could be warm and caring and who had the ability to tease on some occasions.[59]

In 1952 the organization approved a sweeping revision of the code of ethics, the first major change since 1896, when a committee chaired by Isabel Hampton Robb had drafted the original code. In place of a strict code, the committee, chaired by Anna Wolf, presented a complete rewrite, which they called "Some Ethical Concepts for Nurses." The new guidelines expanded the responsibilities of nurses and reordered priorities.[60] The old code began with a subservient section, "The Duty of the Nurse to the Physician," which declared that "a nurse should always accord to a physician the proper amount of respect and consideration due to his higher professional position."[61] The concepts adopted in 1952 affirmed that "the nursing ethics of each nurse are a part of her individual character as a person, manifest in her nursing service and in every situation in which she is identified as a nurse. Her ethics are deeply personal." The report emphasized that ethical decisions were affected by many conditions.[62]

In the new version, nurses' relations with physicians fell under a section called "the nurse's responsibility to her co-workers." The submissive language of the 1896 code was replaced with wording that presented doctors and nurses as colleagues who were both "responsible, legally and professionally," for treatment of patients, though their obligations were different. The nurse was urged to "exercise independent judgment, in appropriate circumstances, with regard to therapy prescribed by a physician" and be willing to take actions that might question the treatment recommended by a physician—a far cry from the 1896 code.[63]

In 1954 the alumnae association produced the first history of the school, titled *The Johns Hopkins Hospital School of Nursing, 1889–1954,* by Blanche Pfefferkorn, 1911, and Ethel Johns, former editor and business manager of the *Canadian Nurse.* The association raised the money to produce the book and the Johns Hopkins Press published and distrib-

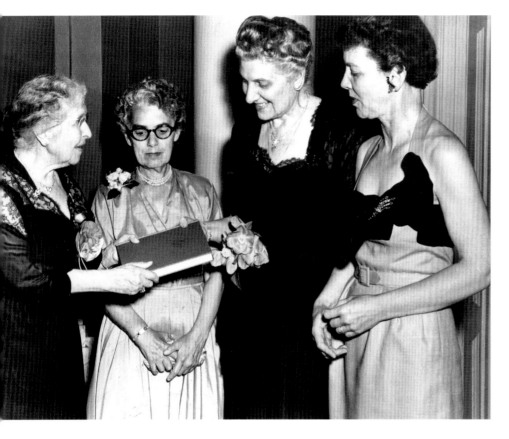

Years of effort and anticipation were fulfilled on May 24, 1954, when Effie Taylor presented Anna Wolf with the first copy of *The Johns Hopkins Hospital School of Nursing, 1889–1949* as Blanche Pfefferkorn (wearing dark-rimmed glasses), 1911, one of the book's authors, and Helen Grose Fallon, 1930, president of the alumnae association, looked on. The Johns Hopkins Press published twelve hundred copies.

uted twelve hundred copies. The project had been under way for several years, so its publication made members of the organization justifiably proud. The book received positive reviews by members of the Hopkins academic and medical community and the wider nursing population. Jessie Black McVicar, 1930, who championed the effort to see the school's history published, wrote an elegant summary:

In this wonderful volume the history of the glorious past, the golden years, has been beautifully described. The present history with its impact of social, economic, medical advances and public health has been related with meticulous care. And the future history of our School will perhaps be written by another generation of alumnae who will carry on the Hopkins traditions. History is being made now; each day, each year. Another volume is in the making. Let us not forget these memorable words, spoken by Mary Adelaide Nutting: History is the past, the present, and the future."[64]

After the book appeared, Johns and Pfefferkorn published several articles in the alumnae magazine featuring data not included in the book.

The annual Roll Call for alumnae support became more prominent in alumnae records in the postwar era and donations grew steadily throughout the decade. While the late 1940s had seen the annual giving to the school drop below $100,000 dollars, by the early 1950s the amount had climbed to over $140,000.[65] Between 175 and 200 members would return for homecoming during the 1950s, to socialize and conduct

The Johns Hopkins Hospital School of Nursing, 1889–1949 gave me a whole new slant on why Miss Wolf was so intense on this collegiate school of nursing. The idea came from Isabel Hampton Robb. Miss Nutting just left, went to Teachers College. Then the vision skipped two generations because Miss Lawler was here for thirty years, and then it was taken up again by Miss Wolf. Miss Wolf really suffered because she was devoted to this and she constantly kept it in front of us and the class before us. There was no doubt that was what she wanted. When she was appointed superintendent, she stated in so many words that this was her goal and they accepted her. Johns and Pfefferkorn did such a beautiful job of getting stories along the way, beautiful characterizations of the personalities of the people. Hopkins came alive again for me. I sure wouldn't give my copy away.

Betty Borenstein Scher, 1950

When I talk up the alumni association, being active in it, to young nurses, I tell them that it's such a pleasure because one of the biggest advantages is you work with wonderful people that you never would have met if you hadn't become active. Helen Wilmer Athey was from a wealthy family. Mrs. Athey had that rare gift of not just being intelligent and getting things done—she loved the challenge. The Gate House Shop was her baby and it was such a success when she was there—but she also had that rare gift of a sense of humor expressed in just a few well-chosen words. She was intelligent, talented, devoted, and had this wonderful wit that you get so rarely. We used to look forward to our alumni association annual reports because they were wonderful. And she was as nice as could be at meetings. She did not take over at board meetings. She listened. She might put in some crucial statement but she didn't throw her weight around.

Betty Borenstein Scher, 1950

Alta Elizabeth Dines, 1914, an instructor of public-health nursing at Teachers College, Columbia University, chaired the Nursing Council for War Service in New York State, which coordinated nursing programs during World War II.

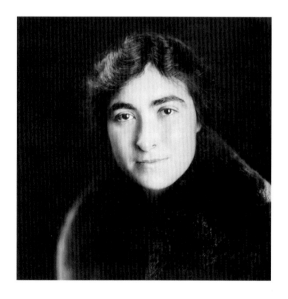

the business of the association. In 1956 attendees voted to revise the bylaws and change the organization's name from the Johns Hopkins Hospital Nurses' Alumnae Association, Inc., to the Alumnae Association of the Johns Hopkins Hospital School of Nursing, Inc.

The Gate House Shop Committee continued its many fund-raising activities into the 1950s. Crucial to its success had been the small group of alumnae who volunteered in the shop, especially Helen Wilmer Athey, 1905, a generous friend of the alumnae association for many years. Graduates donated white elephant items and needlework; even Miss Lawler took up yarn work and made afghans to be raffled from the shop. By the middle of the decade, however, active supporters had begun to die and fewer donations were being received.[66] What had been an asset since the 1920s changed dramatically. Successive annual reports indicated that sales were down and the operation was faltering. By the end of the decade, the toll of age and infirmity forced the committee to seek an end to the arrangement with the hospital, and the resources of the shop were divided between the Women's Board of the hospital and the alumnae association.

In 1958, in honor of the centennial of Adelaide Nutting's birth, the organization produced a special edition of the magazine focused on higher education for nurses and the need for baccalaureate degrees in the profession. Isabel Stewart, who had worked closely with Miss Nutting, wrote about her mentor's philosophy of nursing as it related to the future of the school. Graduates Mary T. Harms, 1932, and Mildred Barnard, 1950, wrote about the value of university programs. Blanche Pfefferkorn reviewed the past efforts by nursing leaders for a university-based nursing education program. Effie Taylor, Virginia Dunbar, and Alta Dines, 1914, also wrote of the issues relating Hopkins to university education for nurses. Director Mary Sanders Price contributed a short article citing the changing delivery system and nursing's role, which required additional education, in the emerging health care scheme. The issue made clear that the nursing community at Johns Hopkins and those concerned about the future knew what was needed.[67] Was the message ever going to reach those in control of the university and the hospital? Not in the 1950s.

The end of the decade seemed like the quiet before the storm. The school was quickly slipping behind national goals established by the nursing profession. The clinical faculty, the facilities, physician participation, and the caliber of the students still attracted to the historic nursing program were maintaining a standard of excellence, but the model was quickly becoming outdated. The adamant demands of Miss Wolf, who desperately wanted the leadership to understand what was ahead, had given way to the quiet, persistent, and determined efforts of Mrs. Price, who strove to get those in charge to see the handwriting on the wall.

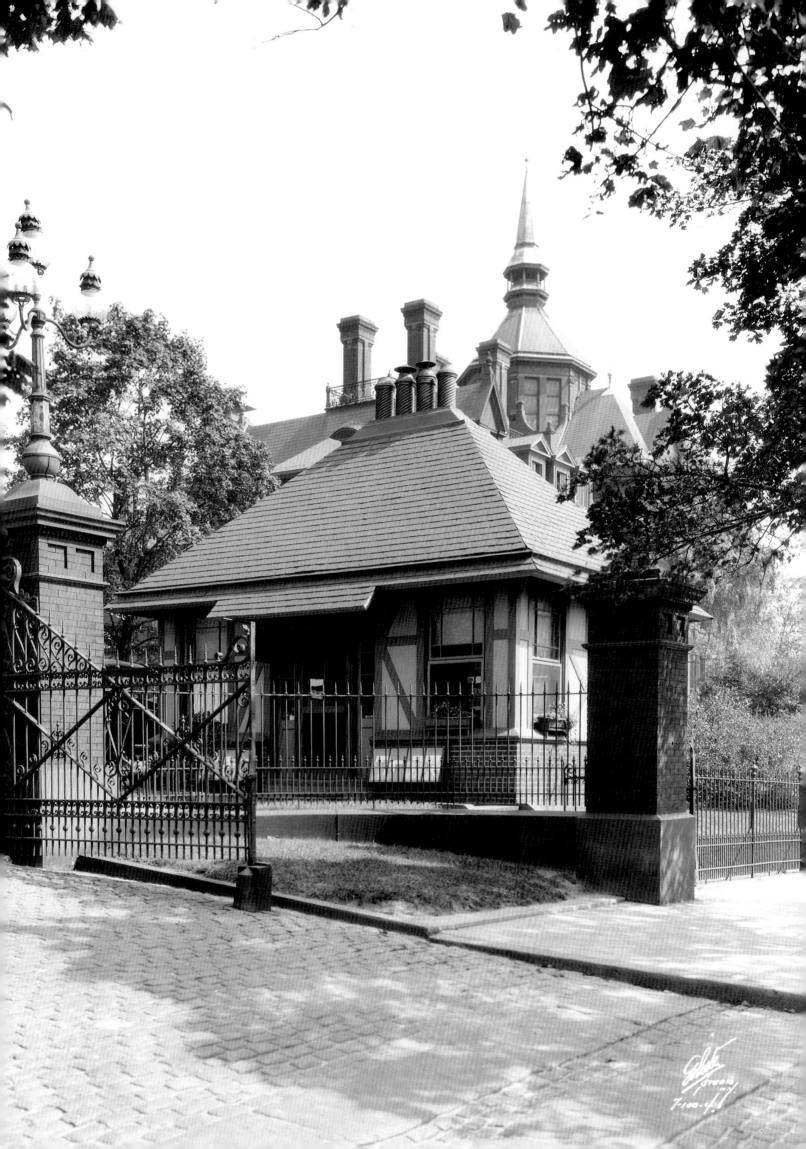

"The Dreaded Uniforms"

Katherine Good Amberson, 1919, snapped her friends during an outdoor break. In cold weather, students wore capes as part of their uniforms. Even after new uniforms were introduced in 1940, capes, made of navy blue broadcloth and lined with lighter blue flannel, remained. Much as members of later classes liked to complain about their "duty booties," these students and their contemporaries wore shoes with much longer laces.

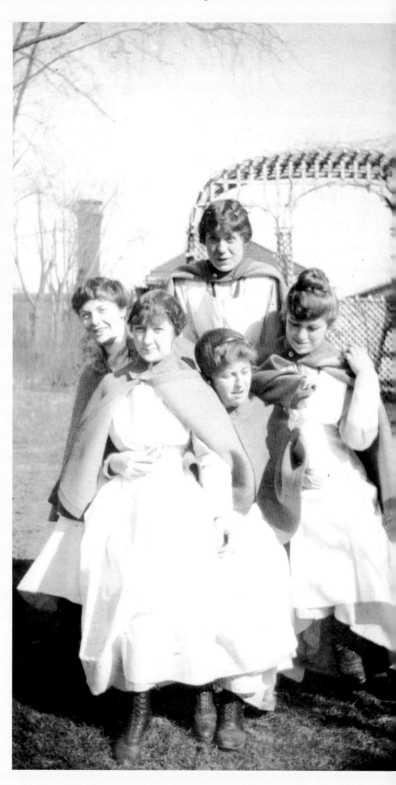

Vashti Bartlett, 1906, caught some of her classmates fooling around, probably in the dispensary. The young woman in the middle looked a little concerned about what her friend was planning to do with the portable electric lamp she wielded, especially since it was plugged in high overhead. Even with their antics, all three were successful in keeping their uniforms pristine, although one had let her apron strap slip off her shoulder.

The class of 1943 was the last class to wear the old uniforms, which had long sleeves. They wore brown stockings and they had a different cap. It was old-fashioned. It had an apron and cuffs and a collar that all detached. The new uniform was all one piece.

Mary Farr Heeg, 1941

First-year students c. 1938 were particularly careful in anatomy classes, held in the medical school's anatomy and physiology laboratory, to keep their aprons and starched white cuffs clean.

We had to wear a lab coat as probationary students. It didn't do much for your self-esteem. We all badly wanted to be nurses and we wanted to look like a nurse and we didn't. In fact, we were often mistaken for housecleaning people. More than one of us walked into a room and before we could even introduce ourselves our patient would say, "Oh, the trash can's over there."

Cathy Novak, 1973

First we wore, it was said to be, a tan lab coat. Well, it was sort of a rosy pink as far as I was concerned. We wore them over our clothes. We all had wool winter clothing and had to wear these lab coats over top of them. I had one cotton dress and I wore it for two weeks. We wore brown stockings and brown oxford shoes. As the years went by it became sort of a source of pride. We understood that there was only one other school in the United States at that time where nursing students still wore the brown shoes and stockings.

Lois Grayshan Hoffer, 1962

We got our BM-brown lab coats that had to be buttoned all the way down, even the bottom button, which we soon lost because sitting in class everybody's popped. Rather than make us sew on another one, the instructors just ignored that we didn't have it. And brown hose and brown shoes and hairnets. If your hair came to the shoulder, you had to wear a hairnet on duty, so we really were attractive.

Betty Borenstein Scher, 1950

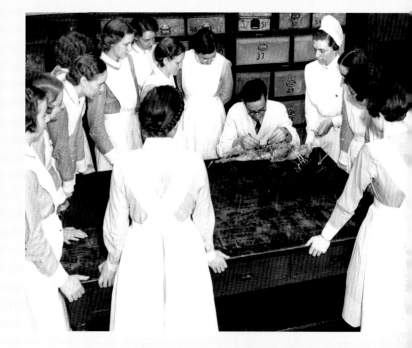

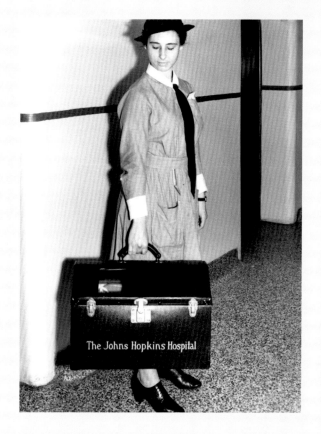

Students wore a different uniform when they went into the community for public-health nursing. The one-piece garment had a white collar and cuffs but no apron. A dark necktie and hat added a stylish touch to their no-nonsense look. The container this student toted was an infant carrier, used to transport premature infants from home to the hospital.

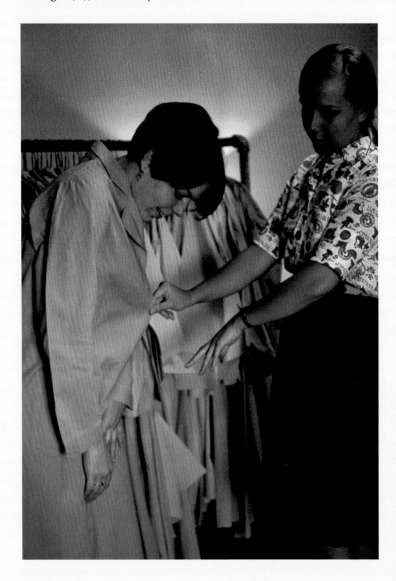

We were given two or three brown lab coats, which were very, very ugly. We were told to bring two pairs of sturdy brown oxfords and hose with seams down the back. For six months we wore the brown lab coat to class and to any clinical practice and everybody, without question, hated what they wore every day. Then in six months we were able to wear our student uniform. Of course, they used the six months to make all the uniforms.

Betsy Mumaw McGeady, 1955

They weren't white lab coats. Oh, no, just an ugly tannish brown. Lab coats distinguished us as being the brand-new kids on the block. We stood out in the crowd with the Buster Brown shoes, which we had to wear. You could change them and most of us did in the second year. Ugly as they were, it was nice. You didn't have to polish them much.

Donna Dittberner, 1966

Most of the fall semester we wore a lab coat that was pretty unattractive, but then we had a capping ceremony sometime in the fall. It was held in the evening in Hurd Hall. We carried little candles. It was very moving. It meant that we had gone through a probationary period and had done well enough to take the next step. From that point on, then, we wore the light blue uniforms with the white cuffs and the brown shoes.

The student cap had a little blue JHH across the top. It was something that we were responsible for keeping clean. It had a little button almost like a staple at the top and you attached it to a little knitted thing that you put on your head. We called it a brain patch. You put a long bobby pin through that little staple and then attached it to this brain patch that you had in your hair. I'm sure that my Big Sister knitted me my first brain patch.

Sandra Stine Angell, 1969, BSN 1977

The candlelight ceremony was rather impressive. It made me realize that this was something really important. When you went to college, no one asked you to make a commitment to what you were going to do. Of course, being able then the next day to go into the hospital with a student uniform on made a big difference to our outlook. We felt like we had some status, low as it was.

Betsy Mumaw McGeady, 1955

Opposite: Beginning in 1941 the candlelight ceremony (here shown in 1952) became a rite of passage for nursing students in the hospital school. It marked the end of their preclinical period and was the first time they wore their new uniforms.

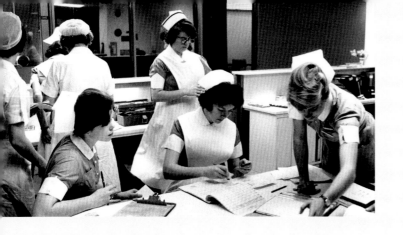

The nurses' station in the new Children's Medical and Surgical Center was crowded in 1964 with students from Hopkins and affiliated schools, who wore their own distinctive uniforms.

We had thirteen uniforms. The hospital did the laundry. You had to make sure you kept your buttons because they had little pins to hold the buttons on. You threw them down the laundry chute. If you did it right, you had six one week. While they were gone, you wore the other six. Then you kept your formal one for teas or formal occasions. If you wore that formal one when you were doing your bed baths with your patients, you had to be careful to not get the sleeves wet. That's why the short sleeves were for everyday wear. You learned how to do it so that you still looked neat at the end of the day. If you messed up and you had to wear your formal uniform, then when teatime came around and you didn't have it, you couldn't go. You couldn't wear a short-sleeved one so you were out of luck.

Trudy Jones Hodges, 1959

Uniforms were eighteen inches from the floor. If you were five nine, you had, in 1963, a skirt that was almost to your ankles. If you were five one, you had a nice short one. Of course, those of us who were tall could not wait until after capping to hem our uniforms but never the dress uniform.

Donna Dittberner, 1966

Our tradition was that you found a student in a lower class and you passed your student uniform on to her. The reason was that the patients, who so often were repeaters, knew that the deeper the blue, the newer the student. So by taking seniors' uniforms, freshmen or incoming students could be given a little bit of the benefit of the doubt.

Betty Borenstein Scher, 1950

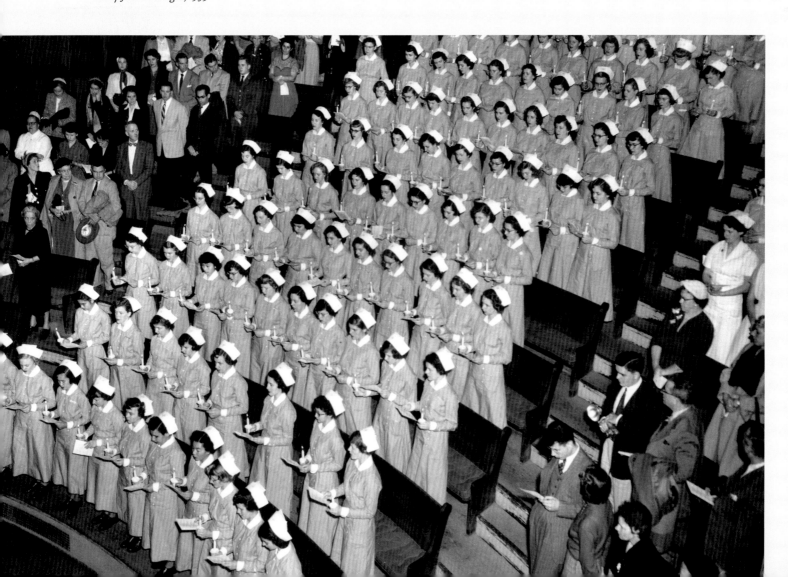

Jean Lashinsky and Claire Lambert were still wearing their student uniforms on graduation day in June 1947, but they had proudly donned their graduate caps.

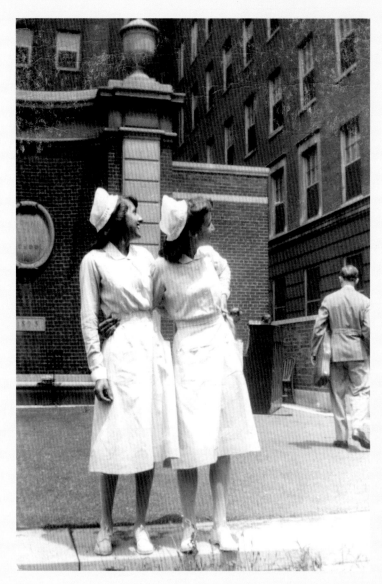

You got taught by your Big Sister how to starch your caps and plaster them up on the marble shower walls. It was this blue liquid starch and you just plunk it in there and you bring it out dripping wet, just dripping with this starch solution. Then just plaster it up there on the shower marble wall. You'd work to get all the wrinkles out so it'd be nice and smooth. Then it would dry. Then you'd peel it off and when you pulled it back to put the little button in, it was this little tri-corner thing and then you'd have the wings. The better starching job you did, the more the wings sat out. None of us liked wearing the caps but if you're going to wear it you wanted it really well starched.

Sue Appling, 1973

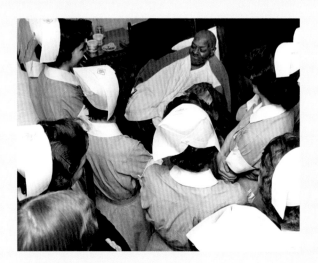

The new uniform, introduced with the class of 1944, included a stiffly starched cap emblazoned with JHH on the center of its rim. Learning to maintain it in perfect condition became one of the first skills new students mastered.

I think that uniform was very important. We did not wear any part of our graduate uniform until the day we graduated. That was the first time we put the cap on; the first time we put on the white uniform with the long sleeves. We wore white hose and white shoes. We looked like nurses.

At that time, the alumni association gave you your first cap. They had a gift shop in the gatehouse. The week before graduation you were given a little slip of paper that said you were worthy to wear the cap. It was thrilling—absolutely thrilling. You really felt like you were a Hopkins nurse. And we got our alumni pin. To have that pin, I had been able to accomplish something that had been my dream as a child. I was really happy.

Betsy Mumaw McGeady, 1955

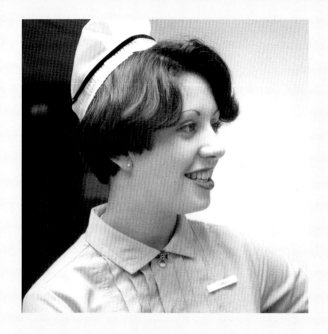

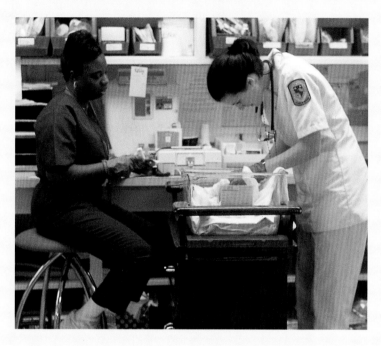

The addition of a narrow velvet band of blue and gold just above the pleated edges distinguished the School of Health Services' Nursing Education Program students' caps from those of the hospital school.

Jim Buzzard, 1995, and Christiani Guerrero, 2001, wore uniforms featuring a badge with the school's emblem as students in the Johns Hopkins University School of Nursing.

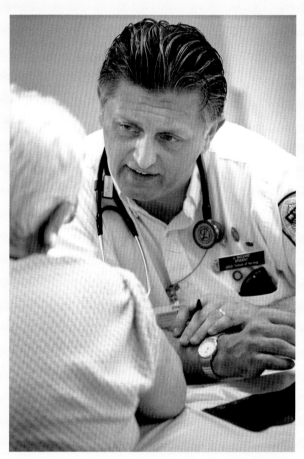

We didn't wear uniforms to class but when we were in the clinical area we had uniforms. They weren't very well liked. I remember one person commenting that we men looked like a bunch of barbers in the uniforms. Now, having met other alumni, nobody's ever liked their nursing school uniform. I think that's one thing that really unifies us all.

Bernard Keenan, 1986, MSN 1993

The dreaded uniforms. And now they have it better than we did. Isn't that always the way? We had lovely, lovely white uniforms that were mostly polyester that you could see right through. You could wear whatever the standard-issue white lovely polyester pants were and this lovely tunic top that, despite the fact that you ironed it, didn't hold a press worth anything. We referred to ourselves as Q-tips because we were white from head to toe. Oh, and mandatory white leather shoes, closed toe of course, and no markings were allowed to be on them. People complained so much that they are now able to wear blue scrub pants with a white polo shirt that has the Hopkins patch on it. As much as I complained about the uniform, in working with students on the floor in a hospital, the white uniform is a good thing. They told us, "You're not going to like it but the whole purpose, basically, is to identify you as a nursing student." And it worked because nobody else is in white head to toe anymore.

Kate Knott, 2002

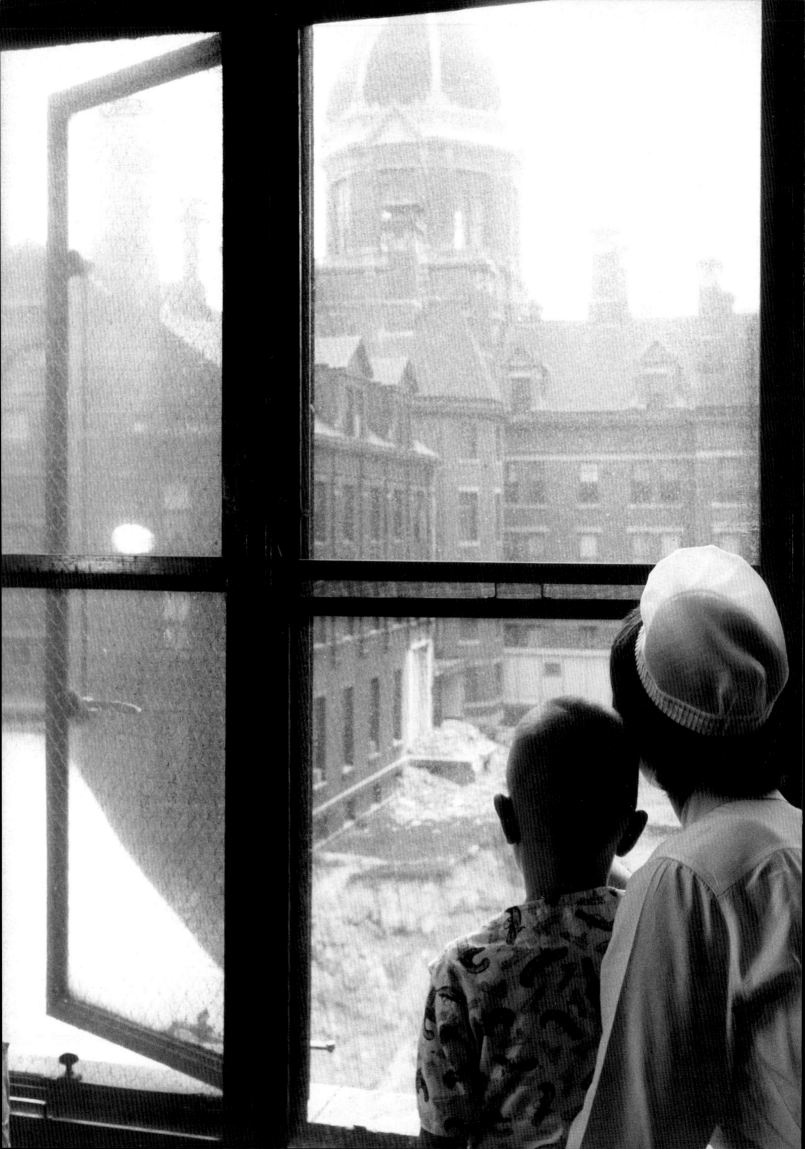

The Handwriting on the Wall, 1960–1970 · LINDA SABIN

4

Jeanne Dougherty, 1960, and a young patient kept
an eye on the early stages of construction of the new
cafeteria and the Children's Medical and Surgical
Center from the third-floor porch of the Halsted
Building in January 1962. At the time, Dougherty was
head nurse in a pediatric research unit.

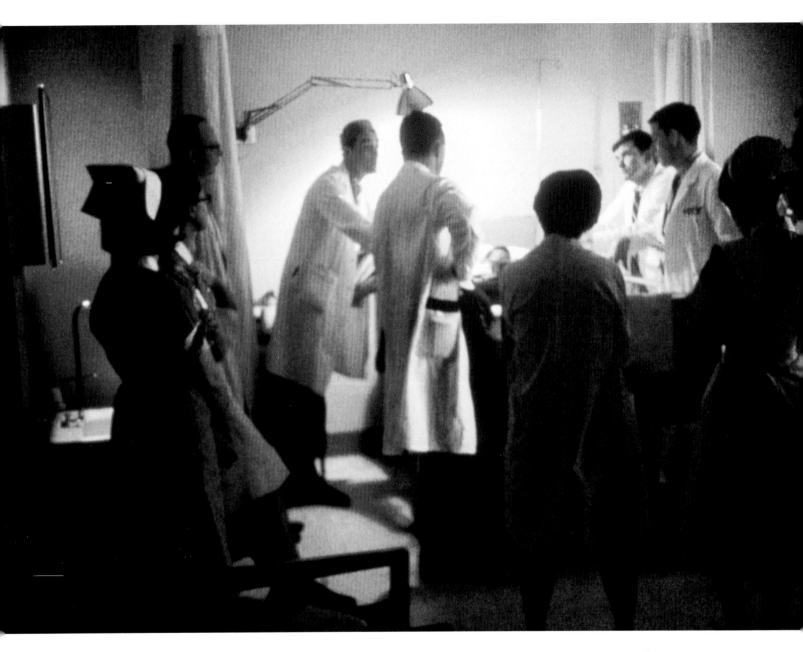

Both Johns Hopkins and affiliated nursing students attended rounds with doctors, nurses, and medical students. In 1967 one student already was on duty without a cap—a sign of changing times and standards.

THE ARRIVAL OF THE 1960s seemed to promise new transitions throughout the social order, and hope for change at the School of Nursing remained high. The postwar period of recovery and redirection was ending, and the American electorate chose a new, young president in November 1960. John F. Kennedy appealed to a new generation to commit itself to service and called for the creation of the Peace Corps. Technological innovations and scientific advances amazed the public on a daily basis. As the 1960s progressed, the era brought revolutions in sexual mores, family structure, and the role of women in society. It was a stressful decade in every way for the Hopkins community and for much of the world. As the School of Nursing was swept along in this accelerated environment, nursing leaders tried to seize the opportunity to achieve the goal of a bachelor's program for the school.

The Johns Hopkins Hospital began extensive building programs in the early 1960s, and the East Baltimore campus underwent dramatic alterations in a short period of time. Old landmarks disappeared. In July 1960 the nursing alumnae's board of directors voted to close the Gate House Shop, which had served patients, visitors, staff, and nurses in the hospital for many years. In 1964 the Gate House building, which had stood by the Broadway gate of the hospital since 1889, was torn down.[1]

The medical unit in the Osler Building was named for Dr. William Thayer and the surgical unit in the Halsted Building was named for Dr. John Finney. At about the same time, several porches in the two buildings were enclosed, adding more beds for both medical and surgical patients, the first expansion since 1931. These new facilities replaced beds lost when the old hexagonal Thayer Building was demolished to make way for the new Children's Medical and Surgical Center.[2] This new children's structure, which opened in 1964, provided eleven stories for clinical care and research laboratories and combined the efforts of four previous pediatric entities: the Harriet Lane Home for Invalid Children, the Robert Garrett Fund for the Surgical Treatment of Children, the Hospital for Consumptives of Maryland (Eudowood Sanitarium), and the pediatric surgical section of the Johns Hopkins Hospital. It was a modern, child-friendly facility, and it provided expanded educational resources for the School of Nursing.

As part of the renovation and building program, the nursing office was relocated in early 1964 to a larger space on the second floor of the administration building; the former location on the first floor had become too small, and the new situation provided workspace for twenty-four administrative staff members. During this same period the Phipps Psychiatric Clinic was completely refurbished to accommodate new approaches and pharmacological therapies.[3]

On December 20, 1960, members of a subcommittee on long-range goals for the School of Nursing issued a report.[4] They sounded a call that would echo through the entire decade as leaders in the school raced against the clock to secure a future for nursing education at Johns Hopkins: "In summary, it may be stated in simple terms that Johns Hopkins must have a university school of nursing with a four year college course leading to a baccalaureate degree of Bachelor of Science in Nursing if this institution desires to adhere to the highest standards as it has in the past."[5] The subcommittee drew up detailed plans based on extensive research and several surveys to demonstrate both the need for the program and its potential cost. Members discussed the types of students who would be attracted to the program, outlined a proposed curriculum and faculty, and considered how federal and regional resources might be used.[6]

The need for nurses with bachelor's degrees was growing; in 1960, when it was estimated that one third of all RNs should have bachelor's

Working in the hospital was challenging. It was stimulating. At times, it was heartbreaking. The camaraderie was extraordinary. We really learned to work with physicians. In fact, physicians took us on rounds. And if you did not ask questions, you were a goner. You were expected to know so many things. You would be asked, "What would you expect the blood chemistries ordered would be? What would you expect the results would be?" It was a very rigorous experience.

The medical students had to put in medications and IVs. It was Maryland state law. The medical students time after time would say, "I don't know why I have to do this. You know much more about pharmacology." The physicians, particularly the residents, were very supportive. We learned how to work together. I remember many a time waking a resident who'd been up all night saying, "Here, have some orange juice, have some coffee, because they're going to be here for rounds in about twenty minutes and you don't want to be on this gurney."

Donna Dittberner, 1966

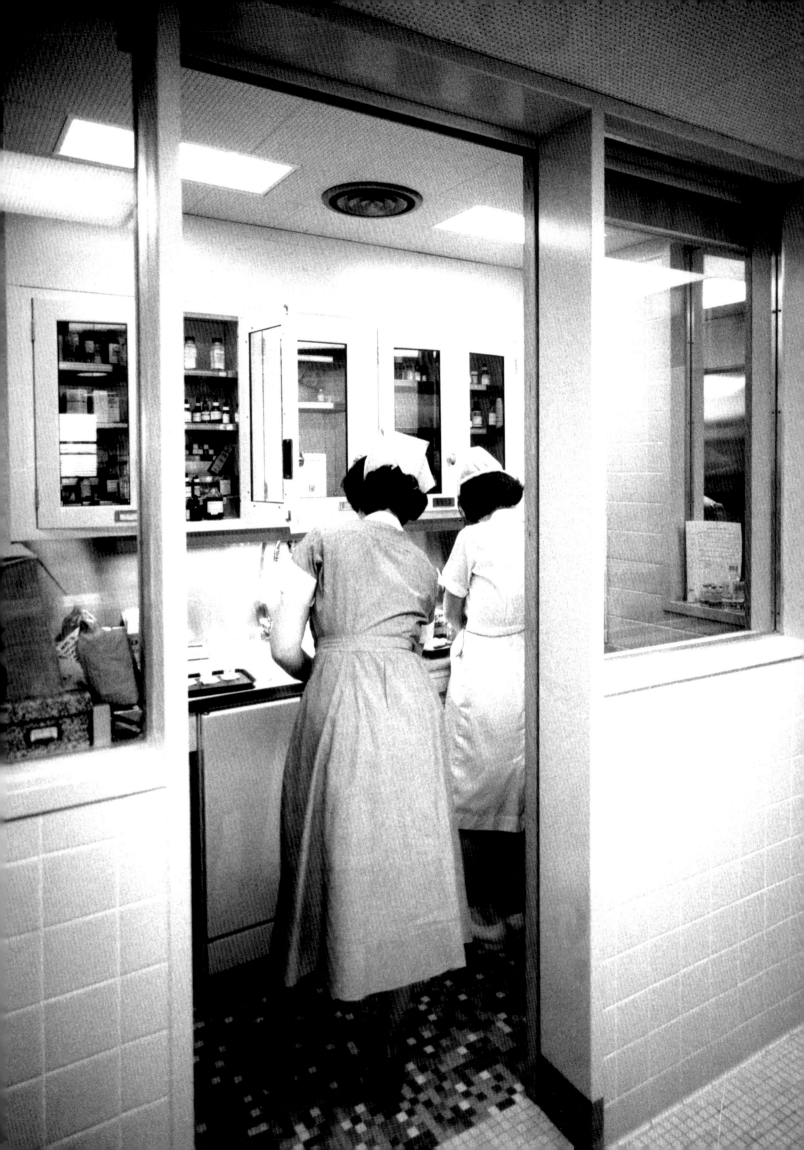

preparation, only 9 percent actually met those requirements.[7] Although there had been little progress in establishing a relationship between the School of Nursing and the university, the issues and obstacles were becoming ever more obvious, and Dr. Russell Nelson, the president of the hospital, was becoming more emphatic and articulate in communicating these issues to the parties involved.

A meeting of the advisory board in June 1960 focused on the future of the school. Issues that affected the school were reviewed from the perspective of both the hospital and the university. The concerns of nursing students and faculty were put forward as the group attempted to obtain a clearer picture of the dilemma they faced. The main obstacles, according to Dr. Nelson, were uncertainties about the financing of a university program and the opposition of individuals in the hospital and the medical school who feared that hospital services and medical school education programs would be adversely affected. Nelson noted that the same concerns had emerged in the 1940s, when Miss Wolf was beginning her campaign for a degree program, adding that the same impediments still existed in the hospital community.[8]

Milton S. Eisenhower, president of the university, was also at this meeting and shared the perspective of his constituency. In fact, "as far as he was concerned, he would be favorable to the Hopkins having a collegiate school of nursing as it has been in the Hopkins tradition to aim for excellence."[9] He warned the group, however, that there were several systemic problems that would have to be addressed:

1. At the university pressures were growing for a decreased undergraduate enrollment in order to focus more on graduate programs and research.

2. The all male tradition at the Homewood Campus creates problems when contemplating a female program such as nursing.

3. The Homewood Campus is already overcrowded and classroom space is very limited.

4. There is opposition to the proposal from the Faculty of Philosophy.

5. The question of funding will be a key obstacle in developing the school, even if the hospital continued to fund the program as it does now.[10]

In this same meeting Dean Richard Mumma, of McCoy College, Dr. Paul Lemkau, from the hospital and the School of Hygiene and Public Health, and the alumnae representative all supported the need for the new program. They cited changing trends in nursing, the difficulty of recruiting strong students, and the lack of accreditation for the current arrangement with McCoy College. Several members of the board addressed President Eisenhower's concerns about the potential nursing program, but Eisenhower apparently was not dissuaded.[11]

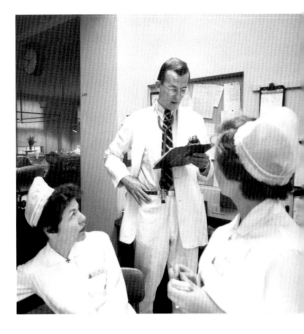

This surgical resident in October 1961 had no expectation that the alumnae working in the nursing station would vacate their seats when he entered. Hopkins students adopted the alumnae's approach, but students from affiliating schools were trained to jump when physicians entered the room.

Opposite: Soundproof medicine rooms, located on each patient floor in the new Children's Medical and Surgical Center, were an innovation welcomed by staff and patients.

So many of them wanted to come to Hopkins because it was Hopkins. Then they found out that they were just going to be an RN so they were pretty unhappy when they finished. Eventually, we were getting younger and less-qualified people because Miss Betzold would say, "You know, we don't offer a degree. When you finish, you're just an RN." The better students were going other places. We couldn't make any headway with the university.

Mary Farr Heeg, 1941

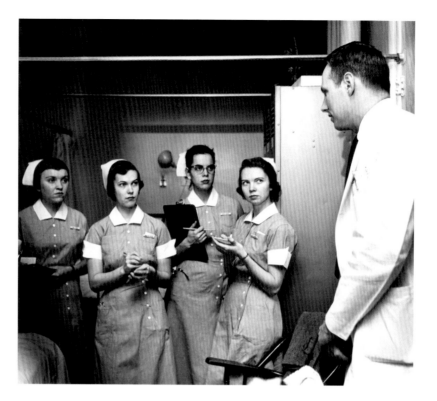

Residents in each department spent time with nursing students like these members of the class of 1960, making sure they understood the complexities of various cases.

As the result of several meetings with Dr. Nelson, alumnae, and nursing leaders, President Milton Eisenhower convened a meeting at Higgins Mill Pond on May 25 and 26, 1963, to explore the possibility of developing a bachelor's program in nursing at the university.[12] Participants included Eisenhower; Dr. Russell Nelson, representing the hospital; Doctors Philip Tumulty, Tommy Turner, Edward S. Stafford, and Barry Wood, representing the School of Medicine; Mrs. Mary Price and Dr. Margaret Courtney, representing nursing; G. Heberton Evans, dean of the Faculty of Philosophy; Richard Mumma, dean of McCoy College; and Wilson Shaffer, then dean of the Homewood Schools.

Milton Eisenhower opened the meeting by acknowledging that establishing a collegiate school of nursing had "been an issue of every president of the university since 1941."[13] Dr. Nelson gave the group a history of earlier efforts to secure collegiate education for Johns Hopkins nurses and summarized the current state of nursing education.

In the past 20 years the quality of the program has declined somewhat, especially since 1945, for several reasons. Nursing has become a complex profession. Trained "aides" have filled up the nursing ranks; there has been a decline in the average age of student nurses and the quality of candidates applying for nursing education; it is difficult to build competent staffs for there is much competition among hospitals for nurses' services. This latter fact, incidentally, is generally related to nursing education programs, for high-quality nurses are most attracted to institutions where the quality of nursing education is superior. Status and prestige are important to them, as to those in other professions. Graduates of the Johns Hopkins

Hospital School of Nursing have often expressed ... their disappointment in not being able to obtain a college degree. They say their opportunities for advancement in the field are limited by a lack of a degree.

Presently, in the three-year diploma School at Hopkins, the women admitted to the program stand high as judged by their achievement on national examinations and other factors. The School offers a distinguished program. Its curriculum is a good one and meets the minimum professional standards of a collegiate program. In other words, the School is meeting the needs of nurses rather than just fulfilling the Hospital's requirements for service to patients. The School has a good faculty, but it must be strengthened if it is to compete favorably with the leading collegiate schools of nursing.[14]

Dr. Mumma described the current relationship between the School of Nursing and McCoy College, which allowed students with sixty credit hours of college work from another institution to complete the diploma program and receive a bachelor's degree. Students could also enter the diploma program and earn the remaining hours for a bachelor's degree from the college. Mrs. Price spoke of the faculty's concern about the affiliation with McCoy College and its reluctance to have the university bestow a BSN degree on graduates of the diploma program. She did not think the relationship with McCoy College should be mentioned in the school catalog and other materials used in recruitment because students would be unable to discriminate between the Hopkins program and a generic bachelor's program in a university. Dr. Mumma expressed a similar concern that the arrangement needed to be reevaluated. The group then spent two days examining what a collegiate program in nursing might be in the Hopkins institutions. The goals of the program, the types of student and faculty that would be needed, what nursing-service problems would be created, and the potential cost of the new program were all discussed. There was general agreement "that plans could be worked out to offer necessary liberal arts courses to nursing students on the Homewood campus."[15]

Following the Higgins Mill Pond meeting, Mrs. Price and Dr. Stafford conferred with the deans of the schools of nursing at Case Western Reserve and the University of Pennsylvania about curriculum, selection of students, and sources of financial aid for collegiate students. Other financial officers at the hospital and university contacted their counterparts at those universities to project the cost of developing the program. A key stumbling block in this process remained the issue of nursing service for the hospital. While the number of actual practice hours for students was dropping, students still cared for patients every other weekend, and the hospital depended on a steady supply of new graduates coming from the large classes in the school. The proposed program could accommodate only a small number of outstanding students

Nursing students in the old diploma school benefited because we had the best teachers in the medical school also teaching us. We went on rounds every morning and we had the experience of watching the house staff and the medical students present, and we were often called upon. We were the ones who had been there all night with the patients; we were the ones who knew more about the patients' social environment or family situation.

You learned early to be prepared. You learned to answer concisely, you knew what the literature was, and you knew data. Rarely was it acceptable to say "well, I think." The expectation was that you would know. You were constantly being asked why. That's the hallmark of a Hopkins education: you're expected to know why. Why is this patient here? Why didn't this patient take their medication? You were constantly being intellectually stimulated and challenged to understand what was going on with a patient and then what you were going to do and why you were going to do it.

Martha Norton Hill, 1964, BSN 1966

I remember one doctor laughed and said, "You Hopkins nursing students are so different. You expect physicians to open doors for you. You don't immediately jump up and give them a seat." I said, "Well, not when I'm busy doing something like charting." We viewed, quite frankly, the visiting students from some of the other hospitals as acting in a very subservient way; they did everything but genuflect before physicians. Hopkins nurses are extremely proud. Some might even say, quite accurately, arrogant when it came to other nursing programs. We really did develop an ability to work with physicians that is sometimes missing in the nurses that I've seen today. They don't know how to work seriously yet collegially.

Donna Dittberner, 1966

Debate and discussion went on all those years until the university started to admit women. Those men were sitting there on the board of trustees, both at the hospital and the university, and they didn't want to have anything to do with women on the Hopkins campus. That was just a no-no. So when they had to admit women in 1971, then we had a little bit more clout.

Constance Cole Heard Waxter, 1944

When I came here for my interview at Hopkins, she said, "Do you understand that the baccalaureate education is the degree of the future and that's not what you will get?" She went through that very carefully and made sure that I really did understand. We were eighteen years old. The future was next week, not five years from now.

Sandra Stine Angell, 1969, BSN 1977

Most schools of nursing had nursing-school pins and we didn't. In order to have the pin, which we all wanted and coveted, you had to be an alumni member. Then you got your little piece of paper that said you officially could spend your money on this pin.

Lois Grayshan Hoffer, 1962

able to meet the university's admission standards, which meant that the hospital would still have to maintain a diploma program—at least in the short term—so it could not help to establish the new venture. Women on the Homewood campus and the shortage of campus housing also emerged as matters for discussion. Milton Eisenhower approached the medical school faculty, which responded positively to the idea of having a small, elite group of students who would be admitted as freshmen and go through a "unique accelerated program with a 'university' as opposed to a 'college' curriculum to complete graduate school." He decided to appoint a committee made up of physicians and nursing leaders to look at this proposal.[16]

Milton Eisenhower reported to the advisory board in early 1964 that, after the Higgins Mill meeting, a matching grant for $1,750,000 had been submitted to the Ford Foundation to provide funding to establish the new program. The grant had been denied, and because the university had no unrestricted funds, there would be no money available in the foreseeable future. Eisenhower then left the meeting, and Dr. Nelson expressed his dismay at the obstacles to developing the collegiate program. He saw no alternative at that point but to continue the diploma program.[17] One can only imagine the disappointment of those in attendance at that meeting, all their work at Higgins Mill (and in many other committees) having proved fruitless.

Numerous questions are left to ponder as to why Milton Eisenhower failed to advocate more emphatically for a professional nursing program at a university that prides itself on its pre-eminence in medical fields. Why was only one funding agency approached? What about the resources available from the 1964 nurse training act, which were aimed primarily at collegiate programs? No one doubted that the cost of establishing the program would be high—far higher than most other programs in the university. Housing needs made the issue of women at the university cultural as well as economic. Johns Hopkins had yet to welcome undergraduate women as full-time students, and even for its undergraduate men, there was limited dorm space. The bottom line for a university president had to be the financial health of the entire system.

The professional issue was more abstract but just as compelling. While the entry of nurses into higher education was well under way elsewhere in the 1960s, the scholarly productivity of nurses and other characteristics of a true professional, as viewed by the men at the Johns Hopkins University, particularly its medical school, just were not very apparent. The Hopkins institutions had little experience of new scholarly disciplines, and they viewed nursing in purely terms of practical service. While the handwriting was on the wall for the leaders at the School of Nursing, many of their counterparts in the hospital and university could not, or would not, read the message.

After meeting with the School of Nursing Advisory Board, Milton Eisenhower formally requested that Dr. Tommy Turner, dean of the School of Medicine, lead an effort to explore the possibility of establishing an elite nursing program under the direction of the medical school. Dr. Turner formed a committee to determine whether a program could be established for approximately twenty-five students who would complete both undergraduate and graduate degrees. In the fall of 1965 Dr. Nelson went to the Advisory Board of the Medical Faculty with Dr. Turner's support and stressed that "one of the strengths of the clinical departments at the founding of the hospital was the superb quality of the nursing service; the establishment of a School of Nursing at a collegiate level appears to be the best way in which an exceptionally competent nursing staff can again be developed." Concern about a nursing shortage was expressed, and Dr. Nelson explained that nurses wanted more than higher salaries; they wanted more education to improve nursing practice. The group generated several new questions about such a program but agreed in principle that "the needs for such a school may be greater than can readily be met in this locale."[18]

Little seems to have come of this proposal. The idea was not well received by the Homewood schools, and the medical faculty advisory board recommended that Goucher College be approached with the concept for an elite nursing program that would provide a AB-MS in nursing. After initial conversations, leaders at Goucher withdrew their interest in the project. The Advisory Board of the School of Nursing returned the idea to the Johns Hopkins University in the hope of establishing this special program totally within the Hopkins institutions. The plan was to admit students to the university at the beginning of their junior year; students would complete non-nursing and medical science courses at Homewood and receive a baccalaureate degree from the Faculty of Philosophy after two years and, after another two years, a master's degree from the medical faculty. The plan was not acceptable to the medical faculty, however.[19]

Years later Betty Cuthbert, a long-term, revered faculty member who was active in the alumnae association and had witnessed many of the changes that came about in the 1960s, reflected:

It's not enough to present a logical, reasonable plan that makes a plan acceptable or not. It's the politics of the situation. I think that's why Ms. Wolf never succeeded in having the school become part of the university. The real answer was money. The bottom line is money. Finances were never discussed in any of the proposals I saw. The fact that the proposals were rejected was probably a direct result of no financial plan. There were no reasoned financial arguments for the school becoming a baccalaureate program.[20]

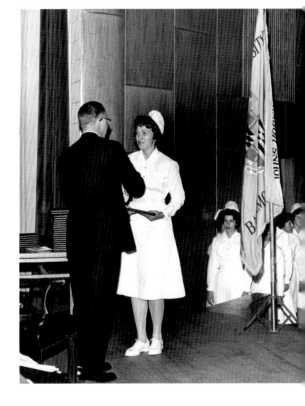

Hospital president Russell Nelson presented Jan Good with her diploma while Lois Grayshan and other members of the class of 1962 waited patiently at the bottom of the steps. The ceremony marked the first time commencement was held in the auditorium of Shriver Hall, on the Homewood campus. Jessie Black McVicar, 1939, wrote in the next alumnae magazine, "One cannot resist the temptation to dream. And to hope that very soon the School of Nursing will become an integral part of the University."

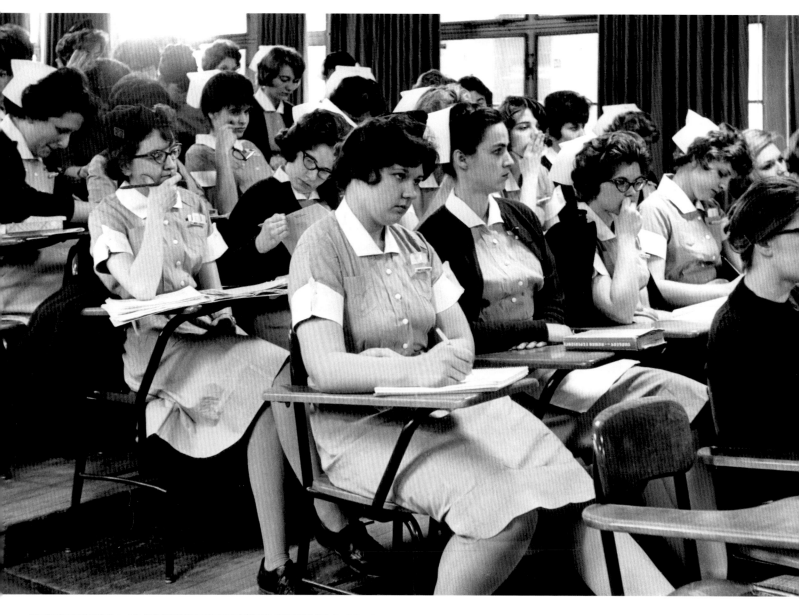

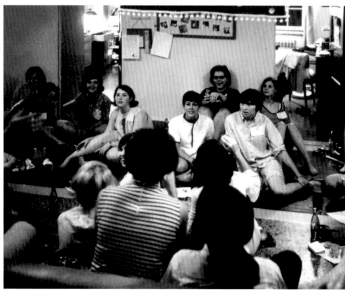

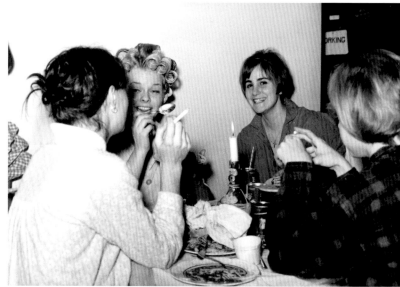

The American Nurses Association (ANA) brought the issue of nursing education to the forefront in late 1965 when it issued a position paper that had a profound impact on diploma programs. The group recognized the changing economic pressures on hospitals and the need for nurses to meet the professional standards typical of other service professions such as social work and teaching. The position paper called for the education of professional nurses in baccalaureate programs in colleges and universities, while technical nurses should be educated in associate, two-year programs in community colleges.[21] This plan left diploma programs out of the professional scheme for education. While the majority of nurses were still coming from diploma programs, this forward-looking view of how things would be in the future created strong reactions among nurses.

The Alumnae Association of the Johns Hopkins Hospital School of Nursing published the position paper in its alumnae magazine.[22] Frances Reiter, 1931, who served on the committee that prepared the ANA's paper, wrote a provocative article discussing the paper's significance. She emphasized the need for Johns Hopkins to change quickly and reminded alumnae that Dr. Richard Cabot had recommended a broad liberal arts and sciences education for nurses in 1901. The position paper, Reiter noted, was a sign of a trend that was picking up speed and transforming nursing education: nurses of the future would be college or university educated. She also pointed out how social work, medicine, and other helping arts had matured within the system of higher education, while nurses continued to be educated using turn-of-the-century methods. And she recognized the dichotomy in the profession in the 1960s: nurses wanted more recognition and reward for professional practice, yet they had strong feelings about the significance of hospital-based clinical experiences.[23]

Students enrolled in the Johns Hopkins program knew that college degrees were desirable and worthwhile—as demonstrated by many of the faculty at Hopkins—and the position paper made an immediate impression on them. The halls of Hampton House were filled with informal discussions about the impact this would have on graduates in the near future. There was also considerable discussion among the faculty and leaders of the school. Mrs. Price brought the position paper to the advisory board. For many students and faculty, this statement from the largest nursing organization articulated what many had quietly wondered about. It was a difficult issue for students and faculty because there was no doubt that the educational opportunities at the Johns Hopkins Hospital and its related agencies were outstanding, and the students excelled at what they did. Yet the idea that a Hopkins nurse might not be considered a professional was hard to accept.

As the clock ticked on the nursing program, another proposal was developed in 1967 under the leadership of Dr. Russell Morgan. President

Marty Hill was very, very bright as a student. She was an aggressive student. She was very highly thought of by faculty because she was one of these "go through anything, get through anything" people, yet very gentle with patients.
Donna Dittberner, 1966

Dr. Mary Betty Stevens was a physician who gave the type of lecture where you sat on the edge of your seat because she was so fascinating. Her subject area was connective tissue disease so she talked about lupus and arthritis. She probably could have talked about the weather and she would have been interesting. She was really dynamic.
Sandra Stine Angell, 1969, BSN 1977

Opposite, above: Little did she or her classmates realize when they attended class during their final year in 1964, that Martha Norton (far right, with an empty desk beside her) would one day be the first alumna dean of the Johns Hopkins University School of Nursing.

Opposite, below: Students during the late 1960s held monthly corridor meetings to discuss issues facing Hampton House residents, including the problems they might face when they graduated without a baccalaureate degree. Concerns were not always serious, however. In 1967 one student found time to curl her hair and share a candlelight supper with pajama-clad friends.

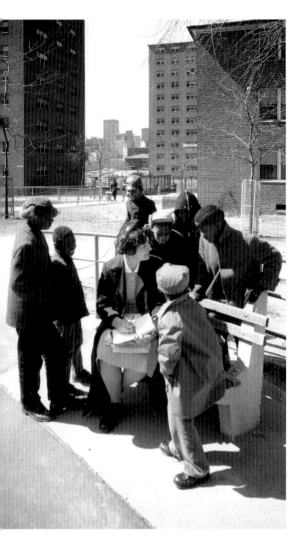

Children in nearby housing projects knew Carolyn Griggs, 1964, as one of many nursing students who provided health care services in their homes. For years students fanned out over the Eastern Health District, a one-square-mile area near Johns Hopkins Hospital. The district was established in 1932 to conduct research on living conditions, general health, and diseases in the neighborhood, especially tuberculosis and diphtheria.

Milton Eisenhower had appointed Morgan chair of a special Committee on Allied Medical Professions, to study the possibility of developing a school for allied health professions on the East Baltimore campus adjacent to the hospital. The committee believed that federal and private funding might be available for programs to provide bachelor's and graduate degrees in newly developing professional fields—in addition to nursing. This idea called for a separate school along the lines of the School of Public Health, which might have departments for nursing, radiology, medical technology, and other allied fields.[24]

Nursing alumnae, including current and former deans of several collegiate programs, expressed concerns about clustering nursing with other programs. There were no other options being considered at Johns Hopkins, however, so this program became the first real attempt to put together a baccalaureate school that included nursing that might receive major funding. This approach would have a major impact on what would happen to nursing education at Johns Hopkins in the 1970s.

The Advisory Board of the School of Medicine and the medical board of the hospital approved the Morgan committee's proposal in principle, but correspondence among alumnae leaders indicated grave concern about the design and the vagueness of the proposal. The retirement of President Milton Eisenhower in June 1967 further complicated the process, and for a time little was done with the committee's ideas. The new president of the university, Dr. Lincoln Gordon, appointed a different committee to fashion a division of allied health education at Johns Hopkins. This new committee consisted of members from the university and its medical school, the hospital staff, and nurses Mary Price and Dr. Ruth Freeman, a faculty member in the School of Hygiene and Public Health.[25]

In the meantime, a task force headed by Dr. John P. Young completed a feasibility study for the proposed "College of Health Sciences," which would be eligible for federal grants supporting allied health professions. After working with various faculty groups and advisory boards related to the School of Medicine, the School of Hygiene and Public Health, and the university administration, Young's group brought a formal proposal to President Gordon. In September 1969 Gordon called a joint meeting of the East Baltimore advisory boards and that of the Faculty of Arts and Sciences.[26] The combined group reviewed the proposed program for "allied health sciences" and agreed to continue to explore options for developing the program since there was no source of funding at that time.[27]

The 1969 proposal included "no separate nursing program or department."[28] Instead, nursing would be assigned to each corresponding specialty in the medical and public-health curricula. This meant that the medical faculty would oversee nursing education in medicine and surgery, and nursing students would experience the public-health portion of the curriculum in the School of Hygiene and Public Health.

Clearly, there had been no nurses on the feasibility committee. The nurses present at the meeting rejected the proposal, pointing out the futility of a plan that disregarded current standards in nursing education. The group agreed to include nurses on the committee in the future.

In October President Gordon spoke to the alumnae association about consultations with Goucher College, which was willing to consider providing the first two years of a nursing program that would be completed at the East Baltimore campus. He cited the changing roles of doctors and nurses and pressure to find innovative ways to produce a practitioner to meet the future needs of society.[29] His presentation was reported in the alumnae magazine: "In the tentative outline of the program, Dr. Gordon said an important share of the academic program should be distributed among professors of the various departments. There is a combined policy group working on an evaluation. The chairman of this group is the provost of Johns Hopkins University. . . . As in the past, Dr. Gordon feels money is a big problem. The Medical School has a deficit of over a million dollars this year." In conclusion, Gordon listed the major points included in the memorandum prepared for the joint meeting of the advisory boards:

1. Any Johns Hopkins program should be designed for students of high quality and directed toward the preparation of leadership groups (whether practitioners or teachers) in new professional categories.

2. The major thrust should be toward innovation in both training programs and the ultimate professional activities of those trained.

3. Market uncertainties make it unwise to begin the program with the establishment of a separate new school of the University, with all the financial and institutional commitments which such an action would imply.

4. It would be undesirable to create two separate Johns Hopkins undergraduate bodies.

5. New Johns Hopkins programs in allied health fields should be closely interlinked with the revised MD curriculum, with masters and doctoral programs in the School of Hygiene and Public Health and postdoctoral programs in the School of Medicine, and with pertinent undergraduate, post graduate and post doctoral programs in the Faculty of Arts and Sciences.[30]

No doubt his audience noted that in his presentation, Dr. Gordon included reassurance that Dr. Courtney, Mrs. Price, and Dr. Freeman would be involved in planning the program along with the School of Nursing's Advisory Board. He spoke of possible funding sources, but the rest of the plan remained vague.

Margaret Courtney was Miss Betzold's assistant and responsible for the school. Dr. Courtney had more to do with the faculty. She was the person who came and sat in on my classes and did an annual evaluation. She had more to do in the day-to-day operation in terms of the curriculum and where the students were and what they were doing.

Stella Shiber

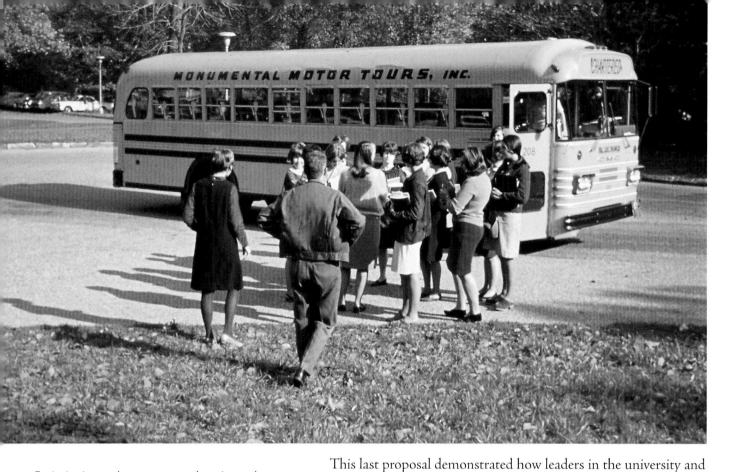

Beginning in 1965, buses transported nursing students from East Baltimore to the Homewood campus, so that first-year students could take courses in science and liberal arts, for which they would receive college credit.

We were the first class actually bused over to the Homewood campus and we took classes there. We took them separately. They certainly didn't want to mix us with any of the men. We took an English course, we took introductory sociology, and I think introductory psychology—fifteen credits' worth of courses during the first year.

Sandra Stine Angell, 1969, BSN 1977

This last proposal demonstrated how leaders in the university and medical communities were struggling with the direction of medical and nursing education in the late 1960s, a period that saw a strong movement toward primary care and the expansion of new health professionals to meet society's needs. Traditional roles related to nursing seemed to be unimportant to the planners. The conclusions of the group that had met earlier in the fall of 1969 reflected the struggles to decide who would do what and how all practitioners would work together in a system that had limited resources. Medicare and Medicaid were less than five years old. These new funding sources were placing a great strain on the health care delivery system, and adjustments had yet to be made to facilitate all the health care professionals who were suddenly needed. At the same time, the costs of both Medicare and Medicaid were exceeding all expectations, so the delivery system was confronted with the dual challenge of providing more and more services at a lower price. This pattern would persist for years. Nurses in the Hopkins community and elsewhere were entering a difficult period as the 1960s closed.

While proposals came and went within the Hopkins institutions, adjustments in the national environment began to take their toll on enrollment in the nursing program. By early 1968 the advisory board was faced with a 20 percent annual decrease in applications for admissions since 1965, and the incoming classes were predicted to be half the size of those admitted in 1960–64. The board looked at all the factors that might have contributed to this drop, including costs and attrition, and concluded that the school could not lower admission standards but would need greater flexibility in admitting borderline students with strong potential. Beginning in 1965, first-year nursing students were bused to Homewood to take arts and sciences classes. There was a feeling among the board members that the hospital would prefer smaller classes of strong candidates to larger classes with students who could not be successful in courses on the Homewood campus and in the nursing curriculum.[31] School administrators and the advisory board agreed to maintain standards in order to support the rigorous curriculum initiated in 1966.

Donna Dittberner, 1966, observed all these forces firsthand. Her class started with 132 students, but only 64 graduated. "It was academically very challenging," she acknowledged. "There were many times that I thought that it would be quite enjoyable to fly for an airline as a flight attendant. That first year was really a struggle in terms of all the new experiences and to me, at times at that age, silly expectations. 'Why do I have to do this?' But I learned to understand and to come to grips. It was a very rapid transition into an adult world. You had to decide whether you were going to sink or whether you were going to swim."[32]

Dittberner came to appreciate the reasoning behind the Hopkins method. "We used to laugh and say that the purpose was to teach us our proper humility. I really don't think that anymore," she said. "I think that the adherence to structure was to teach us to be able to look at a broad picture and see all the specifics and to have a certain grounding, so that later on, when we were making more independent decisions, we would have that structure on which to base them."[33]

By the time someone was a senior student nurse, they knew a whole lot about the operation of the unit and also about many aspects of patient care. When you were charge nurse, you worked alone. If you had an orderly or an aide with you, you were lucky. There would be thirty patients, and this was before intensive care units. Many of those patients were not as acutely ill as the ones we have in the hospital today. But you'd have some very ill patients who needed a lot of attention. The standard of medical practice was extremely high and the standard of nursing practice was very high, and they were totally interdependent.

Martha Norton Hill, 1964, BSN 1966

Below left: Rev. Clyde Shallenberger became chaplain of the hospital in 1963 and a spiritual mentor for many students. He often officiated at events relating to the school, including commencement in 1967. In appreciation for his various contributions, he was named an honorary member of the alumni association.

Photographers for the 1967 *Dome* demonstrated their posing techniques in their official portrait. Publication of the new incarnation of the student yearbook began in 1958, twenty-six years after the last issue of the *Routine*.

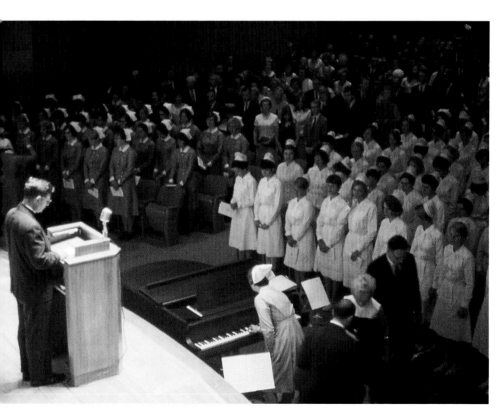

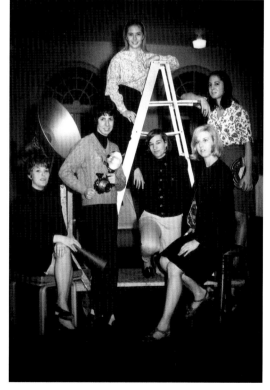

The person who pretty much took care of the school of nursing was Miss K. Virginia Betzold who was Mrs. Price's assistant. Miss Betzold was very precise, very sure about how things should be. She was a strong lady. People paid close attention to what Miss Betzold had to say. They were careful, as much as possible, to follow through.

Stella Shiber

An underground tunnel linking Hampton House and the Marburg Building was part of the initial design, and it came in handy on cold and rainy days. Here, Reverend Shallenberger, Mrs. Price, and Dr. Russell Nelson waited for the elevator in 1967 with four students.

For Director Mary Price and her associate directors, Miss K. Virginia Betzold and Dr. Margaret Courtney, as well as the rest of the faculty, this was a period of mixed blessings. The numbers of students entering climbed quickly as the 1950s came to a close. By the end of 1961, recruiter Dr. Laila Skinner reported that one of the largest classes in the history of the school would enter as the class of 1964.[34] Yet the reality of these mostly younger students with only high school diplomas weighed on the nursing school's leadership and faculty. The Johns Hopkins Hospital School of Nursing was not attracting the more educated students who had come in the past, but the continuing achievements of its students and the excellence of its graduates made it difficult for the school's administrators to convince the university and hospital leadership that the program was in serious trouble. Ironically, the success of the faculty and the arrival of the baby boomers seemed to limit the likelihood of change. Lena Van Horn, 1933, who attended the National League for Nursing's convention in 1961, reported that diploma programs would be under increasing pressure as the number of BSNs and LPNs (licensed practical nurses) climbed—as she predicated it would do, dramatically—in the 1960s.[35]

Mrs. Price worked closely with Dr. Russell Nelson throughout her tenure, seeking to move the school from diploma to university status. Dr. Nelson remained a staunch friend of nursing, working with both the nursing leaders at the hospital and with the alumnae association to move nursing into the sphere of the university. At the hospital, his role and responsibilities were broad and multifaceted. When Dr. Nelson was promoted to president and chief operating officer of the hospital in 1962—after ten years of noteworthy service as director—his roles and responsibilities increased again. He was expected to oversee "future

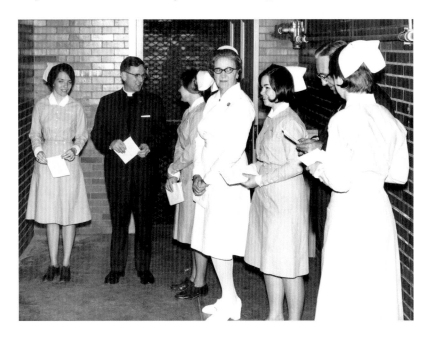

planning of the Johns Hopkins Hospital, including the rebuilding of its facilities; the coordination and development of educational and research activities of the School of Medicine and the School of Hygiene and Public Health as they relate to the hospital; the problems of financing the operation of the Hospital; and, lastly, community relations on a local, state, and national level."[36] With such a broad mandate, which demanded effort and interest in so many directions, it is a tribute to the value of nursing education at Hopkins that Dr. Nelson devoted so many hours and committee meetings to solving this perplexing dilemma. One wonders what role his wife, Ruth Jeffcoat Nelson, 1937, played in this loyalty.

In 1963 Rev. Clyde Shallenberger joined the staff of the hospital as chaplain, replacing Mrs. Price's husband, Rev. Harry Price, the hospital's first appointed chaplain. Rev. Shallenberger came to the hospital with extensive training in pastoral care and counseling. He became pastor to patients, students, and staff. His brief Sunday morning services were popular with many in the hospital community and he provided an enduring presence throughout the tumultuous thirty years he served in this capacity. Chaplain Shallenberger, a pioneer member and leader of the American College of Chaplains, wrote frequently on issues related to the spiritual care of people who faced emergencies and difficult situations. At the close of his career he reflected, "While my responsibilities have been many and varied, there is nothing more satisfying than the privilege of being available to people when they are in the midst of a life crisis, and supporting them and journeying with them through that crisis."[37] Chaplain Shallenberger accompanied many on their journeys and he made an impact on many lives with his presence. He received recognition of his service to generations of students and faculty at the School of Nursing when he was named an honorary member of the alumni association.

As a result of several retirements among her staff, Mrs. Price developed a new leadership team in the 1960s. Miss Betzold retired in 1965, and Dr. Courtney took her place as associate director of the school. A quiet and unassuming person, K. Virginia Betzold was also a stalwart, loyal worker who devoted her life to the school. She worked cooperatively with three very different directors and taught students with precision and compassion. She also counseled many nurses, encouraging them to continue their education and offering them positions after they completed their collegiate work. She traveled frequently to attend meetings and contributed considerable effort to professional nursing organizations. In the closing days of her more than thirty-year career, Miss Betzold wrote a retrospective article for the alumnae magazine chronicling the dream she held dear of a collegiate program for nurses at Hopkins.[38]

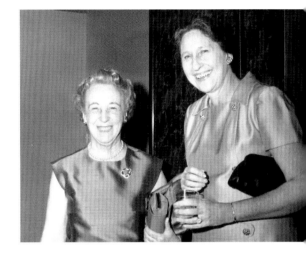

Jessie Black McVicar, 1930 (left), played a prominent role in the alumnae association for many years. Margaret Courtney, 1940 (right), became associate director of the school in 1965, and when Mrs. Price retired in 1970, Dr. Courtney became the final director of the diploma school. "Margaret Courtney was a remarkable woman," remembered Martha Norton Hill, 1964, who was Courtney's student, then her colleague. "She had a tremendous intellect, and was a person of enormous intelligence and integrity and a very funny, outspoken personality. She was a very good mentor and colleague."

Margaret Courtney was the assistant director of the School of Nursing. She and I had conversations over nursing fundamentals, which I found to be exquisitely boring, and my grades reflected that. I remember when she hired me. I was invited to join the faculty in psychiatry. The first day on the job I said, "Hello, I'm Donna Dittberner." And she said, "Well, of course you are." Very dry humor. Terrified us all when we were students. I found when I was on the faculty that she was really a warm, caring, very funny, funny lady.

Donna Dittberner, 1966

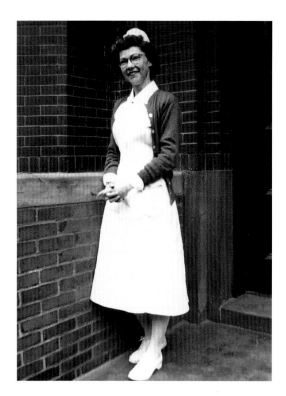

Betty Liggett Cuthbert, 1943, taught psychiatric nursing in the Phipps Clinic. Over the years she became a giant within the alumni association, where she protected not only its historical collections but also the Adelaide Nutting Endowment Fund.

Betty Cuthbert could say "oh" more ways than any human being I have ever met. She'd "Oh?" "oh!" and "oh." We used to laugh about that. She was the school historian from the World War II era. She had been allowed to be married, which was unusual, because he was going off to war. He was a pilot and he didn't make it back. Betty I remember very, very well.

Donna Dittberner, 1966

My first clinic was Halsted, which was surgery, which is still the area I like the best. Sarah Allison was a Halsted instructor. She made you feel comfortable about what you were doing. I always thought very, very highly of her.

Lois Grayshan Hoffer, 1962

Dr. Sarah E. Allison, 1953 (wearing a white lab coat), made a proposal in 1967 to create what would become the Center for Experimentation and Development in Nursing, which analyzed nursing personnel functions.

Margaret Courtney worked at the Johns Hopkins Hospital after her graduation in 1940. She earned her BSN from the Johns Hopkins University through McCoy College's evening program, then secured her doctorate in education from Hopkins in the late 1950s, with the assistance of a scholarship from the hospital trustees. Dr. Courtney had a personality that stimulated strong feelings among students and faculty. Many remembered that she was quite tall and always wore professional suits. Some former students had fond memories of her dry sense of humor while others remembered how difficult she could be in classes and clinical situations. She was an individual with strong beliefs and a quick temper, which could stun students and peers. Some of her former students described being somewhat intimidated by her forceful manner of addressing them in class. Over the years, Margaret Courtney held numerous teaching and leadership positions at the school. She would play a unique role in the school in the 1970s, but her transition to full-time administrator began in the '60s.

In her new role as associate director for the school, Dr. Courtney introduced the History, Trends, and Professional Adjustment course to the third-year curriculum. Students gained a new view of her in this class. She was much more relaxed and informal when teaching seniors than she had been addressing them as freshmen in her psychology classes. She also became an advocate for students. When students requested that they be allowed to wear slacks to the cafeteria when off duty, Courtney responded positively and then suggested that the issue of shorts also needed to be addressed since summers in Baltimore were so hot. While students did not get permission to wear shorts in the hospital, a new cafeteria in Reed Hall was made available to nursing students and shorts were permitted there. Until this time students had been required to wear their uniforms or a dress and hose to meals, even when off duty.

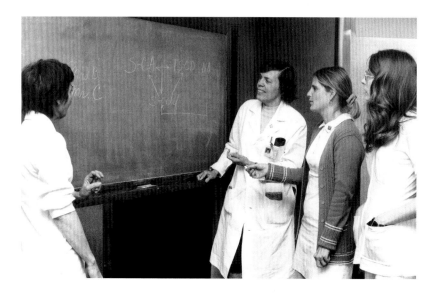

One colleague remembered Dr. Courtney's compassion and sensitivity when a family had to cope with a major crisis related to a student. Although she had initially been reluctant to intervene because of her concern for the needs of the family, Courtney was able to reach out and help the family with skill and competence.[39] Another person who knew Margaret Courtney well described her as someone who could be democratic in her approach to faculty while autocratic about key principles of education. She was a woman of integrity, with unswerving loyalty to Johns Hopkins, who was often frustrated by the rigidity of prevailing standards for nursing education.[40]

The students in this period benefited from an experienced, competent, and caring faculty. Yearbooks regularly featured several faculty members as role models and favorites of the students. Betty Liggett Cuthbert, 1943, who lost her husband during World War II while she was still a student, made her career at Johns Hopkins. Mrs. Cuthbert was a psychiatric nurse who taught freshman. She was known for her low-keyed, often humorous lectures. Mary Farr, 1941, and Esther Jacoby, 1930, served with Mrs. Price in World War II, then returned to their faculty positions at Hopkins. Miss Jacoby directed the nursing service in the outpatient department and taught students there. She was also well known for recounting to students the details of Mary Price's wedding day during the war. Miss Farr was famous for her supervision in the Osler units and her strict concern for the oral hygiene of all patients. She surprised everyone—and stimulated the romantic imaginations of students—in the late 1960s when she and Betty Cuthbert went on a cruise and Miss Farr met her future husband, Tom Heeg. Miss Farr was so concerned about hygiene and cleanliness for her patients that she asked her fiancé to purchase diamond studs for the sleeves of her Hopkins uniform instead of an engagement ring. A wedding shower given by the students was a highlight of that school year. Although Miss Farr became Mrs. Heeg and moved to Maine, she returned to Baltimore for alumni events and meetings virtually every year after her marriage.

Two popular long-term faculty members who were not alumnae were Mary Jane Donough and Ella Rowe. Miss Donough came to Hopkins after World War II and taught continually, except for a short leave to complete her master's degree. Miss Rowe was a Union Memorial graduate who dedicated most of her professional career to teaching Hopkins students in gynecology. Miss Rowe and Miss Donough were honored for their long service to the school and its students with honorary membership in the alumni association.

Sarah E. Allison, 1953, was another Hopkins graduate who not only taught in the school but also brought innovation and growth to nursing clinical practice. After Allison completed her diploma, her goal was

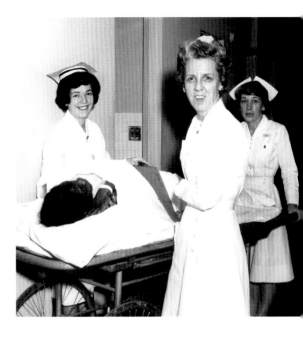

When she returned from a cruise with a serious beau, Mary Farr, 1941 (center), stunned her colleagues and students. After she married and moved to Maine, she remained a faithful participant in many alumni activities.

Mary Jane Donough was not a Hopkins grad. She might have been everybody's stereotype of the perfect head nurse and instructor. She was never caught off guard, never ruffled, never unpoised. She was always a lady and always very appropriate. It was tough to rattle her. She was very well centered in her outlook on things and in her own personal competence. She was an excellent listener, which I found quite a few of the faculty members were. Mary Jane in particular was very objective in her ability to listen to what was being said and to make suggestions. Sometimes she just listened, really didn't actually tell you what to do, but based on her assessment of what you said, you could kind of figure it out. She spent a lot of her career at Hopkins and had an understanding of how it worked and an appreciation of the values of the institution that I think she really carried across without being overbearing or harsh in any way.

Cathy Novak, 1973

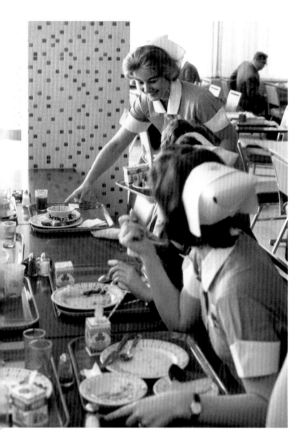

Timing for the opening of the new hospital cafeteria gave Harriet Taylor, 1964, and her friends the opportunity to share a few meals there before they graduated. Nursing and medical students shared the facility with hospital staff and visitors; many doctors preferred the private dining room nearby, which was for their exclusive use.

In the tunnel somewhere there was this little place that was open at night from like nine to ten where you could get sandwiches. Often a couple of us would make a run over there. We were not allowed in the hospital with pants on or shorts. Whatever we had on we would roll up underneath our trenchcoats and make a run over there at night for enough stuff to make sandwiches for a bunch of us. I can remember one year at exams in December going up to the White Castle, which was on the corner of Washington and Monument. They were having an anniversary special and we would bring shopping bags full of those little hamburgers back, just shopping bags full.

Lois Grayshan Hoffer, 1962

to become an educator and a researcher. With the help of a scholarship from the trustees of the hospital, she completed her doctorate at Teachers College at Columbia. After Dr. Allison joined the faculty, Mrs. Price encouraged her to submit a proposal to her and Dr. Nelson to "promote the development and improvement of nursing practice by helping nurses to provide better care to patients and to help make nursing a more satisfying and rewarding career."[41] When this proposal was accepted, in March 1968, the Center for Nursing began pioneering efforts to encourage and develop excellence in clinical practice using the finest educational and research resources.

Outside consultants were invited to participate in shaping the ultimate purpose of the new program. Dr. Allison pulled together a "think tank" of experts from the 1960s, including Dorothea Orem, then associate professor of nursing at Catholic University; Joan Backscheider, assistant professor of psychiatric and mental health nursing at Yale University; Mary B. Collins, associate director of the Mercy School of Nursing in Hamilton, Ohio; Ann Poorman Donovan, a hospital administration consultant from the Indiana State Board of Health; and M. Lucille Kinlein, assistant professor of cardiovascular nursing at Catholic University. This group worked to develop the purpose, organizational structure, and focal areas for research. Once designed, the center became the third unit in the nursing department at the hospital, and Dr. Russell Nelson supported the unit with hospital resources. Dr. Allison became the first associate director of nursing in charge of the Center for Experimentation and Development in Nursing.[42]

This effort was an attempt by nursing leaders at the hospital to assure progress in nursing research and innovation even if there was no university school to undergird those activities. This highly innovative program was designed to encourage creativity and theoretically sound practice among Hopkins graduates practicing in the hospital. The center had two main goals: to develop clinical research, which could then be applied at the bedside; and to assist nurses in practice with consultations and support in solving complex clinical problems. Dorothea D. Orem's model of nursing practice was used as a framework for the center. In the first year of operation, two of the consultants, Joan Backscheider and Mary Collins, were hired to assist Dr. Allison in carrying out the goals of the center. The first area targeted was Osler Medical Clinic. These three nurses worked on the development of the Diabetic Nurse Management Clinic and introduced interventions now considered standard in that field. Within the next few years, successful programs were launched in a nurse-managed cardiac clinic and a comprehensive childcare clinic. This work established Dr. Allison as an internationally recognized Orem Scholar, and she continues to contribute to this approach to solving nursing problems.

For the first two thirds of the decade the nursing program experienced robust enrollments. In 1960 Dr. Skinner, the recruitment director, reported that the incoming class of 1963 had an age range of seventeen to twenty-two and that twenty-six states and two foreign countries were represented. She noted the continuing trend for freshmen:

	1950	1954	1959	1960
High school only	15.3%	59.8%	71.7%	81%
2 years college	52.5%	31.3%	18.9%	15.1%[43]

The number of students with two years of college had dropped so much in the 1950s, that by early 1960, the advisory board accepted Mrs. Price's recommendation that the thirty-two-month option be discontinued, leaving just one curriculum in the nursing program.[44] The high attrition rate was another problem that plagued the student body throughout the decade. A 1962 report described the major reasons students left: dissatisfaction with Johns Hopkins as an institution or with the nursing program, inability to succeed in the program, or marriage.[45]

All students admitted in this era were told during their interviews or in correspondence that the program would not lead them directly to a degree in nursing, yet they selected Hopkins because of its excellent reputation. The performance of the students on licensing exams,[46] the large number who went on to complete bachelor's and advanced degrees, and the career stories of many of the graduates from the 1960s all attest to the quality of their Hopkins education. The leaders and faculty, who wanted something better for the students, still succeeded in giving these novices a sound beginning for fruitful, successful careers. "We were told that we were being trained to be good bedside nurses. I don't think we

They were very, very, very good to us. I always had the feeling that if you made it into the school, they would do anything they could to keep you there. Not that they didn't read you the riot act, because they did. One of the assistant superintendents of nurses, her job was to go through the newspaper every day to see if marriage licenses had been issued to students or if they might be found doing something else in town. Virginia Betzold was the disciplinarian. I'm sure she did other things too but we were told that that was one of her jobs.

Lois Grayshan Hoffer, 1962

Below left: In practice clinics, mannequins were used so that students could learn to work together to move patients safely, both for the patient and for themselves.

Shelagh Hickey and Jean Brinkley, both in the class of 1969, wore scrub dresses as they worked at the desk in a nursing station in 1967. The other students there wore everyday blue uniforms.

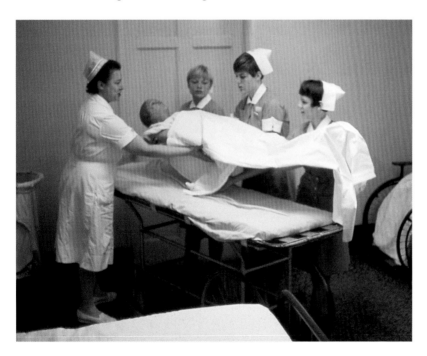

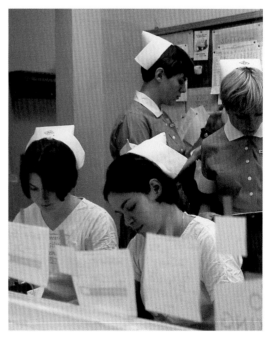

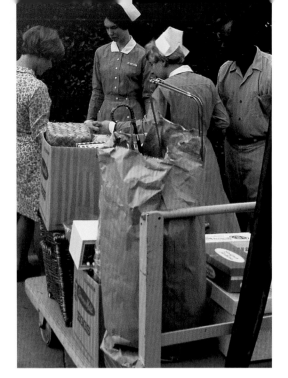

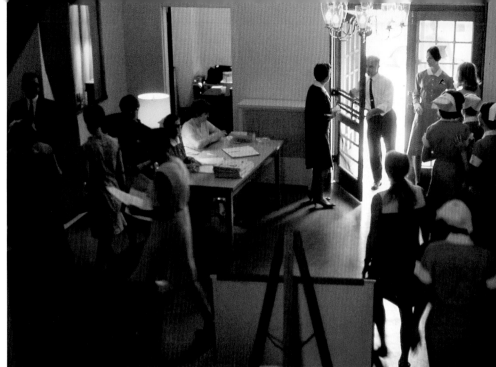

Moving-in day was always a big event at Hampton House. When members of the class of 1970 arrived on their first day, Big Sisters greeted them at the door and helped transport their belongings upstairs. During the first year, Big Sisters kept an eye on them, and when it was time for the candlelight ceremony, each Big Sister taught her Little Sister how to starch her cap and placed the cap on her Little Sister's head for the first time.

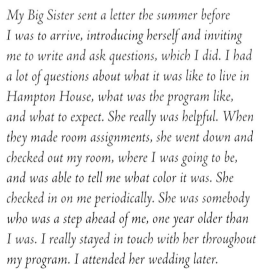

My Big Sister sent a letter the summer before I was to arrive, introducing herself and inviting me to write and ask questions, which I did. I had a lot of questions about what it was like to live in Hampton House, what was the program like, and what to expect. She really was helpful. When they made room assignments, she went down and checked out my room, where I was going to be, and was able to tell me what color it was. She checked in on me periodically. She was somebody who was a step ahead of me, one year older than I was. I really stayed in touch with her throughout my program. I attended her wedding later.

Sandra Stine Angell, 1969, BSN 1977

really were," Donna Dittberner opined. "We were much more trained to be problem solvers, priority setters, educators, and managers."[47]

In an attempt to update the program and meet the needs of the changing population of students, a committee was organized in 1964 to examine the nursing curriculum. In 1966 the Maryland State Board of Examiners of Nurses and the advisory board approved the proposed curriculum, which brought sweeping modifications to the program and increased theoretical education. The length of the program was cut from thirty-six to thirty-two months. The preclinical period was expanded to allow for strengthening fundamental courses. English, psychology, and sociology were taught on the Homewood campus, although classes for nursing students were taught separately. "They certainly didn't want to mix us with any of the men," Sandra Stine Angell, 1969, recalled.[48] Many courses were combined, such as medical and surgical nursing, and public-health and outpatient nursing. This transformation was designed to streamline the program and produce a graduate for the 1970s. There were misgivings about the new plan, which eliminated experiences such as scrubbing in the operating room, but the time had come for change.[49]

Student life in the school adjusted to the times, yet traditions remained a significant part of the students' calendars. Martha Norton Hill, 1964, remembered that she and her classmates regularly attended mixers at Homewood or Loyola. "There definitely were some social mores around medical students and nursing students dating." She noted that "medical students were older and they were all college graduates. Some of my classmates preferred to date people their own age, who were still in college." And there were still restrictions. Life in Hampton House "was a combination of entering a quasi-religious, quasi-military, quasi-college dorm environment. I was coming straight from high school. There were rules and there were curfews. There were very clear

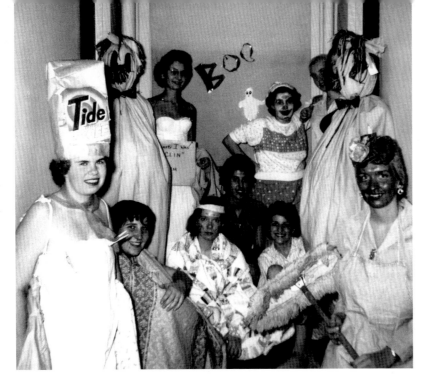

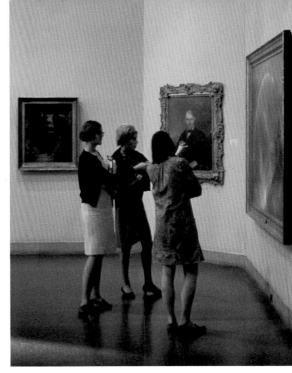

Students were encouraged to take advantage of cultural activities in Baltimore. Martha Norton Hill, 1964, remembered that free concert tickets were often posted in Hampton House or Reed Hall. Here students in 1967 visited the galleries of the Baltimore Museum of Art.

Above left: Silliness ruled on Halloween night in 1960, when students created costumes from whatever they could find in Hampton House. No one chose to disguise herself as a nurse.

Left: Nine hospitals in the Baltimore area had nursing schools in the 1960s, enough to create a competitive basketball league. Some athletes played on the team while others, like these students in 1966, preferred to join the cheerleading squad.

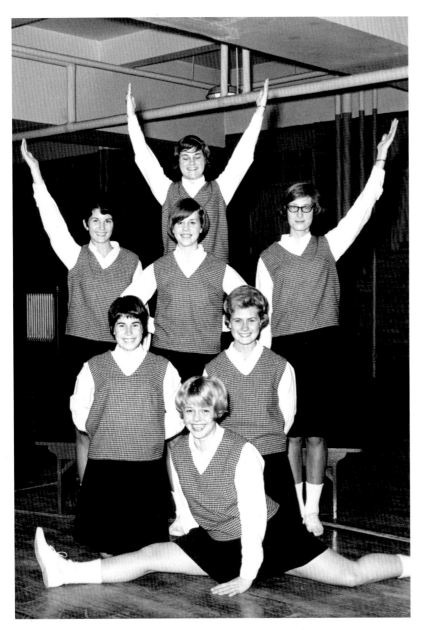

A lot of nursing students started dating medical students and some dated interns. A lot of nursing students dated folks at Homewood. Then a significant number also dated guys down at the Naval Academy. And they would bus us down to the foot of Broadway to Fells Point when the British ships came in and we would hang out with the British sailors. Occasionally they'd bus us out to Goucher, where they'd have mixers with Hopkins and Goucher and us. That was where we had our socializing.

Sue Appling, 1973

expectations in regard to how you dressed, how you would behave, so that the reputation of the school and the university and of yourself would be protected."[50]

One popular feature from the 1950s that continued into the 1960s was the school's basketball team, which competed with other nursing schools in the city. The team also played an annual face-off against the faculty, with each game highly contested for bragging rights for the following year. In 1963 the students defeated the faculty by one point and a fractured ankle.[51] The highlight of the game was the half-time show, put on by faculty cheerleaders who were dressed in army attire and led by Margaret Courtney. The crowd cheered wildly during the performance, which featured a stunning ballet, as Miss Farr's fox terrier stole the show.[52]

Changes in society had a profound impact on the culture of Hampton House residents. The birth control pill became available, and with the coming of the Vietnam War, marriages before the end of school became more common. Marriage for students was still discouraged, but admission of married students began in 1964, with Mildred Rogers and Erika Glaser, both of whom successfully completed the program. The Vietnam War and developments in the civil rights movement were constantly in the background as the 1960s advanced. Students watched the city of Baltimore erupt after the assassination of Martin Luther King Jr. on April 6, 1968. National Guardsmen became sentries on the roof of Hampton House and for a time, regular activities were suspended. Sandy Angell remembered that it was an exciting time. "I guess when you're nineteen, you're less concerned about your personal safety than perhaps you should be. We certainly didn't try to get through any barricades to go where we weren't supposed to be." Instead, she said, students watched from windows high in Hampton House as fires burned in several businesses along Monument Street. "I was very naïve about the anger and, certainly before I came to Baltimore, very naïve about any of that. It was a time of great

Pointing her camera out of a window in Hampton House, Peg Cushman, 1969, photographed smoke billowing into Monument Street. This may well have been one of the fires set after the assassination of Martin Luther King Jr. in 1968, which stirred some frustrated and angry mourners to set buildings near the hospital ablaze. Students' movements were severely restricted during the crisis.

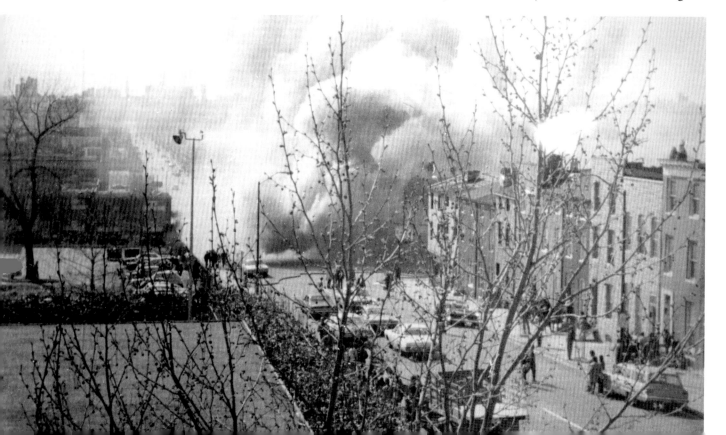

change. It was also the era of Vietnam, so there was just a ton going on."[53]

New traditions were established to celebrate various transitions in student life. Seniors began hanging their brown shoes on the fence in front of the residence when they donned white uniforms and shoes for graduation. The senior class would march through the dorm in a noisy procession, announcing their new status by pounding on metal trash-cans and clanging pan-lid cymbals. It was not unusual for the class to end up in the new swimming pool located behind the residence.

The turtle derby endured but took a decidedly modern turn as the themes began to reflect current events such as hit movies, the U.S. space program, and newly developed sex-change procedures. Nursing students participated in the annual derby band and in fund-raising activities. One year the post-derby party culminated in a full-blown panty raid on Hampton House by medical students and house staff. Nursing students prodded the event along by tossing out marked undergarments of their classmates. Those who lost underwear spent considerable time retrieving it from Reed Hall residents who had gathered up the treasures during the raid. Needless to say, Chaplain and Mrs. Price, who resided on the first floor of Hampton House, were not impressed with the behavior of any of the participants.

Students still had holiday duty in this era, so special Christmas celebrations were important. Alice Kiger, 1964, reported in the alumnae magazine:

Something new was added to Christmas this year for the girls who would not be going home. On Christmas Eve we hung Supp-hose in the lounge and each of us helped to fill all of them. Christmas morning we got up at five-thirty and went down to the lounge in our pajamas to take down our stockings and sing carols. Mrs. Eisner had coffee for us and at six fifteen, Mrs. Price joined us and we had prayers. At noon, we had our own special table in the cafeteria, complete with tablecloth, candles, and centerpiece and Mrs. Ensor acted as hostess. All in all, most of us felt that it was the nicest away-from-home Christmas we could have had, and we especially appreciated the contributions of Mrs. Ensor and Mrs. Price.[54]

The candlelight ceremony remained a major event for freshmen. The strengthening of the "Big Sister–Little Sister" program enhanced the ritual in 1961, when Big Sisters began capping their Little Sisters as the younger students dressed for the occasion.[55] The class would congregate in the lounge of Hampton House and then proceed to Hurd Hall in the hospital. The program planned by the student association included speakers from the upper classes and a nursing leader. The class then lit their lamps and accepted the code of honor for the School of Nursing: "We will maintain the highest standards of professional honesty and personal integrity. We, with our co-workers, will assume professional responsibility for our patients. We will abide by the policies

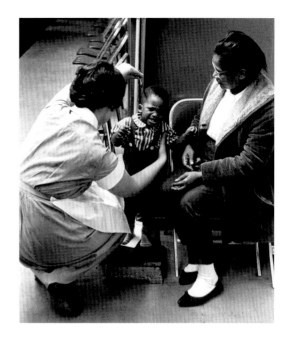

Not all patients who came to the pediatric outpatient clinic were happy to be there. This student in 1964 had her hands full as she tried to measure and weigh a crying toddler.

It was like slave labor. We got very good at taking what they now call power naps. We'd be up at 6, eating breakfast, and on duty at 7. We worked P.M.s, we worked Saturdays, sometimes Sundays. We did not work nights in my class. We were the first class that came in that didn't do nights. So we populated the hospital quite a bit.

Donna Dittberner, 1966

Mary Price was very stern, but I always felt there was a softness about her too. I really liked her, and her husband was an absolute sweetheart. She and Harry lived in an apartment in Hampton House. You would see her coming and going and she would always nod or acknowledge you, maybe not by name, but you always felt like she was watching. She was tall and very straight and trim and stern.

Lois Grayshan Hoffer, 1962

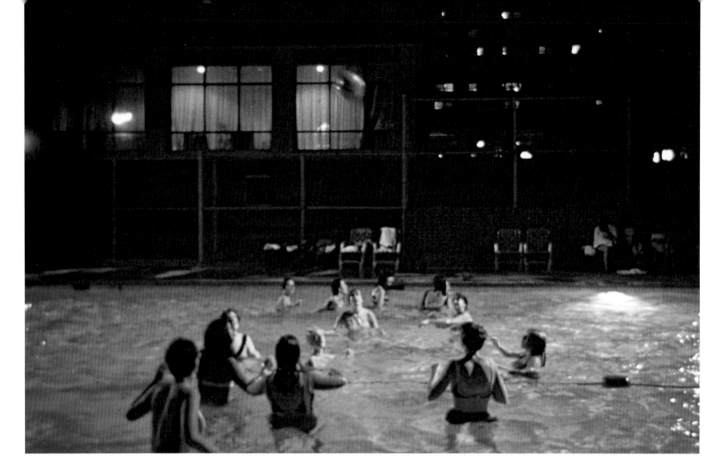

An Olympic-sized swimming pool opened behind Hampton House in July 1961, giving nursing students yet another opportunity to mix with medical students who lived in nearby Reed Hall. The opening of the pool provided an alternative to the cottage in Sherwood Forest, which had become a problem owing to its segregated setting.

That's when we had to give up Sherwood Cottage. Integration was taking place and it was decided that we couldn't keep the cottage because Sherwood Forest was segregated and Hopkins didn't feel they could get into a problem with that.

Ethel Rainey Ward, 1947

Sunbathing on the roof of Hampton House was still a popular pastime, but once the pool opened, students often preferred to relax there.

outlined by the school of nursing. We hereby pledge ourselves to abide by these principles."[56]

The students benefited from the opening of the new Olympic-sized swimming pool in July 1961. This facility, located behind Hampton House and next to Reed Hall, was available to the entire Hopkins community. The nurses' alumnae association, the Women's Board, the Turtle Derby Committee, the university, and many individuals helped to fund the pool. In 1965 the Dick Cottage in Sherwood Forest was sold because students no longer used it often enough to justify maintaining it and the vehicle they used to drive out from the city. Students preferred the convenience of the pool, which made the sale of the cottage both easy and timely. While the School of Nursing had integrated in the 1950s, Sherwood Forest remained a segregated community.[57] This development brought a treasured facet of the school's history to an

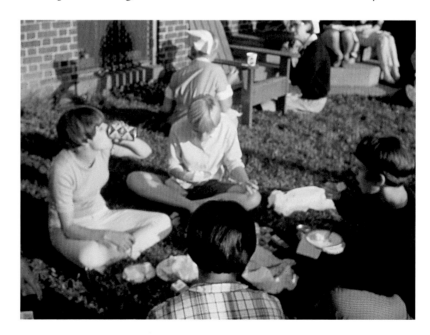

end; the cottage on the Severn River, where generations of students had enjoyed taking breaks, had been hospital property since 1916.

As the 1960s progressed, the number of clinical hours decreased in response to new National League for Nursing rules regarding educational practices in diploma programs. Night duty for Hopkins students ended in 1965 as the result of the inability to recruit an instructor for that time period. Students still worked weekends and evenings in various rotations after their freshman year.[58]

A new group of students began coming to Johns Hopkins in the early 1960s. These short-term students were registered nurses seeking additional education under the Professional Nurse Traineeship Program sponsored by the U.S. Department of Health, Education, and Welfare. They were learning the latest pediatric theory and practice in order to qualify as pediatric nursing supervisors. These intensive, one-month programs attracted nurses from more than twenty states.[59]

A dramatic development occurred in 1968 when Herb Zinder and Jim Levya joined the student body—the first male students to attend the Johns Hopkins Hospital School of Nursing. The following year, two more men registered for classes, but Zinder and Levya were the only men to complete the diploma program. Zinder remembered that the school was generally unprepared to accommodate them. No thought had been given to what kind of uniforms the men would wear, and they were quickly dressed in "blue pants, white-buck shoes, and a Dr. Kildaire–type smock that buttoned down the side."[60] Because no one else in the hospital wore similar garb, patients and staff were often at a loss to understand exactly what the male students' role was.

Levya and Zinder were not allowed to care for female patients, and they were asked to leave the room when their fellow students were taught breast self-examination techniques. Even more challenging, unlike generations of female students who had gone before them and unlike their classmates, the male students had no role models to identify with. "When I did rotations in the recovery room or operating room, I would go into the doctors' locker room to change into a scrub suit and all my classmates would go into a nurses' locker room to change into a scrub suit," Zinder recalled. There were both benefits and complications with this arrangement, however.

The male doctors interacted with me more than they interacted with my classmates, and the female nurses interacted with my classmates and not so much with me. Even though I was a nursing student, I was treated almost as a resident or a medical student. It had some benefits but it also caused some jealousy too. I could go into the doctors' locker room and ask questions, where my classmates really couldn't do that with medical doctors. There were plenty of female physicians around, but I'm not sure that they really interacted that much with student nurses. It was a unique, long three years.[61]

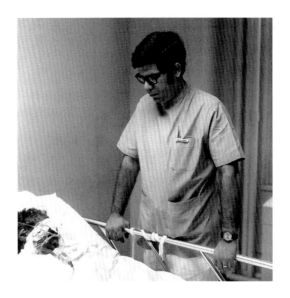

The arrival of Herb Zinder, pictured here, and Jim Levya in 1968 as the first male students to attend the Johns Hopkins Hospital School of Nursing marked a major turning point. Their graduation in 1971 required the alumnae association to become an alumni association.

I went to the School of Nursing. I remember walking in. I can't remember her name but she looked at me like I was from Pluto. She said, "We've never had male nurses here." I said, "Well, I wouldn't mind studying here at Hopkins." She was really flustered. To make a long story short, they did, in fact, accept me into the School of Nursing. I was ten years older than all my classmates. The first day of school they had a parents' meeting. Well, my wife went to the parents' meeting. The girls all lived at Hampton House, and I went home. I have to stress that there were people at Hopkins who were very supportive. They knew that I was making a lot of sacrifices, financial and otherwise.

Herb Zinder, 1971

When I was on the faculty, the last year we had two males, so we had two male graduates of the Johns Hopkins Hospital School of Nursing. They had to pick a patient to do their clinical paper on. Herb Zinder said, "Can I pick anybody?" I said, "Sure." He said, "Can I pick a female? I've never really had female patients. They always sort of have me with men." I said, "Well, then this is a wonderful opportunity."

Donna Dittberner, 1966

Following in the tradition of their predecessors, alumnae provided leadership in education, administration, and practice. They were frequent keynoters at candlelight and commencement ceremonies, furnishing inspiration and serving as role models for students and new graduates. Ethel A. Brooks, director of the Hartford Hospital School of Nursing and Nursing Service, underscored the need for reform in nursing and nursing education in her address to the graduating class in 1962. She pointed out that the profession was facing "a three-pronged dilemma. It is caught between the complexities of hospital administration, the demands made by rapidly expanding medical science, and the needs of the patient for nursing care."[62]

Several older graduates completed their careers in the 1960s, including Lucile Petry Leone, 1927, and Frances Reiter, 1931. By the end of the decade, most alumnae from the early years of the century, including some who led and served during World War I, had died. Elsie Lawler, 1899, Helen Wilmer Athey, 1905, Alice Fitzgerald, 1906, Effie Taylor, 1907, and others of that early generation were gone. The ties with the beginnings of the program were loosening.

Alumnae practicing in the 1960s experienced the changes that Medicare and Medicaid brought and learned new approaches to documentation and accountability that came with third-party reimbursement from the government. As the delivery system became more complex, the pressure for continuing education and for nurses to complete degree programs increased. The alumnae magazine was filled with notices and reports of graduates returning to school for undergraduate and graduate degrees.

Distinguished Hopkins graduates were reaching the peaks of their careers and receiving recognition for excellent service. Margaretta Craig, 1925, was honored in 1960 with the Florence Nightingale Medal from

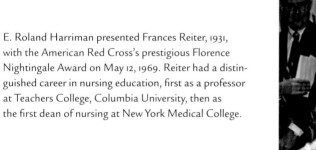

E. Roland Harriman presented Frances Reiter, 1931, with the American Red Cross's prestigious Florence Nightingale Award on May 12, 1969. Reiter had a distinguished career in nursing education, first as a professor at Teachers College, Columbia University, then as the first dean of nursing at New York Medical College.

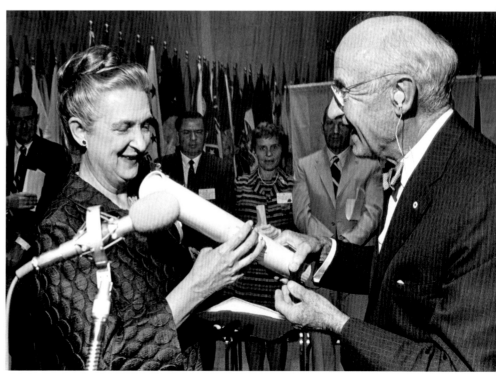

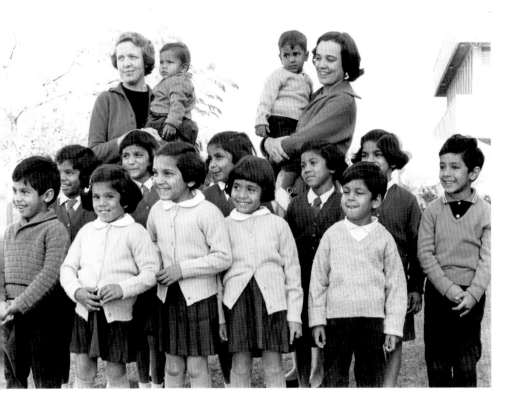

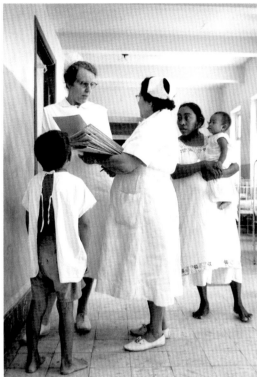

Alumnae continued to spread out across the globe. Jacqueline Liechty and Laurel Gene Long, members of the class of 1953, worked with children in India. Elva McMahon Legters, 1935, was a missionary nurse in Merida, Mexico, where she shared her expertise with a local woman and a fellow nurse in 1961.

the International Red Cross. The award recognized Craig's efforts to establish two modern nursing schools in India during her long commitment to missionary nursing as well as during her tenure as the principal of the New Delhi College of Nursing.

Many of the baby boomers who populated the school in the 1960s completed advanced and doctoral degrees. Their roles expanded with the demands of the health care and higher education systems in the country. In 1997 Dr. Martha Hill, 1964, became the first nurse and the first nonphysician to serve as president of the American Heart Association. Today she is the third dean and the first alumna to lead the Johns Hopkins University School of Nursing. Other graduates are deans, department heads, researchers, educators, advanced nurse practitioners, entrepreneurs, governmental leaders, and policymakers. Many have also committed time and effort to their professional organizations and honor societies. Like generations who came before them, the alumnae of the 1960s continue the Hopkins heritage of excellence.

Donna Dittberner found much to be grateful for in her Hopkins experience, both as a student and as an alumna.

There's a sense of pride that I feel every time I see that Johns Hopkins has been named number one institution in the country. It brings back all sorts of memories of clinical fun. You know, silly times. Remembering being on the medical unit with just two students and slipping in some spilled water with my cap flying and trying to stop these little old ladies from getting out of bed to help me. It brings back memories of the collegiality. We were taught to be independent thinkers. We were forced to be decision makers. I feel very good about what has occurred in my career in nursing and I attribute that to having a jump start from Johns Hopkins.[63]

We began to have Spanish patients and I thought, "I'd better learn to communicate with these people." I went to the university to take Spanish. I thought, "While I'm doing that, I might as well matriculate and see what is necessary."
I just started to take courses. It took eleven years but I finally got a BS at McCoy College.
In fact, Martha Hill and I sat in one or two sociology classes together. But she went on and got her PhD and I stopped.

Constance Cole Heard Waxter, 1944

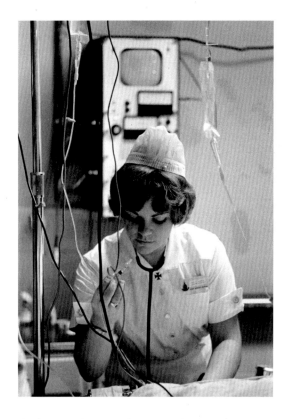

As the 1960s drew to a close, many dramatic changes were taking place. Not the least was the decision by some nurses to abandon their hard-earned graduate caps when they worked in the hospital. Susan Dieterle Cook, 1967, proudly wore both her cap and her alumni pin on duty in the intensive care unit in 1970, but Jeanne Regan Aronson, 1969, abandoned her cap when she worked on Osler after graduation.

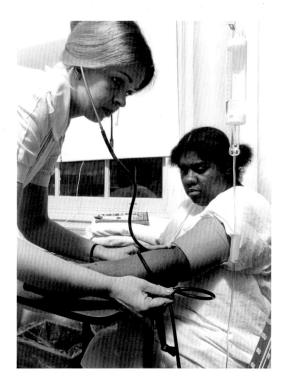

The alumnae association maintained its mission to help members and students be successful. Herb Zinder thankfully recalled a career-saving loan provided by the association as he struggled to keep his young family afloat and make ends meet during his second year in nursing school. He went to the alumnae office (which, upon his and James Levya's graduation would become the alumni office) and admitted, "I'm not able to continue unless I can tap into some fund. There's just too much financial pressure." He was given a grant of $500. "That," he said, "was the pivotal moment that I knew that I was going to finish this program. Five hundred dollars is not that much today, but back then, I knew that with that five hundred I could finish. Without it, I probably would have quit."[64]

As the decade progressed, the drive for the collegiate program became a priority for more alumnae and the association intensified its efforts. On September 9, 1960, Mrs. Price and the association's executive committee met with President Nelson, who described his efforts since 1956 regarding future options for the school. He had conducted interviews with university officials, educators, doctors, and nurses to develop the goals of a collegiate nursing program at Johns Hopkins to delineate how such a program would differ from the diploma program. He reported considerable interest in developing an integrated collegiate program in nursing at the university, but he warned the alumnae group that many questions had to be answered and problems solved before the goal could be achieved.[65]

After attending the first School of Nursing graduation held in Shriver Hall on the Homewood campus of the Johns Hopkins University in 1962, Jessie Black McVicar, 1939, admitted: "One cannot resist the temptation to dream. And to hope that very soon the School of Nursing will become an integral part of the University. Johns Hopkins surely intended that the Nursing School would be a vital part of the Hospital and the University, for these institutions of higher learning are so closely related that one can hardly separate the Nursing School and the Medical School from the Hospital and the University."[66]

The highlight of the alumni association's seventy-fifth anniversary celebration was a symposium on university education for nursing, particularly as it would relate to Johns Hopkins. Dr. Sarah Allison, the alumnae representative to the Advisory Board of the School of Nursing, requested in 1966 that funds from the Mary Adelaide Nutting Endowment Fund be used, and the idea received support from the board. In preparation for the program the alumnae association devoted an entire issue of its magazine to a discussion of baccalaureate education for nurses at Johns Hopkins. Lucile Petry Leone wrote the central paper, followed by a series of articles by leaders in the school. In her article "Progress or Decline?" Betty Cuthbert depicted the changing student body and considered what those modifications meant.[67] Perhaps the most poignant article came from K. Virginia Betzold, who had witnessed the efforts of three directors to establish an advanced educational system at the school. She traced the efforts of every director since Nutting to maintain the school's excellence through improved educational standing. "It is regrettable that in this Seventy-Fifth Anniversary number of our magazine we should be describing the fruitless efforts of fifty years to turn a dream into reality," she lamented. "None of us can predict what tomorrow holds.[68]

The symposium was called "Response to Change in Health Services," and health care and educational authorities from across the country presented papers. Issues covered included current nursing education, the university and health professions, the responsibility of nursing for patient care, and collaboration between doctors and nurses. Of all the presentations made that day in 1967, Case Western Reserve University's Dean Rozella M. Schlotfeldt's words probably rang most prophetically in the ears of the nursing leaders and their supporters at Hopkins:

The educational preparation of both nurses and physicians must provide them opportunities to gain knowledge and understanding essential to their practice, skills unique to their professions, and values and commitments appropriate to professionals who serve others.

Nursing is one field that, to date, does not uniformly fulfill expectations properly held for a learned profession. The reason can be found in the historical fact that nurse training programs were initially developed in service agencies and over three-fourths of them are still almost completely isolated from the scholarly influence of the university. Patients are now suffering from the effects of failure to develop a scientifically based and theoretically oriented system of professional nursing education within universities and from tardiness in the development of programs of nursing research.[69]

Dr. Schlotfeldt pointed out how the first president of the Johns Hopkins University, Daniel Coit Gilman, had missed the opportunity to conceptualize nurses as collaborators rather than assistants to physicians. She reminded the audience that both doctor and nurse have spheres of care that require different preparation and that each is critical to the well-being of the patient.

During the association's business meeting in 1967, the group ratified a resolution calling for a university-based nursing program at Johns Hopkins, increased support from alumnae and a shift in the control of the finances of the program from the hospital to the university. It is clear from the resolution that the alumnae saw a major role for Hopkins graduates in the effort to secure a quality program that would lead to a bachelor's degree. As the anniversary celebration concluded, Dr. Morgan's committee was still working on the proposed School of

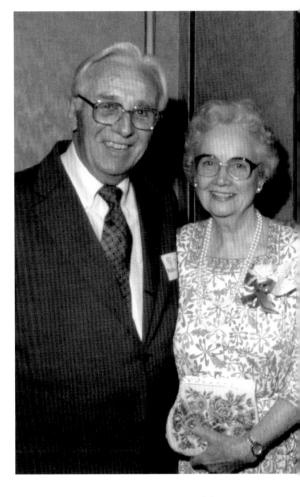

Hospital president Russell Nelson was a solid supporter of nursing education at Johns Hopkins. He backed the alumni association's efforts to see the school become a degree-granting division of the university, no doubt with the encouragement of his wife, Ruth Jeffcoat Nelson, 1937.

I was so poor. I remember learning that the alumni association had a dedicated bed at the hospital for a graduate. I'm thinking, "I am so poor if I get sick I'm going to need that bed."
Herb Zinder, 1971

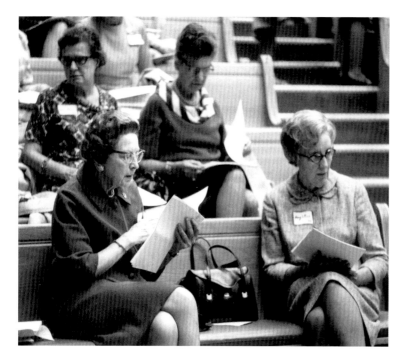

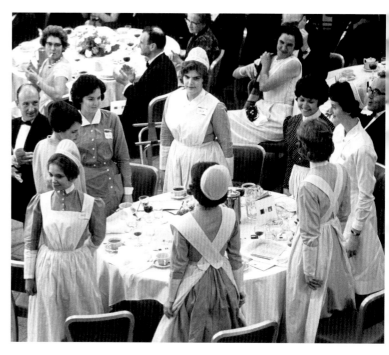

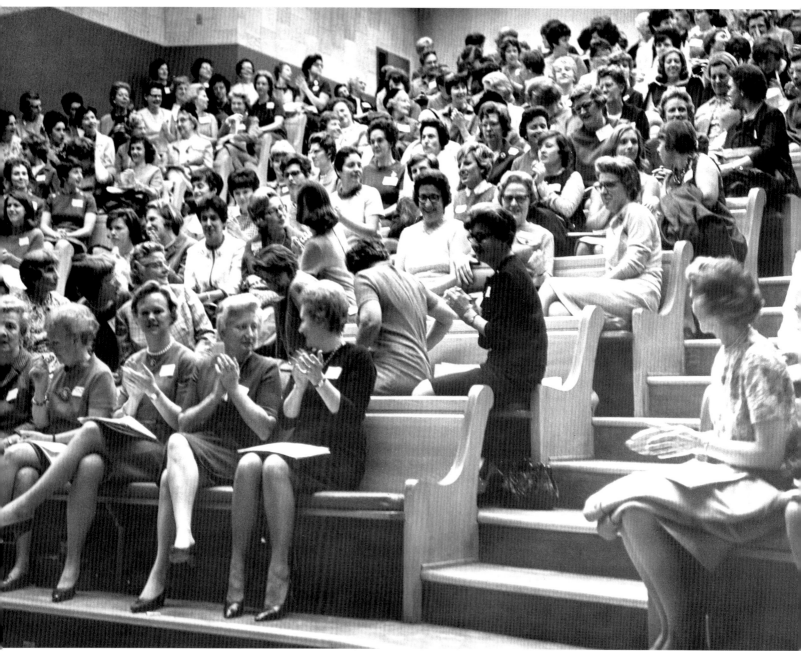

Allied Health Sciences, but the alumnae knew that the problems were mounting and that time was running out for the diploma program at Johns Hopkins. The drop in applications and student enrollments was openly discussed. Over the next few years, officers of the association spent many hours in meetings, making an effort to stay in communication with university and hospital leaders and expressing their willingness to help.

The alumnae association created a committee on nursing education in the 1960s to lobby for support for the bachelor's program at the university. Members were not deterred by the numerous setbacks and problems with the various ideas and proposals that poured out of appointed committees within the university and the medical institution. One problem that hindered the association was the limited understanding some members had about what it would take financially to establish a baccalaureate program. Even in the 1960s, nursing education was relatively inexpensive because of support from the hospitals. Many alumnae had become nurses for very little money. It was difficult to understand that the Nutting Fund, although it was worth about half a million dollars by the late 1960s, would provide just a fraction of what it would take to establish a university-based program.

The dream of this program, which was first described by Isabel Hampton Robb and Adelaide Nutting and argued for so strenuously by Anna Wolf, had not been popular with many diploma graduates in the early years. Now that the nursing world was shifting in that direction, even reluctant members wanted to keep up and remain "professional"—yet few truly understood what this was going to take. Alumnae leaders like Margaret Courtney and Sarah Allison tried to alert the members about the need for ongoing commitment to the endowment fund, but there were few contributions in this period. Little did most alumnae realize that the struggle to keep nursing education at the Johns Hopkins institutions was about to reach its climax.

I'm very fortunate that I'm local. I think alumni activity adds enrichment to your life, a connection that goes back from the time that you were a student, an appreciation of the advancement that has gone on and the development of the nursing school itself. I liked the association with the other nurses, not necessarily my classmates—all the Hopkins nurses. I was on several homecoming committees and the membership committee.

Betsy Mumaw McGeady, 1955

We were very conscious of our heritage in terms of what was expected of us. Usually 100 percent of students from Hopkins pass the state boards on the first attempt and students from Hopkins are expected to become leaders. I think there was a certain amount of smugness attached to being a Hopkins student, as opposed to being a student from one of the affiliate hospitals who came to Hopkins and lived in Hampton House for a few months to do clinical rotations, and a certain sense of superiority. I don't think the alumnae fostered that, but somehow it got filtered down from one class to another.

Sandra Stine Angell, 1969, BSN 1977

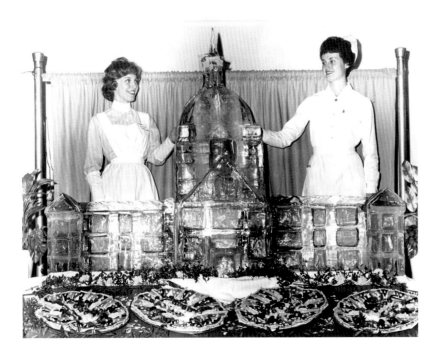

Opposite and left: Members of the alumnae association were hopeful as they gathered in 1967 for a symposium honoring the seventy-fifth anniversary of the organization. The subject was university-based education for nurses. K. Virginia Betzold, 1933, and Mary Sanders Price, 1934, sat just in front of Mildred Struve, 1926. Current nursing students, who modeled school uniforms through the years, attended the dinner. The centerpiece for the occasion was an impressive ice sculpture of the Administration Building.

LINDA SABIN

"We Had a Good Time"

We came in September and we had a total of three months off in a three-year period. In our first year, we had two weeks at Christmas and a month in the summer. The second year we had a month sometime from May to September. We didn't all have vacation at the same time, with the exception of that one two-week period at Christmas.

Lois Grayshan Hoffer, 1962

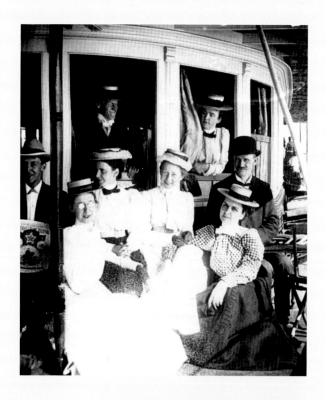

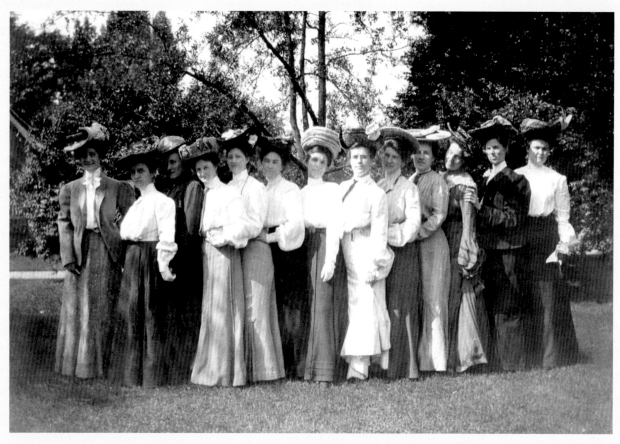

Above: Nurses and students took advantage of what little time they had away from the hospital. Charity Babcock, 1897, took this snapshot of friends "one pleasant day" on the Chesapeake Bay.

Below: Vashti Bartlett, 1906, and some of her classmates dressed in their finest garb and most stylish hats when they made an excursion to Washington.

"Nurses class day 1906" reads the legend by this charming scene around an ornate silver punchbowl. One happy nurse and her friend lifted their cups to the photographer.

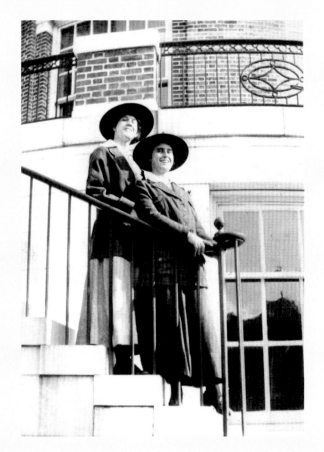

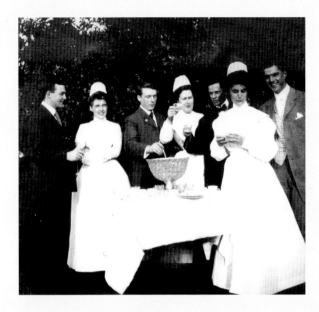

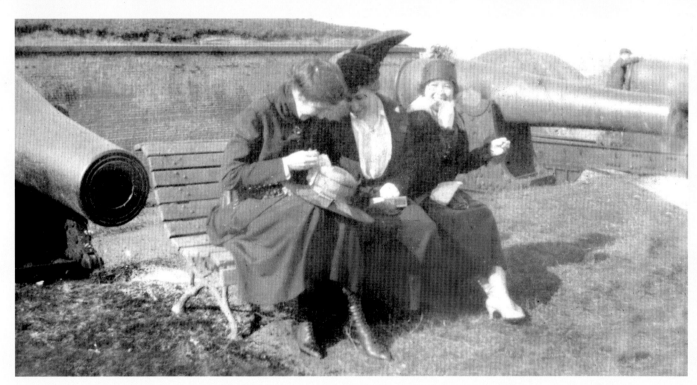

Above: Three off-duty nurses with an interest in American history took in the sites at Fort McHenry in 1916.

Above right: Two students took a jaunt to the new Homewood campus of the Johns Hopkins University, four miles away from the hospital. They posed on the back steps of Gilman Hall, which was dedicated in 1915.

Students took advantage of a warm day c. 1917 to read
their mail in the garden area near the Main Residence.

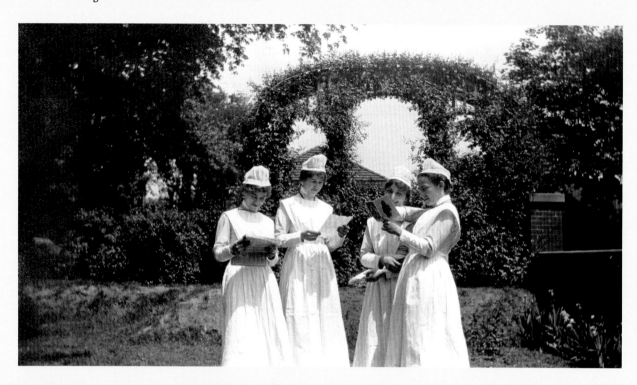

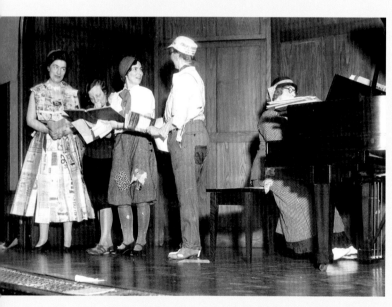

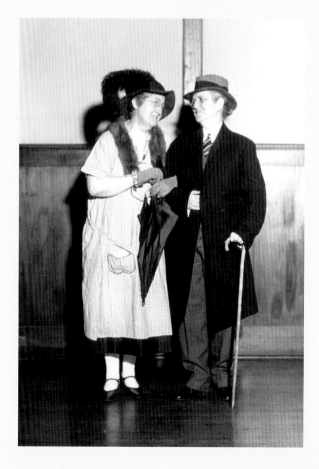

The Great Depression inspired a "poverty party" in
1932, where everyone donned outfits appropriate to the
circumstances. One student wore a dress made of
newspapers. Even Elsie Lawler (holding an umbrella)
and Christine Dick (with a cane) joined the fun.

Students who played table tennis on the top floor of
Hampton House in 1939 also got a great view of the
hospital and the city when they looked out the windows.

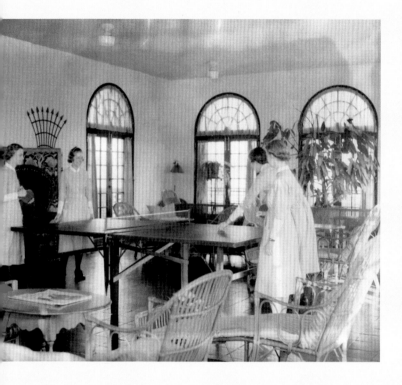

Miss Wolf wanted us to have many interests. We had
symphony tickets tacked on the wall of the bulletin
board of the elevator in Hampton House. You didn't
have to apply; you just took them. We had teas. We
were encouraged to go to the museum. I remember as a
senior student walking through the corridor and Miss
Wolf was coming toward me. She said, "Oh, Miss
Borenstein, what are you reading?" I said, "Textbooks,
Miss Wolf," and she went "Tsk, tsk. What are you
reading for pleasure?" She wanted us to be very broad
people so that we could be excellent nurses.

Betty Borenstein Scher, 1950

Below left: The State Theater at the corner of Monument
and Castle Streets, photographed in 1934, was just a
short walk from Hampton House. A wide array of foods
was available next door at the Northeast Market.

Below: A quick game of cards in the sitting room on
the fifth floor of Hampton House made for an easy way
to relax in 1939.

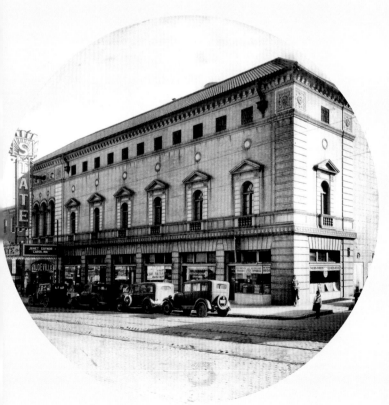

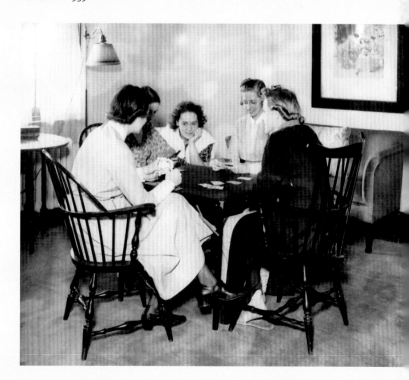

"Hoptown" was fondly remembered by students from all eras of the diploma school. Levinson & Klein's furniture store, pictured here in 1937, was the source for furnishings for many nurses after they graduated.

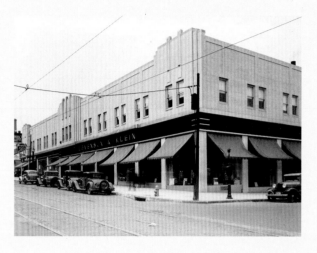

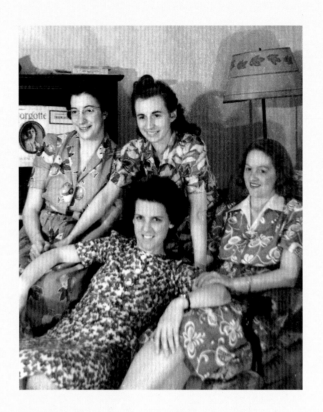

Graduate nurses Mary Farr, Lucy Greenfield, Buelah Mae Sheets, and Mary Keeler rented an apartment on the second floor of a row house at 1042 North Broadway after they graduated in 1941. "The last one in slept on the couch," remembered Mary Farr Heeg.

Down Monument Street where the market was and the stores—that was called Hoptown. I lived in the 2700 block of East Madison Street. If I went home while I was a student I could walk. My mother shopped at the Northeast Market from the time I was a little girl. They had dress shops, hat shops, drug stores, bakeries, shoe stores, a bicycle shop, barbers, and hairdressers. Up closer to the hospital were the more commercial blocks. You could buy anything along Monument Street.

Betsy Mumaw McGeady, 1955

We had a wonderful officers club in Australia. We'd go out on the town. The dentists would rent a cottage and we'd go down for overnights and dinner parties, a lot of us or some of the friends that we'd made. We had a good time.

When I was leaving, I remember Dr. VandeGrift saying—he was in charge of the lab and he was also in charge of all the alcohol at the parties— "Well, this calls for a party." There were thirty or thirty-five of us who went home on the next ship.

Mary Farr Heeg, 1941

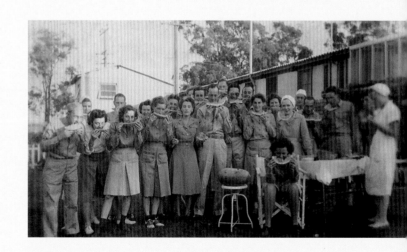

Mary Farr was relaxing at an oyster roast in Baltimore when she got news about the attack on Pearl Harbor. Right then, Farr decided, "By golly, I'm going to go." Here she and her friends in General Hospital No. 118 enjoyed a watermelon party in Australia.

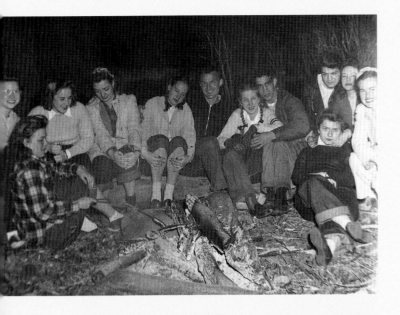

During their last six months of training, students and their beaus in 1946 huddled by a campfire at Perry Point Psychiatric Hospital.

Center: Students from the classes of 1948–50 enjoyed the fresh air on the porch of the Sherwood Forest cottage.

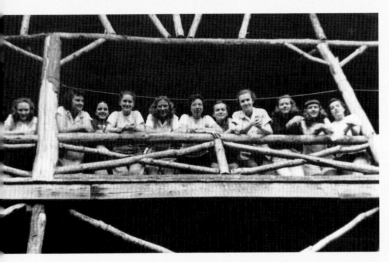

There was a cottage at Sherwood Forest. It was on the Severn River and there was a little station wagon. Dr. Hugh Young had given the cottage for the student nurses. When we had some free time occasionally we could go there. It was bare bones but a beautiful setting. I remember going there when it was cool. We would put the wood in the fireplace and then it would die down and you'd wake up cold. They had a little store not too far away, so when you went in you bought some groceries. It was kind of roughing it in a way. I remember about ten or twelve being there at one time, sleeping here and there. Usually you had your own little group going but sometimes there'd be another group there too.

Ethel Rainey Ward, 1947

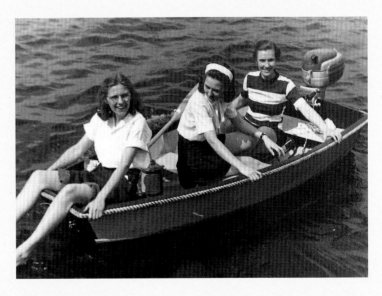

A small dinghy was available for adventurous students to take out on the Severn River when they visited Sherwood Forest in the late 1940s.

Left: Betty Borenstein, 1950, noted in her scrapbook that this picture was taken "our first time at Sherwood."

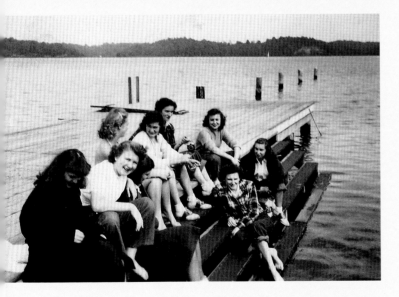

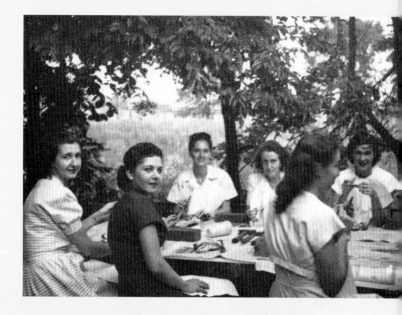

*Many of the girls who were from out of the area had
an alumna in the area assigned to them as a friend,
somebody to help you see a little bit more of Baltimore,
to help you navigate through some of the ins and outs
of the school, to give you a different perspective on
things, and to just help you escape out of the school for
a period of time. There were some really great relationships. That was a really nice concept.*

Catherine Novak, 1973

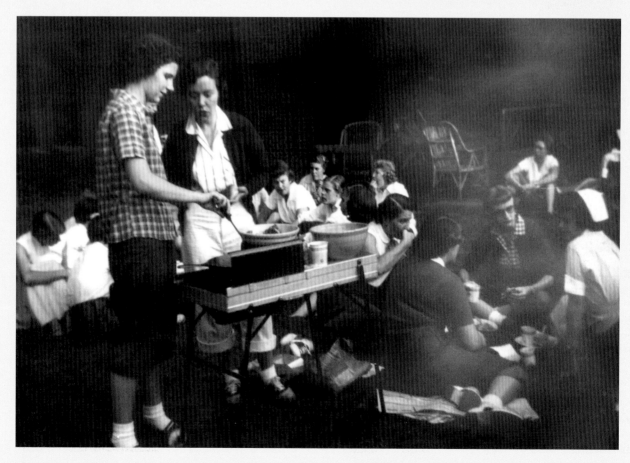

The roof of Hampton House provided the setting for
this cookout in 1952. Bobby socks and saddle shoes
apparently were the order of the day.

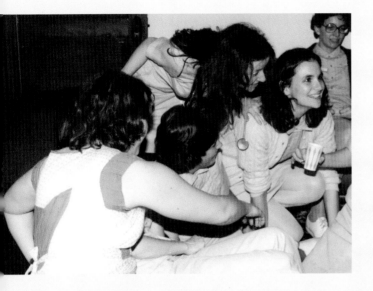

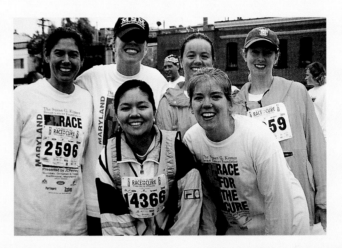

The Race for the Cure in 1999 was an opportunity for students of the university school to burn off frustrations and energy for a good cause.

Students from the Nursing Education Program in the School of Health Services in 1978 found a few minutes to fool around between classes.

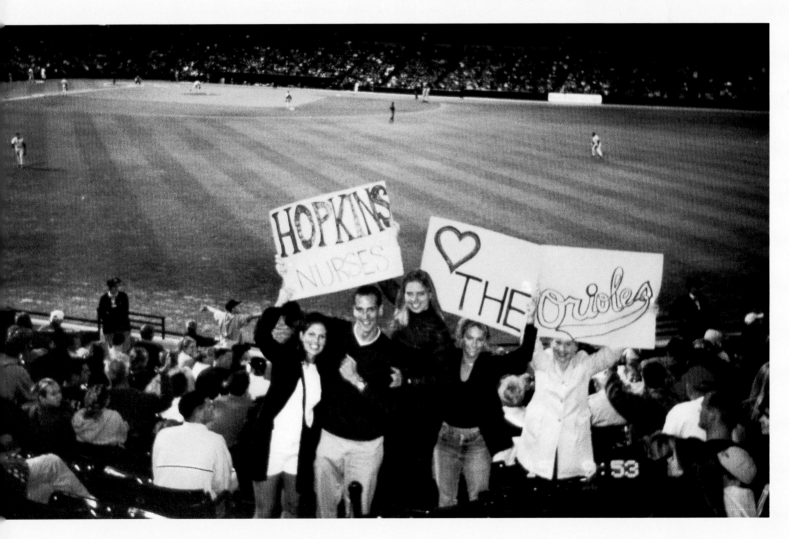

An Orioles game at Camden Yards inspired a handmade display of affection for the team from five Hopkins nurses.

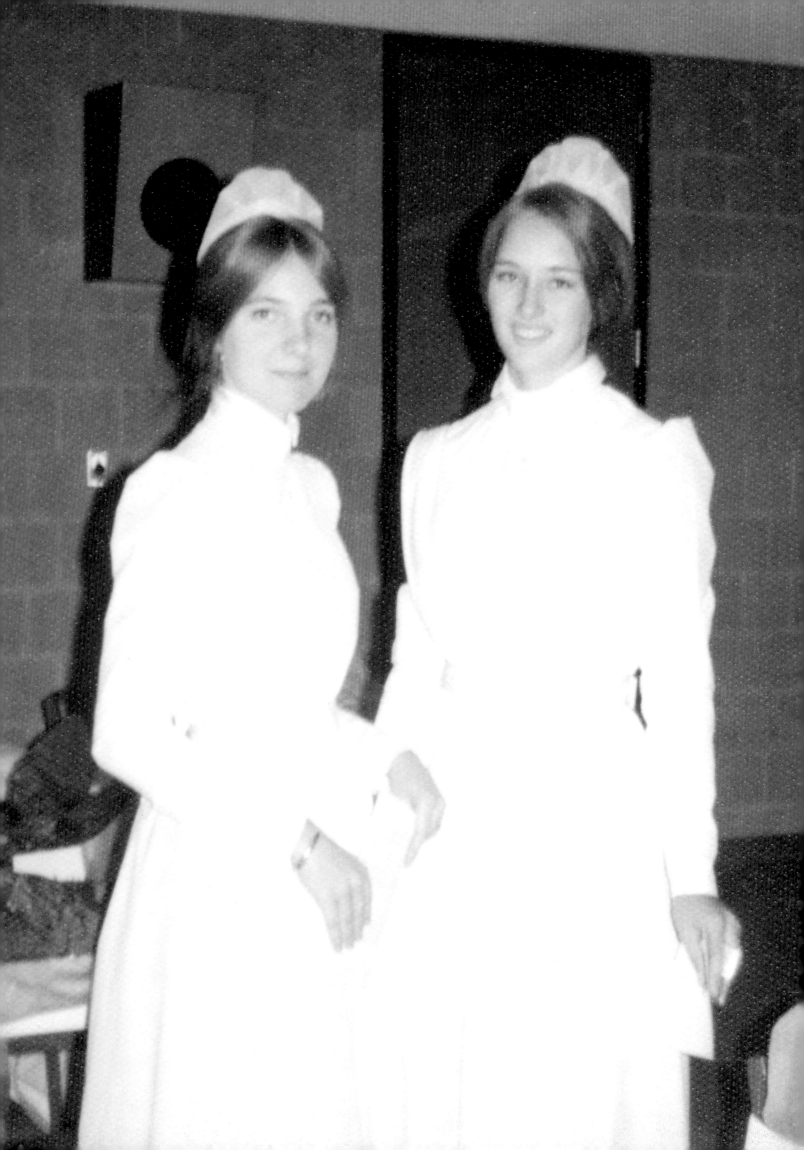

Tension and Triumph, 1970–1979 · MARY FRANCES KEEN

5

Adelaide Nutting's assertion that "history is the past, the present, and the future" seemed particularly apropos at commencement in 1973, when students donned uniforms modeled on those of the first graduates of the Johns Hopkins Hospital's nursing school. Angela Diggs, left, and Marlene Kazamek were in the final class to receive diplomas; they achieved their goal at a time when their profession was in transition, however, leaving them to face uncertain futures.

THE 1970S UNFOLDED as a decade of extreme turmoil. Developments in nursing education and changes in the status of women at home, in the workplace, and in academia had profound effects on the Johns Hopkins Hospital School of Nursing. In March 1970 a report entitled "The Future of the School of Nursing," prepared by Director Mary Price and Associate Director Margaret Courtney, was circulated to members of the school's advisory board for discussion at their April 1 meeting. The report clearly identified several factors that necessitated a serious look at the future of the school. The factors included:

1. the number of applications, admissions, and graduations had declined—coupled with an increased attrition rate due to academic failure;

2. recruitment of competent faculty was becoming increasingly difficult, especially in light of the increasing number of community college programs;

3. the cost of operations continued to increase and was becoming more of a problem with fewer students;

4. major renovations in educational facilities and equipment were needed;

5. a national trend away from diploma education was impacting the number of applications and admissions of qualified students.[1]

Two alternatives were set forth in the report. One was "to admit and make every effort to graduate 100–125 *average* high school students a year"; the other proposed "that the Johns Hopkins Hospital discontinue the School of Nursing and make its contribution to nursing education in cooperation with other institutions through the provision of clinical facilities and a limited number of supporting services."[2]

TO BE OR NOT TO BE

As one would expect, there was little or no support for the first proposal, which would have changed the Hopkins image and which did not really address any of the factors that had led to the present dilemma. The general feeling of the advisory board was that no school was preferable to a second-rate one; the board was also aware that the decision to close the School of Nursing might serve as an impetus to Johns Hopkins to establish a university-based nursing program. The second proposal was unanimously supported by the advisory board members and was subsequently recommended to the board of trustees of the hospital by Dr. Russell Nelson, president of the hospital. The trustees were well aware of the importance of their decision and the need for a full review and discussion. At the May meeting, after considerable discussion, tentative approval was given to close the school after the June graduation of the class of 1973.

On May 18, 1970, Dr. Nelson met with the board of directors of the alumni association and stated that he would welcome any feasible

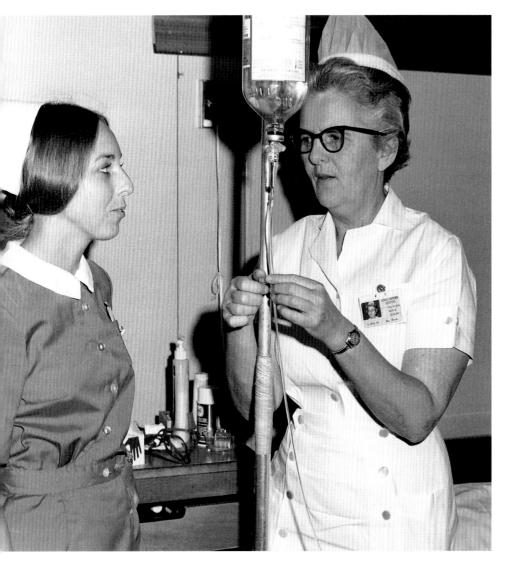

Ella Rowe reviewed procedures with Bonnie LeHew, 1973, as they checked an intravenous line at a patient's bedside. Rowe graduated from Union Memorial Hospital's nursing school in 1936. The Johns Hopkins Nurses' Alumnae Association named her an honorary member in 1968, in gratitude for her years of teaching at the hospital. LeHew wore the last version of the hospital school uniform, which no longer included starched white cuffs on the sleeves.

alternative for a university nursing program and that he would personally convey the proposal to university President Lincoln Gordon.[3] However, a press release dated the same day clearly described the conversion of the nursing education program from a three-year diploma school to a cooperative program with other academic institutions.

The School would accept its last class this fall, and close following the class's graduation in 1973. The Hospital, however, would continue to offer an affiliating program in pediatric nursing for the diploma nursing schools of Church Home, Maryland General and St. Joseph's Hospitals. As the School phases out, the Hospital will develop cooperative arrangements with universities and colleges having baccalaureate and graduate degree programs in nursing, Dr. Nelson said. In addition, the Hospital will expand activities with associate degree (two-year) nursing programs of the junior colleges in the immediate metropolitan area.... The Hospital Trustees are hopeful that the Johns Hopkins University will include one or more programs in nursing education in its planned program for a College of Allied Health Sciences. Dr. Nelson said the Hospital will establish immediately

Faye Spring, who had her doctorate and was at the University of Colorado, Denver, got up and made a motion "that before the hospital closes the School of Nursing, we should recommend the closing of the School of Nursing because it will not live up to the standards that we prefer." But Miss Betzold got up and she said, "Oh, no, no. That wouldn't be ladylike." I kid you not. There was a discussion. If there were 500 people in the room, the vote was 498 opposed and 2, Fay Spring and me, for. I don't think Miss Betzold, to her credit, ever realized her influence. All she had to do was stand up at any meeting and say something and everybody would go that way. The next year the board voted to close the school.

Betty Borenstein Scher, 1950

a new Department of Education and Training. This department will carry out the joint efforts with education institutions and develop in-hospital training programs for several types of health workers.[4]

In response to Dr. Nelson's request for proposed alternatives from the alumni association, Sarah Allison, 1953, and Betty Cuthbert, 1943, submitted a report to the school's advisory board. The proposal called for the development within the Evening College of an upper-division basic baccalaureate degree program that could also lead to a master's program. The first two years of liberal arts and prerequisite college courses could be taken in any accredited junior or four-year college. The program of clinical nursing courses would be provided in East Baltimore while other required upper-division courses could be taken through the Evening College at the Homewood campus. The advisory board expressed concern about maintaining excellence and not condoning halfway measures; the proposed program was seen as a possible interim or transition step if not adopted as a permanent arrangement.[5]

The advisory board had no authority to recommend the alumni proposal to the university; it could only refer the proposal for examination through President Gordon to the Evening College. Dean Richard Mumma of the Evening College pointed out that financing could be a problem, especially since the Evening College was self-supporting on a fee-per-course basis, and that full-time faculty members with academic rank would be required, of which there were none in the Evening College. Another potential obstacle was accreditation from the National League for Nursing. Allison and Cuthbert were well aware, perhaps more than others, of the inherent difficulties in having such a program adopted by the university.

One of the basic difficulties, often not recognized by those outside the Hopkins family, is that the University and the Hospital are two separate institutions, with separate boards of trustees. They are linked by mutual concerns rather than administrative structure. Therefore, the Hospital, and nursing within it, can in no way dictate to the University that it should establish a program of nursing within the University. The most that any organization or individual outside the University can do is offer suggestions and ask that they be considered.[6]

Administrative changes in the School of Nursing accompanied planning for the short-term future of the school. Mary Sanders Price retired in July 1970, at which time the decision was made to separate the School of Nursing from the hospital's nursing service. Dr. Margaret Courtney, 1940, became the seventh and final director of the school and Doris Armstrong, formerly assistant director of operative and acute care services, became the director of the nursing department of the Johns Hopkins Hospital.

In those days, you sent a letter off and asked for information. I got a packet right away from Hopkins that went through the history, what the goals of the school were, and laid out the program of study. I read that and I just knew that's where I needed to go. My parents were a little concerned that it was not a university-based program. Their concern was heightened after the announcement came out that my class would be the last class. That didn't deter me.

I was invited to interview. We met with Betty Cuthbert. She was very lively but very direct. She said, "You know your record's really quite good. You could easily get into a university program." I told her that what Hopkins thought nursing was—and the caliber of nurse they produced—matched what I wanted. She acknowledged that they had a standard and did not expect to waiver from that standard. She helped allay my father's concerns. They'd already thought out how the school was going to downsize. There would be some attrition of the faculty, but instructors would be available to fill the slots of those who might leave. She did go through the course of study and was pretty clear about what was required. That total immersion concept just thrilled me. That was exactly what I wanted.

Cathy Novak, 1973

On December 18, 1970, the university announced the formation of the Center for Allied Health Careers in an effort to solve the nation's problems of health care delivery. The Johns Hopkins institutions were attempting to determine the extent to which Hopkins should be involved in the allied health sciences as a part of its health care delivery system. A series of faculty and administrative committees recommended that a specially qualified group study all aspects of the subject. The university and hospital boards of trustees, upon the recommendation of the Medical Planning and Development Committee, approved the appointment of Dr. Dennis G. Carlson as director of the center and Dr. Moses S. Koch as the deputy director.[7] The study conducted by the Center for Allied Health Careers entailed traveling to similar schools across the country and conducting interviews to determine what was being done elsewhere.

Members of the alumni association were uncertain whether or not their concerns were being heard, so on April 16, 1971, the association sponsored an all-day small group conference of nurses and nurse educators to develop recommendations for the future of nursing education within the center. Dr. Koch was among the conferees. A report with recommendations from nursing was written, approved by the board of directors of the alumni association, and sent to Dr. Carlson. The report was also circulated to the director of the School of Nursing and the advisory board. Recommendations from the report were expansive:

1. A nurse educator should be appointed to the staff of the center as soon as possible to serve as a consultant and planner. The nurse educator should be chosen by a search committee with nurses composing at least half of the committee.

2. The commitment of the program should be as broad as possible to serve national health needs and the national needs of nursing education and practice. The extended role of the nurse as an independent practitioner or in primary care outside the hospital setting must be a major consideration. The current and future systems of health care delivery must be outlined and serve as the framework for all health professions and job levels.

3. The finished product should be a professional nurse who can design, plan, and evaluate the health care provided by him or herself and other nursing personnel in a setting where health care is required. The primary role of the nurse will be to help people adjust their behavior to the extent necessary for them to maintain their health or assist them in illness. This nurse must be able to work in a wide variety of situations, with new concepts of health care delivery and within a continually developing profession.[8]

Other recommendations suggested that the curriculum include courses in assessing, designing, planning, and evaluating outcomes to help graduates determine the effectiveness of their efforts, as well as

HARBINGERS
OF FUTURE DIFFICULTIES

Doris Armstrong is a very competent, capable, caring person and really able to wend her way through most of the politics of Hopkins. We worked well together. It was right in the midst of really trying to implement a new approach to nursing care and delivery there, trying to introduce a stronger role for clinical specialists, trying to encourage and support the nurses in clinical decision making, and trying to strengthen their role and, in quality assurance, taking on more responsibility in a proactive way for how they were looking at their patient care.

Kay Partridge

Doris Armstrong became director of the nursing department in the Johns Hopkins Hospital when Mary Sanders retired in 1970, the only time the trustees separated the leadership of nursing services from that of the school. Armstrong played an important role as plans for the Nursing Education Program in the School of Health Services evolved. Greatly appreciated by her colleagues, members of the alumnae association welcomed her as an honorary member in 1970.

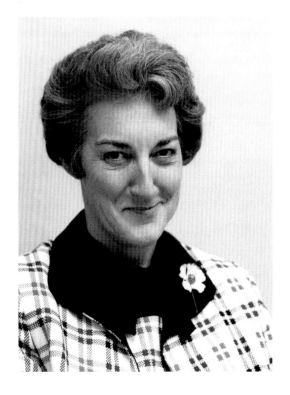

When new enrollments ceased, parts of Hampton House became administrative offices for the School of Health Services. The usual bustle of dormitory life slowed enough for members of the final diploma class Geri Byrnes, Carolyn Kirby, Bonnie LeHew, and Sue Newpher to sit undisturbed during their quiet conversation in the corridor. "I can't help but think that I chose the path less traveled," observed their classmate Deborah Chadwick Holmes. "My three years at Hopkins enriched my life, opened many doors for me, and enabled me to be a better nurse, person, mother, wife, and friend."

When the hospital diploma school closed it was a difficult year, and a very lonely year, for the students, the last class. It was a very hollow Hampton House and sometimes the students reflected that. They had so many feelings about being rejected, about the diminishment of Hopkins nurses. Frankly, the faculty had difficulty too, aside from the fact that we'd have to find new jobs. There was a great loyalty to the program within the faculty. That was a difficult year.

From an alumni standpoint, we fought for so many years to get a baccalaureate program. We would have liked to see the transition into a baccalaureate program. It was almost immoral for an institution such as Johns Hopkins not to have a nursing component, and the new School of Allied Health Sciences was not the answer. Nursing is a separate entity. It is not just an allied health.

Donna Dittberner, 1966

Wendy Weissman, 1973, used her less than sterile teeth to hold the cap of the needle she used to inject classmate Chris Komoroski. Sue Appling, 1973, recalled that clinical made up the bulk of their training. "You came out able to hit the ground running. You didn't need mentoring; you were ready to rock and roll."

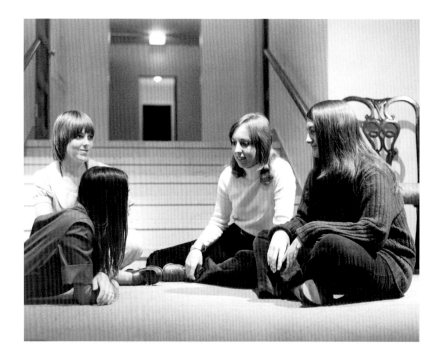

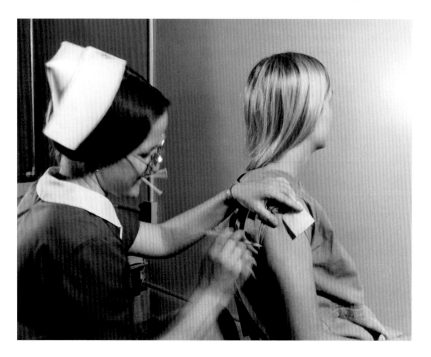

courses pertaining to health assessment and preventive health care and the counseling role of the nurse in health promotion and health care. The report also recognized the need to address the issue of financial support for the center in the event of the loss of federal or other grant funds. In today's context, none of these recommendations seems startling; however, the recommendations were made in 1971. The nurses writing the report were clearly forward-looking for their time and in tune with the future of health care delivery.

The direction of the Center for Allied Health Careers was of concern to others besides nurses. On December 19, 1970, one day after the announcement of the establishment of the center, Dr. Ridgeway Trimble and other influential physicians from the hospital sent a fiery letter to President Gordon requesting a baccalaureate program for nurses.

The reason given for the closing of the Nursing School is that there are insufficient numbers of qualified candidates applying for training. We have learned that sufficient numbers of qualified candidates could be obtained if nurses, after four years of study and training, were awarded a baccalaureate degree in nursing by the Johns Hopkins University. In any merit system today a baccalaureate degree is a prerequisite for advancement. Therefore, programs giving this degree in nursing offer the only direct route for those who wish to advance in public health nursing, clinical specialization, leadership roles in nursing practice, and later teaching and administration. Candidates for all these positions are required in ever increasing numbers for our expanding patient care programs and for national needs.[9]

Although the letter was somewhat simplistic in its recommendations, and its signatories were seemingly unaware of the possibility of a baccalaureate nursing program within an allied health professions school, the letter clearly indicated a high level of support for the School of Nursing from some of the medical staff.

In May of 1971, five months after the creation of the committee, Dr. Carlson submitted its final proposal to three advisory boards of the university for approval. On September 13, 1971, the Board of Trustees of the Johns Hopkins University voted favorably on a series of recommendations that approved in principle a school that would have a nursing program, "it being understood that the entire cost of developing and maintaining such a school is contingent on obtaining funds for that purpose." Further, the board authorized the president "to establish the nucleus of what will become the advisory board of the school, to seek funds toward the establishment, and initiate further detailed planning for the school's development in cooperation with the advisory board. The final plan for the school and its official name will be submitted to the Trustees for their approval at a later date."[10]

Following the approval, in concept, of a school of allied health that would include nursing, interim university President Milton Eisenhower immediately appointed the nucleus of an advisory board for the proposed school, consisting of seven physicians and one nurse—Doris Armstrong, director of the hospital's Department of Nursing.[11] In Eisenhower's letter to the members of this committee, he stated that the board's primary mandate was "to work out the specifics of a curriculum for the proposed new Division. Other matters on the agenda for this year include formation of a search committee for a new dean, policy recommendations on the raising of outside funds to support the Division, formulation of criteria for the selection of faculty and students, and the

It's not that they were disrespectful of authority, but you didn't get anywhere with a Hopkins nurse by just telling them they had to do something because there was a rule that said you did it or some group that said it had to be that way. They wanted to know the whys and the wherefores and then, if they agreed with you, they'd do it. They were irreverent. There's just something about having gone through that program. I have been told I'm a snob because of it, and we all laughed about that when we were going through. We knew it was happening to us. I try to be gracious about it by saying that there are other really good nursing programs in the world, but I know what I got from the program. I went on to the University of Virginia and embarrassed myself terribly. I remember my first day. I was really trying to understand how the hospital was laid out. I was on a ward that had a medical floor here and a surgical unit here and a urology unit down here and I didn't really understand. I said, "Well, where exactly is the medical building?" The supervisor just started laughing and said, "Cathy, you're not at Hopkins."

Cathy Novak, 1973

Hopkins taught you that your opportunities were endless. You didn't have to just be a staff nurse, although all of us wanted to be the best staff nurses we could be. We were taught early on that we could be leaders. That was the whole thrust of the program. We saw many different models of nurse leaders. While in school we were taught to be team leaders, told to expect to be charge nurses, and groomed to be directors of nursing. These were things we were told to shoot for. The models of women who went before us were amazing.

Cathy Novak, 1973

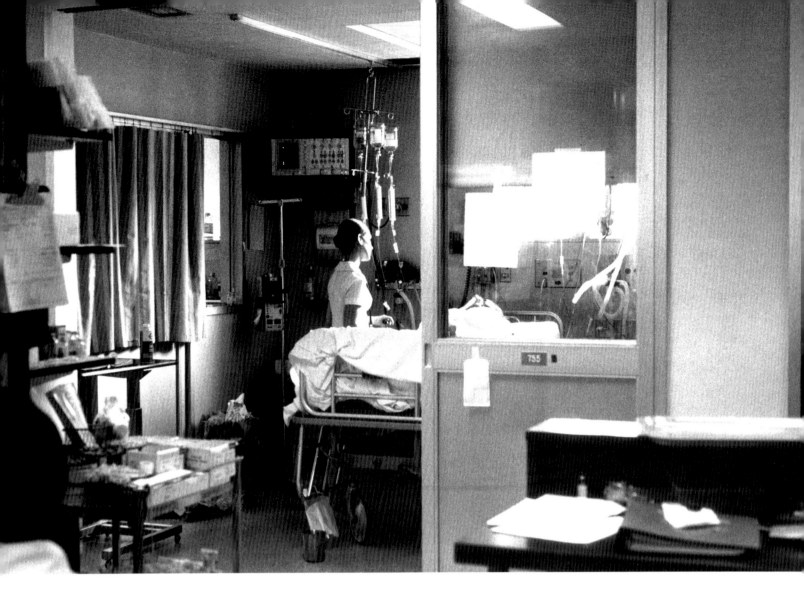

Even with the arrival of the first class in the Nursing Education Program in 1975, staffing seemed sparse in the mid-1970s, compared to previous decades, when dozens of diploma students cared for patients in the hospital.

That second year you really had to buckle down. That's when you got the heavy-duty medsurg, pediatrics, and maternal-child health, and there was a lot of work associated with it. You were also seeing more and more serious medical problems and conditions. You were really around people who were having difficult times. Not to use a cliché, but there were life and death issues and that certainly changes you. When you were the one responsible in the second year for someone's care at that level it became different.

Cathy Novak, 1973

development of policy for the relationship of the new Division to the established Divisions of the University."[12]

At an October 7, 1971, meeting of the advisory board to the hospital School of Nursing, members expressed concern about the continued limited representation of nurses on the proposed advisory board for the new school. They called attention to the failure of Dr. Carlson's group to include a nurse educator in drawing up their proposal on matters concerning nursing and nursing education, even though the alumni association had offered financial assistance to provide consultation from a nursing educator knowledgeable about baccalaureate and graduate degree programs. The concerns of the board were transmitted to Dr. Steven Muller, then provost of the university and chair of the advisory board for what would become the School of Health Services.

In December 1971 a newly created nursing subcommittee submitted a proposal to the Advisory Board of the proposed school. Members of the subcommittee were Doris Armstrong; Dr. Margaret Courtney; Dr. Kay Partridge and Dr. Anna Scholl, both assistant professors in the School of Hygiene and Public Health; Nell Kirby, an instructor in surgery; Mafalda Lochow, assistant director of nursing for outpatient services at the hospital; and Lois Ann Furgess, 1959, president of the alumni association.[13] Even though representation by nurse educators was limited to Dr. Courtney, the subcommittee developed two proposals, one of which was very enlightened for the time. One proposal called for a program that would confer the master's degree as the first professional degree, while the other, more traditional proposal called for the development of an upper-division baccalaureate program. While the master's degree was the preferred option, the committee was aware of how nontraditional this degree would be, especially in the tradition-bound academic setting of Hopkins; the baccalaureate program was offered as the more viable option.

Physician Malcolm L. Peterson was named dean of the emerging school for nursing and other health services on March 9, 1972. Since 1969 Dr. Peterson had been director of the Johns Hopkins Health Services and Research Development Center in the Office of Health Care Programs. The center was federally funded and its goal was to examine and evaluate the performance of physician extenders. Dr. Robert Heyssel, who later the same year would take over Dr. Nelson's position as administrative head of the hospital, had recruited Dr. Peterson for Johns Hopkins. Heyssel and Peterson had been together on the house staff at Washington University in St. Louis and were friends for many years. Before coming to Hopkins, Dr. Peterson did research on manpower use, information systems, and the shortage of medical doctors. He held joint appointments as associate professor of medical care and hospitals in the School of Hygiene and Public Health and associate professor of medicine in the School of Medicine.[14]

As planned, the new school would initially offer three upper-division programs at the baccalaureate level: nursing, health associates (non-

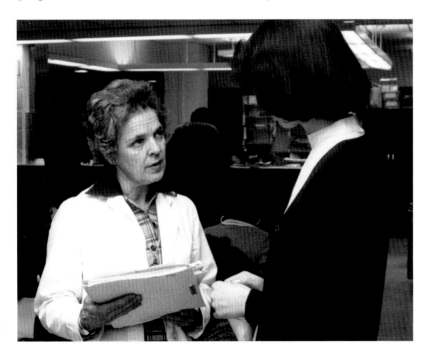

Mafalda Lochow, left, assistant director of nursing for outpatient services, served on a subcommittee that attempted, in 1971, to make innovative recommendations for the Nursing Education Program.

Suddenly, all the doctors were on our side, all the doctors who couldn't be bothered before—except for Philip Tumulty and Philip Wagley. There may have been others, but I know that those two championed us all along.

Betty Borenstein Scher, 1950

There were two degree programs and a couple of certificate programs in the School of Health Services. The overall mission of the school, which absolutely amazes me, was to educate a new kind of professional. That's not nursing. It never was nursing and nursing did not fit in the mission. It seemed like, "Well, if we're going to have this new school and they're going to educate a health professional, we'll stick nursing in there too."

In the administration of the School of Health Services, the dean was a physician. The director of admissions, the associate dean for financial aid, and the two or three associate deans, none were nurses. None of them knew anything about nurses. They were in the School of Health Services to educate this new kind of professional and as far as they were concerned, we were going to fit into their mission and purpose—or else.

Stella Shiber

The School of Health Services was a vision of the dean, Dr. Malcolm Peterson. He was discouraged by both medicine and nursing. His idea was to create this health associate program, which he compared to the barefoot doctors in China, a primary care, holistic approach. They were not envisioned initially as a physician's assistant. It was supposed to be a worker who was partly medicine, partly nursing. I think they needed a nursing program because that's where there were more students. The nursing program legitimized the school because everybody knows what a nurse is, but they didn't know what this health associate person was.

The idea was that the health care worker from that school was going to be a primary care worker. That's why the nurse practitioner programs fit well with that image. The students who went through the nursing program had many experiences in the community and in primary care and much more extensive physical assessment, interviewing, and so forth than was then in most baccalaureate programs.

Maureen Maguire

We had a big faculty and I think that was one of the problems—it was expensive. And it was a demanding program, when you realize these people had to find clinical placements, establish those relationships, do curricula, interview students, and prepare their coursework. They had to get ready for accreditation. They had to get ready for the nurse examiners. Plus, we're saying, "Would you please do some research?"

Kay Partridge

Dr. Nelson was the best of the old time physician-administrators, a gentle soul and very capable. It was a sea change when Heyssel came in. It was reflective of what was going on in health care at the time. Hopkins had to come in to be a full player in that scene.

Kay Partridge

physician providers of primary care), and clinical laboratory sciences. The base of operations would be in a renovated Hampton House and the target starting date was September 1973. A "core curriculum based on the biomedical sciences, with strong emphasis on the behavioral sciences, and methods of health care organization" would be common to the three programs. Teaching of combined student groups was envisioned as an opportunity for students—"physicians, nurses, health associates, clinical laboratory and radiology technicians"—to share experiences and to learn to work together as a team. The intent was "not to solve manpower problems within the Johns Hopkins Medical Institutions, or in the nation, by the production of numbers"; rather, the objective of the new school was to develop and demonstrate models for educating, training, and staffing health services.[15] Some who reviewed the plan did not regard a baccalaureate program in nursing favorably because of the university's reputation as a research university, and nursing research at that time was truly in its infancy. A program that would educate nurses with a greater focus on ambulatory care and physical assessment skills utilizing faculty shared with other programs was viewed as an appropriate compromise.

In April 1972 the Board of Trustees of the Johns Hopkins University approved the naming of the new division the School of Health Services. In presenting preliminary plans for the school to the board, Dr. Peterson stated that "the School of Health Services will educate young men and women to deliver direct patient care in both office and institutional settings. They will fulfill many of the functions which usually have been carried out by nurses and primary care physicians." In addition, the school would prepare students for careers in the management and administration of health care services. "Persons who understand the complexities of the health care field and newly emerging forms of health services organization are in very short supply, and they are being educated now at the baccalaureate level."[16] These statements were harbingers of some of the difficulties that would plague the school in later years: the lack of a clear delineation or understanding of how nurses differed from other health care providers, and the failure to distinguish what constituted undergraduate and graduate fields of study.

Administrative changes that would affect nursing were also taking place throughout the Hopkins system. In October 1972 Dr. Russell Nelson retired as president of the hospital, Steven Muller became president of both the hospital and the university, and Dr. Robert Heyssel assumed the position of executive vice president and administrator of the hospital. Nursing lost a strong supporter with the retirement of Dr. Nelson. Both the players and the administrative design would be important to the future of nursing within the institutions.

The official closing ceremony of the Johns Hopkins Hospital School of Nursing was held on June 15, 1973, and speakers included Lucile Petry Leone, 1927, Associate Professor Emeritus I. Ridgeway Trimble of the Johns Hopkins School of Medicine, Dr. Russell A. Nelson, and President Steven Muller. The speeches observed the closing of the School of Nursing, but the speakers, in their comments, also acknowledged changes within the system. They used the occasion not only to mark the closing of the school but also to forward their own agendas for the future of nursing within Hopkins. Dr. Trimble spoke highly and poignantly of Hopkins nurses. He was also intent on delivering his message that he could not understand why the university had not fulfilled its years of "promises" to have a baccalaureate school of nursing.

Dr. Nelson was emphatic about his view of the future of nursing education at Hopkins within the university:

The principles that must buttress our new school are clear and all important. It must and will be in and of our University, hopefully its nonmedical as well as medical parts. It must be part of the broad work we do in health, but be independent and free to chart its own course. It must aspire to the very best students and faculty, and it must have imagination and do research. It must encourage teamwork with other health professions and it must not, especially in its formative years, be too large and although it must do its teaching and research in patient care settings and all must be real practicing professionals, it must not be bogged down by too much routine and service obligation.[17]

Dr. Muller's remarks appeared somewhat inappropriate given the setting and circumstances; he was clearly not fully cognizant of the tensions involved in the closing of the School of Nursing and the opening of the School of Health Services. He spoke of the work of the search committee looking for a director of the nursing program and of how, although numerous persons had applied, one had become available as a candidate only within the past two months. He also spoke to the credentials of specific nursing alumni to serve as faculty, but he identified no one by name. Confident that students would be admitted to the baccalaureate program in September of 1974, he also spoke about nurses being recruited into the Health Associate Program.[18]

The first class of health associate students entered the School of Health Services in the fall of 1973. During the same academic year, a search committee continued its work to select a director for the Nursing Education Program. Committee members Doris Armstrong, Dr. Turner Bledsoe, Dr. Arthur Bushel, Dean Marion Murphy from the University of Maryland, Dr. Kay Partridge, Dr. Malcolm Peterson, Dr. Henry Seidel (chairman), Dr. Mary Betty Stevens, Dr. Jean Straub, and alumni association representative Genevieve Wessel, 1963, also sought to delineate the nature of the nursing program. At the same time faculty

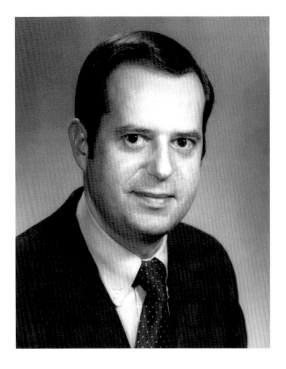

Steven Muller arrived at the Johns Hopkins University in 1971 to serve as provost. Less than nine months later, he was named president of both the university and the hospital, the first person to hold both titles since Daniel Coit Gilman. Although slow to appreciate issues enveloping nursing education at Hopkins, Muller later became a strong and essential advocate for a baccalaureate nursing program.

Malcolm Peterson, a physician who was the dean of the School of Health Services, was very public about being antinurse. He did not want a nursing curriculum. He was creating these new roles of health associate and health assistant. My understanding is that Steve Muller told Malcolm Peterson, "You've got to put a nursing program in there. I'm getting beaten up all over the country by the alumni of nursing and medicine. What do you mean you're starting this whole new school for these barefoot doctors but you don't even have any nursing education?"

Martha Norton Hill, 1964, BSN 1966

At Hopkins, physicians are God. It's just a fact of life. At Hopkins, it just never really dawned on them. They assumed the doctors could take care of everything. It was their world and their resources. It was just like breathing in and breathing out to them—not a whole lot of malevolence involved at all. It's just how they viewed the world and that was one of the ongoing struggles for Doris Armstrong. She was such a diplomat and she really achieved a great deal. That was a hard period. She really had a sense of nursing and its significance.

Kay Partridge

Coincidental with the hospital diploma school's closing, the growth in associate degree programs was taking place—which changed the way hospitals were able to recruit and to treat nurses. Generally, with your own school, you didn't have to care whether people stayed or not because every year you had a new crop coming out that were oriented to your way of doing things. That changed considerably. No longer could hospitals take nurses for granted and say, "We don't care whether you stay or not. You can take our salary and benefits and these hours or else, because we have a whole new class about to graduate. We would just as soon hire them anyway."

Stella Shiber

from the Nurse Practitioner Program, begun under the auspices of the hospital and the School of Public Health and later moved to the School of Health Services, began developing a baccalaureate curriculum in nursing education.

The Academic Council of the School of Health Services, composed at that time of members of the Health Associate Program faculty, asked that the search committee "provide a statement regarding the nature of a program in nursing." The committee responded that the nursing program should encompass the following broad objectives:

1. to prepare students at the baccalaureate and graduate level for a wide variety of nursing roles and specialties . . . ;

2. to insure that a sound academic base is closely linked with a strong practicum in a variety of health care settings utilizing clinical and behavioral skills . . . ;

3. to create a curriculum which has sufficient flexibility . . . ;

4. to relate education in the nursing arts and sciences with the education of other health professionals . . . ;

5. to prepare students to satisfy licensure requirements;

6. to allow the institution to satisfy state and national accreditation requirements.[19]

Dean Peterson appointed Dr. Kay Partridge director of the Nursing Education Program in September 1974. Partridge had a BSN with honors from the University of Colorado, an MPH with honors from the University of Pittsburgh, and a DPH from the Johns Hopkins School of Hygiene and Public Health. She began her career at Hopkins as a faculty member in the School of Public Health and then Doris Armstrong recruited her to be assistant director of the Woman's Clinic; Armstrong later recommended her for the position of director of the Nursing Education Program. Armstrong recalled Partridge as a bright, young, vigorous nursing professional "who got along well, at least as I determined it, with Malcolm Peterson and the other physicians in that program. I thought she could promote nursing within allied health."[20]

Before Partridge's selection, she was a member of the search committee. Someone had been selected for the position; however, at the last minute, that person elected not to come to Hopkins.[21] "They were down to the wire and that's when people began to turn to me to do it. I was there. I had most of the basic qualifications. I loved Hopkins and it was an honor to be able to step in and try to make a contribution to keep nursing alive," Partridge remembered later. "We had one year to try to put things together. It was hard to hire a faculty, find the students, get a curriculum together, and arrange clinical placements. It was ridiculous."[22]

A new era in Hopkins nursing education began in the fall of 1975, when the first students arrived for the School of Health Services baccalaureate program. The class of 1977 had thirty-two members, including four men, and ranged in age from nineteen to forty. The faculty was also nearly thirty-two in number, including both full-time and part-time members; several were graduates or faculty of the former Hopkins diploma program. The basic curriculum was an upper-division program founded on a liberal education encompassing the natural, social, and behavioral sciences and the humanities. Students would complete their first two years of prerequisites at any university or college and then attend Hopkins for the last two years of course work necessary to complete the bachelor of science in nursing degree.

Plans for the Nursing Education Program included the development of a part-time program, which would begin admitting students in September 1977. However, this plan was never realized, owing to internal problems in the School of Health Services. In June 1977, Dr. Peterson asked for Dr. Partridge's resignation as director. Reasons cited by the university for the dismissal were low student numbers and a curriculum that was not accredited because of its deficiencies. Associate Provost Richard Zdanis said, "It seemed to us that the only effective way to get a substantial change [in the curriculum] was to have a change in the director."[23] Dr. Peterson explained further that "the current as well as the proposed curriculum has not been noteworthy for innovation."[24]

Partridge recognized early on that "it was going to be a tough, tough sell." As she acknowledged years later, "the placement of nursing education in the School of Health Services was fatally flawed. First of all, the Health Associate Program and its culture and way of living and doing wouldn't have made so much of a difference except it was the antithesis of nursing. The problems they were trying to solve were the exact opposite of what nursing needed to do. They were trying to create a more humane bedside communicative deliverer of health care. Nursing has that. They're [nursing] trying to establish themselves as a profession that is worthy of receiving recognition and respect from other professions in its own regard." She continued, "It was an unhappy placement. To us, in nursing, it just didn't make sense." Partridge explained that the choice "most of us faced was, is it better to do something and get launched and at least have a presence and do the best we can versus doing nothing? The alumni certainly didn't want to do nothing."[25]

By calling for the resignation of Dr. Partridge, the university further delayed the accreditation of the program. The faculty had anticipated applying for accreditation during the summer of 1977, following the graduation of the first class and full approval by the Maryland Board of Nursing, both prerequisites for accreditation. That process was then delayed because the National League for Nursing (NLN), the nation's

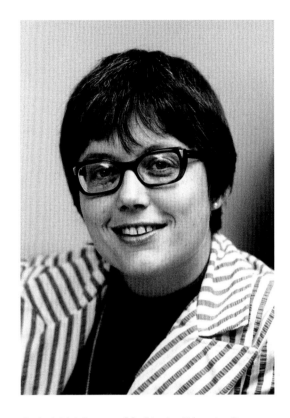

As the initial director of the Nursing Education Program, Kay Partridge hired a faculty, recruited students, developed a curriculum, and found clinical placements for students. "Our goal was to prepare a nurse to work effectively in whatever setting of health care there was, whether it was industry, public health, community, or hospital, and to give her the tools to get the job done," Partridge recalled. Her position reported to physician Malcolm Peterson, dean of the School of Health Services, who was less than supportive of the role of nursing within the division.

Kay Partridge was pretty accessible. She was a strong public-health nurse presence. Public health and research were part of the school's identity. They are a really important piece of nursing, but those who were expecting a more traditional nursing experience didn't really understand. For those students who had two years of college, which was probably half the students, nursing meant that you take care of patients and you learn all these skills and you give medications, give IVs, things like that. But the program was a little more community-focused than that.

Susan Carroll Immelt, 1977, PhD 2000

I really love nursing. I believe in nursing. I think it's truly the most significant thing that happens in health care, no matter what kind of health care. Nurses are responsible not only for hands-on care, but they're for the coordination, the communication. They're the ombudsmen. That's what's desperately needed. You talk to families and they're grappling with all this stuff. They can't penetrate the system. That's really what nursing is about— to make patient care happen in a way that is productive for the individual and the family.

Kay Partridge

Being that second class after the hospital school closed was a heavy weight on our shoulders. We weren't liked very much because we were representing this "new breed." Many times on the floors it was like, "These are the nurses who didn't go through the hospital school. Look at them. They obviously may have book knowledge but they don't know what they're doing." And it was true, because it was a very different way of nursing education. We weren't taught how to make a bed. We were taught how to make a bed with someone in it but not a bed by itself, so our beds weren't perfect. We never really felt welcomed. It was like, how are we ever going to measure up to the great Hopkins nurses from the old school?

Benita Walton-Moss, 1978

Student uniforms in the Nursing Education Program permitted some variety. Women could choose short or long sleeves on the white blouses worn under jumpers or sleeveless tunics. Linda Billman, 1977, hemmed her skirt above the knee, while Joan Wiener, Pat Sullivan, and another classmate preferred slacks. Andre Poe, one of four men in the class, wore a white necktie and trousers. Duty booties were history: evidently, students could wear whatever footwear they preferred.

only accrediting body for nursing programs at the time, required that a permanent director be in charge of the program. Since accreditation could be only eight months retroactive, this placed the graduates of 1977 in the dilemma of graduating from an unaccredited program, which could potentially hamper their efforts to pursue graduate education or a career in the military.

The faculty of both the Nursing Education Program and the Health Associate Program responded rapidly to Dr. Partridge's dismissal by giving an overwhelming vote of no confidence in Dean Peterson and demanding his resignation. Dean Peterson submitted his resignation but President Muller did not accept it, and Peterson remained in his administrative position. Faculty stated that a central issue was not the dismissal of Dr. Partridge but dissatisfaction because of Peterson's failure to consult with professors before making important decisions that affected the

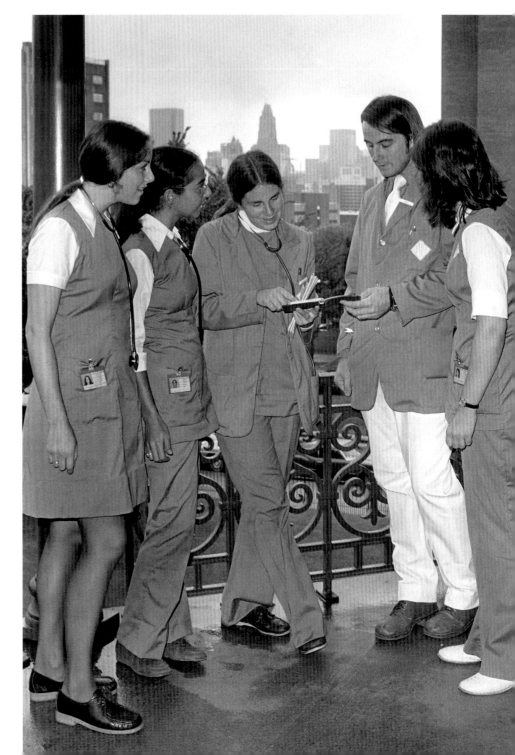

quality of education, including appropriations, promotions, and program evaluations. The faculty also pointed out that the nursing curriculum was developed by and belonged to the faculty and that the director should not be seen as wholly responsible for the curriculum.[26]

There was speculation among faculty that a comment by Carolyne Davis, a 1954 graduate of the hospital School of Nursing and associate vice president at the University of Michigan, had weighed heavily in the administration's decision to ask for the resignation. Dr. Davis stated during a meeting of the Visiting Committee, which Dr. Partridge had convened, that the nursing program as it existed in April 1977 would not be accredited. Davis acknowledged having made the comment but said this "was only one individual's opinion" and she doubted that the university's decision to ask for Dr. Partridge's resignation would have been influenced to a significant degree by the remarks of an outsider called in to evaluate the program.[27] Years later, Davis acknowledged that President Muller had asked her opinion as to the financial viability of the school and what to do about the nursing program. Muller, she said, was "very troubled" and had to make a decision. Although the school had received large sums of money from foundations,[28] it did not have any "hard" money, and schools at the very decentralized university did not borrow from one another. Likewise, Davis felt that the school could not ask the hospital for money because of its community emphasis; hence, the school was seen as a "non-fit." She said simply, "the program had wonderful faculty, wonderful students, and no money, and I could see no way to get them money." She also was "not sure they would get through the next round with the NLN. There was no choice but to close the school."[29] Following a conversation between Provost Richard P. Longaker and Davis, the provost noted that Davis had opined that it was difficult to recruit faculty to the program because there was no autonomy in the nursing program, the school was almost totally dependent on soft money, the financial picture was bleak, and there was not a university-wide commitment on the part of administration, which would be reassuring to those being recruited.[30]

Doris Roberts, a member of the Visiting Committee and chair of the committee's April meeting, observed that "the pragmatic, traditional focus of the curriculum described in the self-study [for NLN accreditation] was in sharp contrast to the innovative, experimental program we had discussed in earlier meetings. . . . In short, the Committee's criticism was essentially with the self-study packet which we felt represented an early draft but needed considerable refinement in order for it to reflect the nursing education program as we understood it to be functioning." A delay in the NLN accreditation visit was suggested, coupled with additional outside consultation. "This is not infrequently found in young programs preparing for their first national

The students and the faculty were good. In the faculty, I looked for clinical and academic competence and teaching experience. And you needed somebody who was willing to take a risk—it was a new program—people who are interested in creating rather than maintaining. It was a very unusual collection of faculty. The students were a wide range of what early-'70s young people were for the most part.

What you had to get were risk takers, who cared enough about nursing and really wanted to do something new. It gave us a chance to do something different within the limits, obviously, of the larger nursing-education world. They wanted to come. You did gather people who, for whatever reason—some good, some not so good—would be willing to participate in the adventure.

Kay Partridge

The faculty members hired for the School of Health Services were good people. One is now the dean at the University of Florida and president of the American Association of Colleges of Nursing. The dean at the University of Pittsburgh, who just retired, was an office mate of mine for a while. They were the kind of people that you would want to have on the faculty. They were knowledgeable, talented people. They were in a no-win situation but the students actually got a quality education.

Stella Shiber

To learn at the end that Carolyne Davis and the dean from Virginia had gone to Steven Muller and talked to him, to me was a betrayal of the worst sort. That's fine if they want to go to Muller and raise whatever concerns they had, but they owed it to their job, to their responsibilities, on that visiting committee and to our program to raise those concerns with me first. I never knew a thing about it. To me it just reflected the worst side of what happens in nursing, and it probably happens elsewhere.

Kay Partridge

We were all pretty saddened with the closing of the diploma school but we weren't going to give up. Then when the university decided it was Dr. Peterson who was going to do that BS program in the School of Health Services, I can tell you most of us weren't that happy. This was a physician who was going to do a baccalaureate nursing program. I guess it was probably a good idea that it happened, but we were disappointed. There were some very good students who came out of that program so that made you feel better, but then the program closed.

Ethel Rainey Ward, 1947

accreditation," Roberts pointed out. "The Committee's review and recommendations were intended to be wholly supportive of Dr. Partridge, the nursing faculty and the developing nursing education program."[31] Dr. Roberts was well aware of the "many ramifications of discord with potentially grave consequences to the nursing program," and she shared these concerns with Dr. Peterson following the resignation of Dr. Partridge.[32]

The resignation was greeted with dismay among faculty, alumni, members of the local and national nursing community, as well as nursing associations and organizations. Many wrote to President Muller to express their concern and support of Dr. Partridge and the program. Muller's response was consistent: the university remained committed to the continuation of the baccalaureate program in nursing education.

In searching for an acting director for the Nursing Education Program, Dr. Peterson suggested Becky Winslow, 1967, a nurse practitioner who co-directed a four-month adult nurse practitioner certificate program with Dr. Peterson from 1973 to 1976. He acknowledged that her administrative background was weak and that she was philosophically at odds with the majority of the faculty, but she was a graduate of the hospital School of Nursing and had many friends within that group. Clearly, Dr. Peterson was concerned about the response of alumni to Dr. Partridge's departure. Dr. Jean Johnson, professor and director of the Center of Research at Wayne State University, who was slated to fill the M. Adelaide Nutting Chair, was suggested as another possible candidate, with Winslow serving as interim director until Johnson could take the position.[33]

On June 22, 1977, the provost announced that Dr. Margaret E. Courtney would serve as acting director of the Nursing Education Program. "Johns Hopkins is totally committed to a baccalaureate program in nursing," pledged Provost Longaker. "We are determined that we will continue to make a substantial contribution to nursing education, and we will do so in a manner that assures a program of the highest quality." In addition to serving as the new acting director, Courtney continued her responsibilities as advisor for registered nurses and coordinator of the baccalaureate program in the Evening College, a position she had held since 1973, when the diploma School of Nursing, which she had overseen, closed. From 1973 to October 1976 Margaret Courtney was also director of continuing education for the nursing department at the hospital.[34] In selecting Dr. Courtney, the university chose someone with extensive administrative experience who was well versed in the history of the hospital School of Nursing, the Evening College program, and the School of Health Services and who was well known and respected by members of the university administration as well as the faculty and alumni.

In January 1978 the Board of Trustees of the Johns Hopkins University, acting upon a recommendation from the university administration, voted to close the School of Health Services on June 30, 1978, with the last class graduating in May 1979. At the time there were thirty-five full-time and forty part-time faculty members for a student body of 120 students in both the nursing and health associate programs. (The clinical laboratory sciences program never materialized.) The school had amassed a $700,000 deficit in fiscal year 1977, and a similar loss was anticipated for fiscal year 1978. President Muller regretted the closing, but financial constraints left the university with no alternative. Reasons given for the deficit included the absence of an endowment for the school, the high cost of education for primary care, a change in attitude by potential sponsors toward the need for allied health professionals (i.e., health associates, nurse practitioners) when some analysts were forecasting a physician surplus, and the difficulty of supporting undergraduate faculty from research grants. Faculty members raised issues of financial mismanagement, an extremely high faculty-student ratio, overreliance on soft monies, and the reluctance of Hopkins physicians to support the concept of health associates or physician assistants; however, the administration never officially addressed these concerns.

While Dr. Peterson was frequently viewed as nonsupportive of nursing, he recognized that at least a fair portion of the financial difficulties of the School of Health Services were related to the Health Associate Program. In a memorandum to Provost Longaker dated January 18, 1978, Dr. Peterson suggested that the School of Health Services be renamed the School of Nursing and Health Services, effective July 1, 1978, at which time a nurse would become the acting dean. He further suggested that the academic council of the school approve "in principle of the concept that the baccalaureate program in nursing will be terminated and a post-baccalaureate doctor of nursing three-year curriculum will be developed and planned." The doctor of nursing option would be in keeping with trends and recommendations of that time. Despite Peterson's support, the postbaccalaureate degree in nursing never came to fruition, although the academic council unanimously approved a motion to explore its creation on January 24, 1978.[35]

When President Muller formally announced the closing of the School of Health Services in February 1978, he declared, "An immediate planning effort will be launched to honor the University's commitment to nursing education by establishing a financially viable nursing program at the post-baccalaureate level. We regard this transition as a positive development for the profession and for the University and will, therefore, begin to plan such a program with enthusiasm and without delay."[36]

One of the tragedies of Margaret Courtney's life was that she got her doctorate at a time when few nurses had doctorates, and she came back to Hopkins assuming that they were going to move to collegiate education. That was clearly the expectation, that Dr. Courtney would be the person to head that effort. Then she got stuck with closing the diploma school and also they got her to close the School of Health Services. That had to be a terrible disappointment for her because she clearly loved Hopkins and expected that if and when they ever moved to a baccalaureate program that she could be the dean. She spent her whole life here and it never happened. That she was the one to close two of the schools of nursing is a remarkable irony.

Stella Shiber

The dean decided that he wanted the nursing program to go in a different direction. He wanted it more primary care and not as much in the hospital. He didn't like our whole approach. He had this vision of this new health care worker. He asked Kay Partridge, the director of nursing, to leave and planned to replace her. When she did leave, most of us also left. That's when Dr. Courtney came in to take over. She had been director of the diploma school. She recognized that the handwriting was on the wall over there, but because she was a Hopkins person, she would fill in the gap.

Maureen Maguire

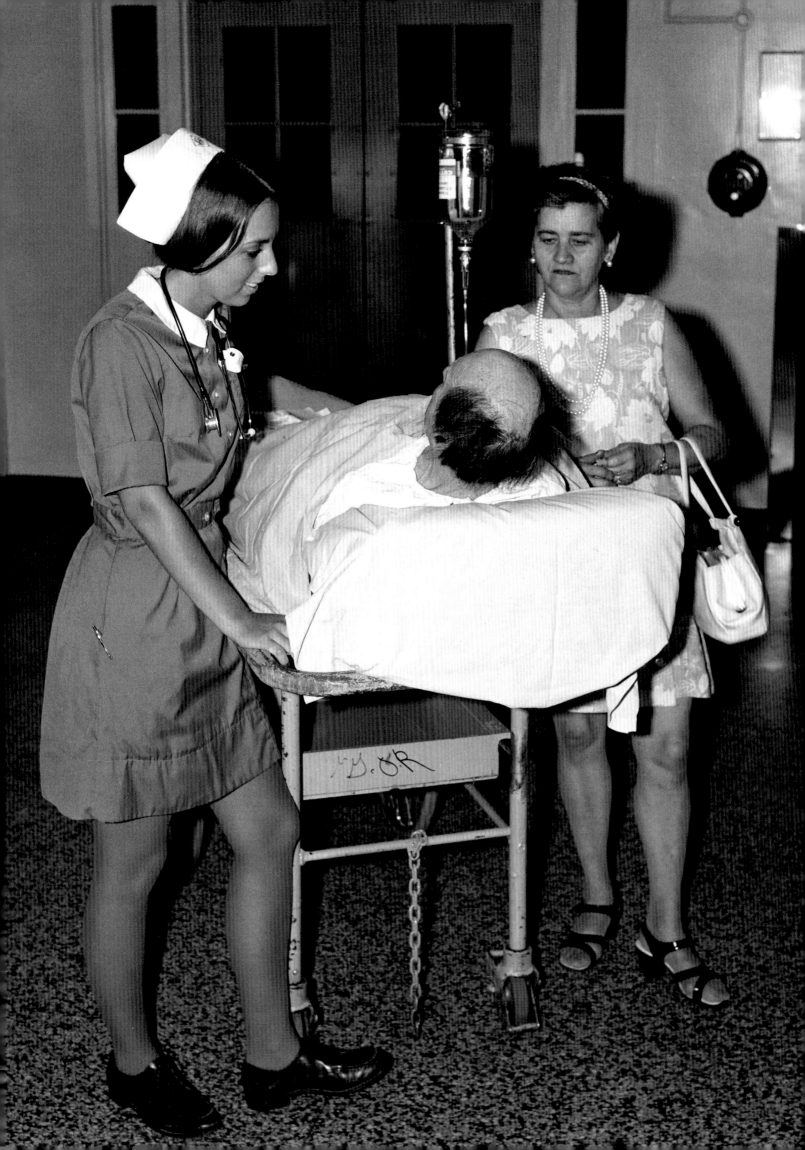

On September 8, 1970, fifty-four students entered as the last class of the Johns Hopkins Hospital School of Nursing, the class of 1973. Their experiences as students would be unlike those of any student who preceded them. This class had witnessed turmoil on college campuses, in American cities, and around the world during the 1960s. The Homewood campus was admitting its first class with undergraduate women just as the School of Nursing was closing. Students in this class, and many in preceding classes, had been clearly told about the trend toward baccalaureate education and been encouraged to consider such a program. Most students who selected Hopkins did so because of the Hopkins reputation for excellence and their desire to have an outstanding clinical experience from the outset of their education.

Life in Hampton House began as it had in years past with sign-ins and sign-outs, limited overnight passes, and no men above the first floor except on selected visiting Sundays. As the last class progressed through the program, the rules became less and less rigid, in part because no one was enforcing them and in part because there were no

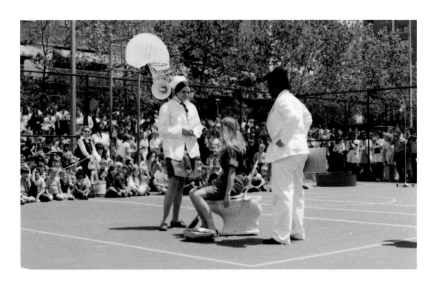

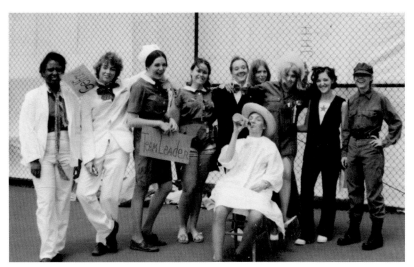

I recall that the person in admissions who was doing our interview said, "Now you know, Miss Appling, you should probably be going to a baccalaureate program." She did not say they were closing at the time but they strongly urged me, and other people within my class, not to come there but to go to a baccalaureate program. They were being very ethical. I was clueless. I just said, "Well, that's not what I want to do. I want to find out right away if I want to be a nurse." But they were very clear that there were other, probably better, alternatives.

Sue Appling, 1973

We were in a tough period. It was a tumultuous time and here we were in this program that had a curfew, for crying out loud. We couldn't go out at night. Curfew had been extended to midnight but it was originally ten o'clock that we had to be back in the dorm. We were allowed a certain number of overnights per month. That meant you had to get permission to go out and stay with even a family member. Meanwhile on the campuses there were coed dorms. It was a chaotic time.

Cathy Novak, 1973

Above: As the final days of classes approached, students in the last diploma class joined in turtle derby festivities on May 11, 1973. Patrice Sturm (wearing her cap) consulted with classmates Judy Jacoby Wickson (sitting on the "throne") and Joyce Williams, in a skit performed on the hospital tennis courts.

Below: The antics—and the costumes—got sillier that day as Joyce Williams, Susan Appling, Patrice Sturm, Robin Rennoe, Dawn Miller, Kathy White, Mary Ann Piper, Nancy Jenkins, and Judy Wickson lined up behind Karen Wolf.

Opposite: Bonnie LeHew, 1973, conversed with a patient as he waited on a gurney. Stella Shiber, a faculty member at the hospital school, recalled that students provided the lion's share of direct nursing care. "They had a number of classes, but the largest part of their time was spent working on the units with the patients."

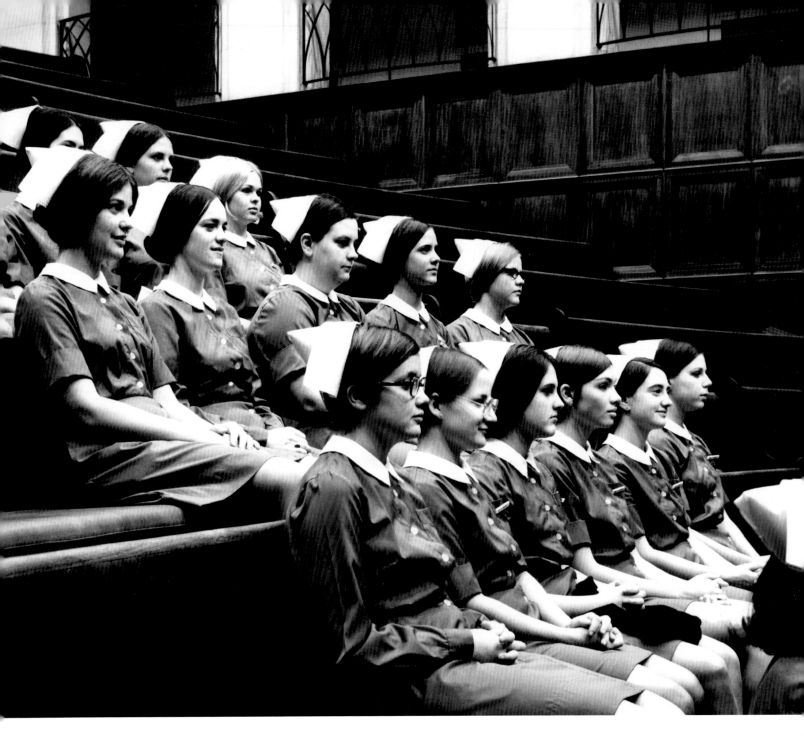

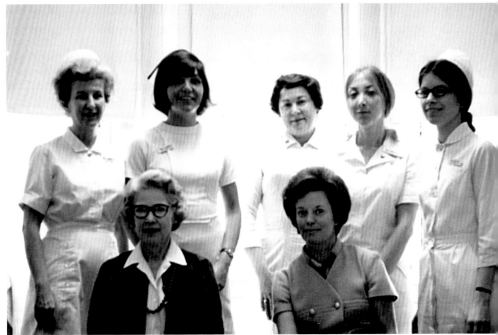

I remember Dr. Courtney telling us when we came for the freshman orientation to look on either side of us because, in three years, one of the three wasn't going to be here. At the beginning of the senior year Dr. Courtney welcomed us back, congratulated us on being in the third year, and said, "You're nine months away from your diploma but you're still nine months away from your diploma, so don't think that you can slack up now. Now's when it really gets tough because you have to put everything together." And she was right.

Cathy Novak, 1973

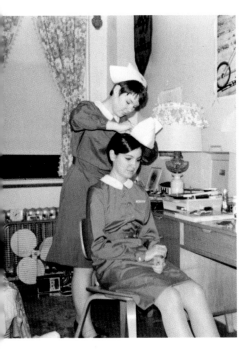

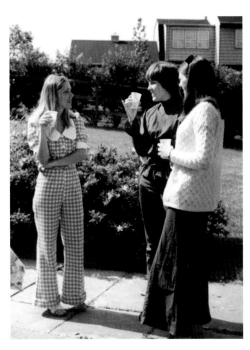

Marty Hill was one of our first-year instructors and then she moved over and taught medsurg nursing and team nursing. She was a very clear, everyday model of someone who is well informed, assertive about patient care. Joan Sutton was also a very good teacher. What made them really outstanding was not only their knowledge and expertise but also their ability to help the students figure out for themselves what they needed to do. If someone tells you constantly "Change this, fix this," you learn, but you don't learn in a way that you can think for yourself.

One of the best skills that I got out of Hopkins was, how do you sort your way out of this problem, especially if you're going to be the leader of the team. They taught you how to think your own way through a situation—how do you figure out what the priorities are, how do you put them in order, what do you use, how do you use the information around you, how do you collect it to begin with, what's important, what's not, what do other people know, how do you keep the communications going—it's very challenging. Their expectations were very high. They believed that you could perform in this manner and they expected it. Anything less was just not good enough. You were constantly being asked to give your best. There was no coasting in the program.

Cathy Novak, 1973

Opposite, above: Members of the classes of 1972 and 1973 gave their full attention to a speaker in Hurd Hall. Most wore their hair straight and their skirts short.

Opposite, below: Even faculty members became more relaxed about their uniforms. Betty Cuthbert (seated, wearing a dark sweater), 1943, was bareheaded when she posed for a group portrait for the yearbook, but her colleague Martha Norton Hill, 1964 (standing, far right), proudly wore her alumna cap.

underclassmen to indoctrinate. Students had pets in the dorm, and room inspections belonged to another era. "It felt odd and empty and a little bit sad because there were fewer of us in the dorm," recalled Cathy Novak, 1973. "We didn't have the pleasure of passing on some of the traditions, and I think we would have liked that. I think we would have made good Big Sisters."[37] Time with faculty was more frequent and more intimate than in years past. Some instructors invited small groups of students to their homes for dinners or picnics, and Ira Morris, an Osler resident, became the "patron saint" of the class.

Dr. Margaret Courtney, director of the school, was seen as an authority figure, someone to react against simply because of her position. Mary Jane Donough, associate director, was truly middle management, often serving as the buffer between the students and Dr. Courtney. As director, Courtney continued to teach a Trends in Nursing course in the senior year. Susan Appling, 1973, remembered the class being taught in the lobby of Hampton House in a relaxed atmosphere with all the students in a semicircle around Dr. Courtney. "She was very knowledgeable and did not seem the threatening, autocratic person we had heard about."[38]

The students were certainly aware of their place in history as the last class to graduate from the Johns Hopkins Hospital School of Nursing. The twenty-sixth and final candlelight service was held on November 30, 1970. (In 1945 the candlelight service had replaced the capping ceremony after the completion of the probation period.) The occasion marked the first time each student wore a blue uniform and cap and pledged to abide by the honor code. During this last candlelight service, senior Barbara Bernhard, 1971, was selected to make remarks. She

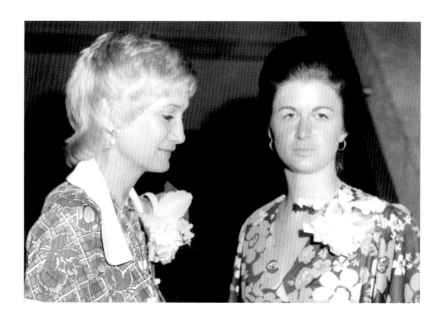

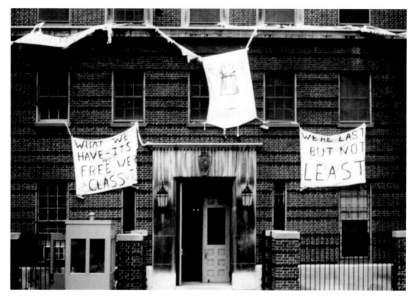

Hospital trustees honored the school with two formal events in 1973: the final commencement on June 16 and a ceremony the day before to observe the formal closing.

Above right: Genie Lipa Wessel, 1963, left, who had just completed her term as president of the alumni association, and Jean Stauffer Roberts, 1968, the current president, found little cause for cheer at the ceremony.

Graduating students had a very different perspective. *Below right*: They plastered the front of Hampton House with banners announcing their pride in being "last but not least." *Opposite, above*: Graduates seemed very pleased as they posed in the rotunda of the Administration Building. *Opposite, below*: Belying their prim attire, Rosemary Waites, Kathy Nix, Karen Nelson, and Debbie Chadwick gleefully "revealed" their joy at having survived three years at Hopkins.

acknowledged that members of this last class might have "an especially difficult task in maintaining a tradition that seems to be dying. But when you feel discouraged or sad about this, let the knowledge of your position, privileged and last, lift your spirit. As you light your candles tonight, may they keep burning as a personal inspiration to each of you in your search for responsibility, knowledge, and honor within the horizons of nursing.[39]

Cathy Novak, 1973, reported in the student news section of the alumni magazine in 1972 that it was becoming very hard to avoid the reality that the school was going to close the following year. "The floors of Hampton House were beginning to be consolidated and students were required to move down to lower floors." She noted that plans were already under way to make the final graduation special so that "the closing of the School will be as significant and memorable as the opening."[40]

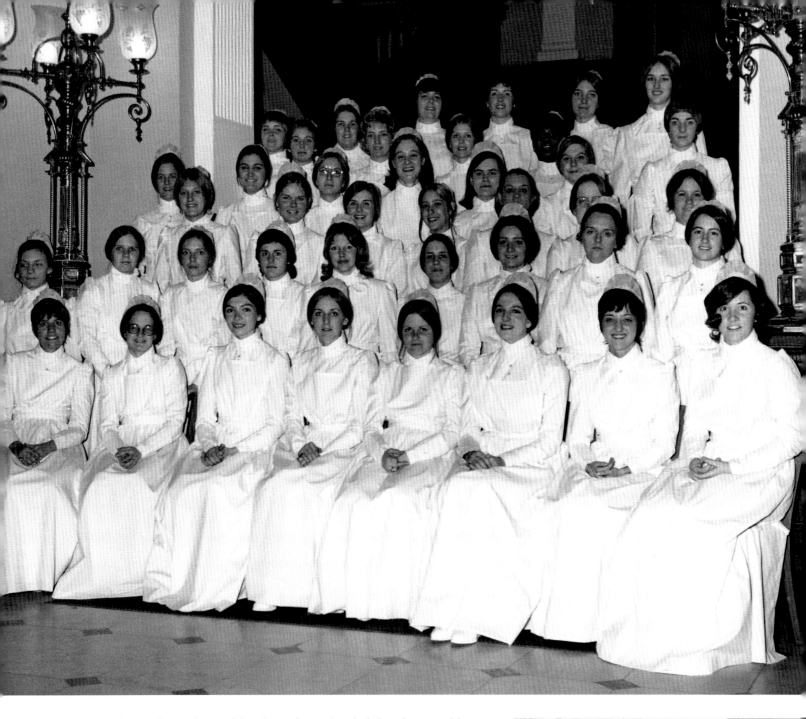

To that end, members of the class of 1973 decided that they would wear replicas of the original Johns Hopkins School of Nursing uniform, a long white dress covered with a long white apron. The graduation uniforms were a joint endeavor of the class of 1973 and alumni from previous years. Susan Appling developed the pattern for the uniform by piecing together commercial patterns and drawing other pattern pieces. Alumni assisted with pattern development and sewing for those students who could not sew, in addition to providing funds to purchase the material for the uniforms. Novak fondly reminisced:

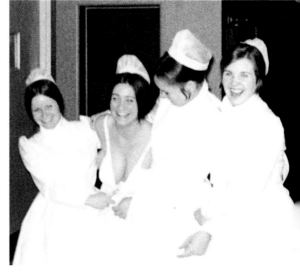

One of the things I think I'm most proud of was the suggestion to graduate in the uniforms of the early graduating classes. We felt the weight of it, I think, in that last year and the finality of it and the sadness of it. Yet, we felt triumphant. We wrestled with how do we do honor to ourselves and do honor to the school. A lot

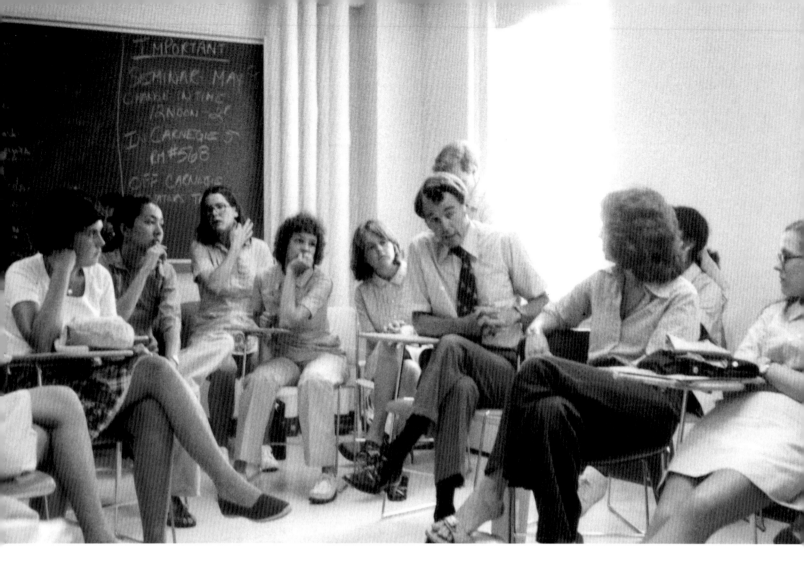

Students in the Nursing Education Program in the School of Health Services could wear whatever they liked to class but uniforms were required for clinical time in the hospital. The dean of the school, Malcolm Peterson, taught some classes to nursing students as well as to health associate students. Susan Carroll Immelt, 1977, PhD 2000, remembered that Peterson "taught a fluid electrolyte class. It was very clever but sort of shallow. He was very friendly and good looking and interested in getting to know us."

I can't specifically remember what our complaints were, but we did end up going to the provost of the university and complaining about the education we were getting in the program. It had to do with not getting enough hard science to support our clinical work. In retrospect, with my experience teaching nursing, we really didn't get very much science, certainly not anywhere near what we expect of nursing students now. Also, we were not accredited until after we were finished. That was a really big source of anxiety.

Susan Carroll Immelt, 1977, PhD 2000

of us felt it was the right thing to do but it just felt insurmountable. The alumni helped and our families helped and our friends helped and instructors helped. It was a very full time, and it was very bittersweet.[41]

Graduation day, June 16, 1973, was sunny, hot, and muggy. Each graduate received a bouquet of long-stemmed red roses from the Johns Hopkins Medical Association as she entered the door of Turner Auditorium. (Members of the first class had also carried bouquets of roses—a gift from Dr. William Osler—at their commencement.) Leading the students into the auditorium, dressed in the blue student and pinky uniforms of 1915, were the new president of the alumni association, Genie Wessel, 1963, and the immediate past president, Jean Stauffer Roberts, 1968. Miss Wolf sent her own alumni pin to Cathy Novak, president of the class and recipient of the Anna D. Wolf Award. By the end of the ceremony, many had tears in their eyes—graduates, faculty, alumni, family, Hopkins family, and friends.[42]

While participants in the Hopkins diploma program had been a largely homogeneous group, the students entering the new Nursing Education Program in the School of Health Services in 1975 were extremely diverse. Some were upper-division college students who had completed their first two years of liberal arts and sciences requirements at Hopkins or other institutions, while others already had baccalaureate or master's degrees and were married or divorced with children. Some had served in the Peace Corps, been active in local politics, traveled extensively, or been community activists. They came to the program from varied backgrounds and had differing ideas about nursing, about their potential careers in the profession, and about how Hopkins would prepare them for that career. Susan Carroll Immelt, 1977, recalled that members of her class "tended to be sort of nontraditional, ex-hippie type of people, vegetarians, very interested in alternative health. That was a great experience, getting to know different kinds of people and working with them. There were four men in our class. They fit in very well. We were all friends and in it together."[43]

Gale Reikenis and Linda Benson, members of the class of 1977, wrote in an article in a short-lived alumni newsletter that they expected to be prepared to operate as fully functional nurses in their selected area of specialty immediately after graduation. In addition, they believed their class would be familiar with methods of nursing research and able to carry out a professional research study. While these statements may simply indicate the naiveté of undergraduates, they may also be indicative of the faculty's confusion as to what level of practitioner they were preparing and the

We thought it was important that students know what happens at the change of shifts, so they had to be there at seven in the morning. Unheard of. Nursing education didn't do that, see. They didn't like that but it happens to make a difference, as a clinician, to know what happens. We had them do some time in the OR. Unheard of. They criticized it. It just makes a difference if you have seen a doctor leaning back on his heels with that retractor on somebody's abdomen, holding wide an incision. It's important, when you're taking care of someone who's had surgery, to have some appreciation of what those people have undergone in the OR. They need to have that exposure.

Kay Partridge

Like generations of nursing students before them, Jeanne Borowicz, Dana Cohen Dias, and Karen Shank Santmeyer, members of the class of 1978, found time for high jinks, even in the hospital.

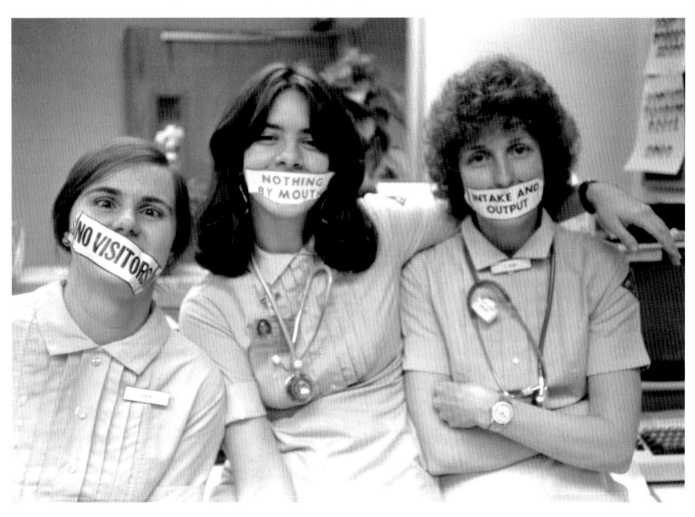

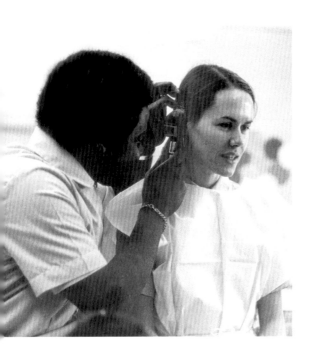

Wendell Street and Katherine Boyle demonstrated, for children at a Head Start center in 1977, how a doctor or a nurse might examine a patient. Kay Partridge, who directed the Nursing Education Program in the School of Health Services, had a strong public-health background and she wanted students to have exposure in that field. "Nursing was the arm that was closest to the community and to the families," she stressed.

students' need to defend the program to the diploma-prepared alumni. Reikenis and Benson also emphasized the number of clinical hours (1,540 hours in the two-year program) in their article—an important factor that would not go unnoticed by Hopkins graduates.[44]

Despite the problems inherent in any new program, graduates fondly recalled faculty members committed to helping students become exceptional nurses with excellent clinical experiences at Hopkins Hospital and surrounding city and county health departments, and they commented on the satisfaction of succeeding at Hopkins. Alumni of the Nursing Education Program went on to become nurse managers, clinical specialists, nurse practitioners, university educators, administrators, and health policy analysts. Eileen Gallagher Leahy, 1978, went to the University of Virginia as a new graduate on a cardiology floor. An attending physician looked at her school pin and said, "Thank goodness there is a Hopkins nurse at Virginia. Nurses from Hopkins know how to run things." From that point on, Leahy felt she "was part of something special."[45] Even though the School of Health Services' Nursing Education Program was short-lived and fraught with difficulties, its graduates were well prepared as leaders in nursing.

Some of the younger students in the program lived in Reed Hall, the medical student dormitory, while most of the older students lived outside the East Baltimore area. The heterogeneity of the student body and the dearth of shared living spaces perhaps contributed to the difficulty students may have had in forming an identity with Hopkins and the nursing students who had gone before them. In addition, the concept of "Hopkins nursing" was foreign to many members of the faculty, few of whom were graduates of the hospital diploma program. While some wanted to maintain the heritage of the hospital school, others felt that the best way to shape a new type of practitioner was to establish distance from that history and from historical images of women and nursing. In the end, though, even absent student homogeneity and a shared heritage with the faculty, the Nursing Education Program students elected to keep the Hopkins graduate cap, adding a blue and gold velvet stripe to identify the baccalaureate graduates. The students also elected to keep the blue enamel Maltese cross pin, with the letters *JHU* in place of *JHH* in the center, adopting the alumni pin as a school pin.

The first class of students to receive a bachelor of science in nursing degree from the Johns Hopkins University graduated in 1977. Each member of the class received a red rose from the alumni association, recalling the tradition that had been reestablished with the last class of the diploma school. By the time the School of Health Services closed in 1979, it boasted a total of seventy-one alumni. The class of 1977 graduated with thirty members; the class of 1978 produced twenty-six; and the class of 1979 claimed fifteen members.

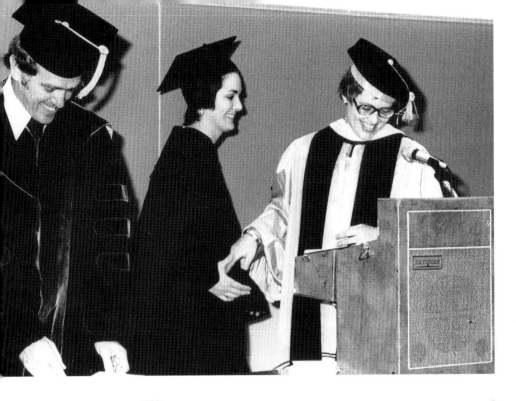
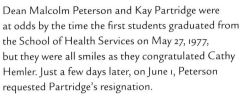

Dean Malcolm Peterson and Kay Partridge were at odds by the time the first students graduated from the School of Health Services on May 27, 1977, but they were all smiles as they congratulated Cathy Hemler. Just a few days later, on June 1, Peterson requested Partridge's resignation.

Many School of Health Services graduates have made a significant contribution to the profession. There were only three classes. They had some unfortunate things happen while they were there, but I never ever would back off from saying they got a quality education. They were extremely well prepared and they've made significant contributions. And I think they realize that now. In large part, they have gone on to do some remarkable things against a lot of odds.

Stella Shiber

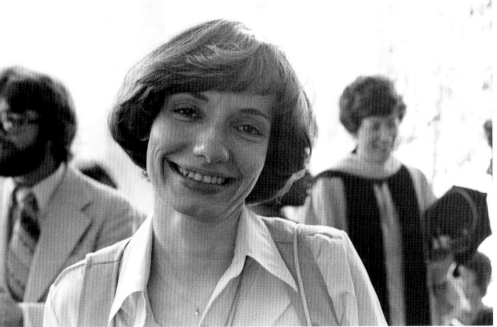

Left: Fran Keen, 1970, who taught in the Nursing Education Program, watched the drama of its gradual collapse. Still, she managed an enthusiastic smile at graduation in 1978.

Members of the class of 1978, the second to earn baccalaureate degrees in nursing from the Johns Hopkins University, posed for an informal group portrait for a class yearbook that was never published. Only one additional class would graduate from the School of Health Services before it folded.

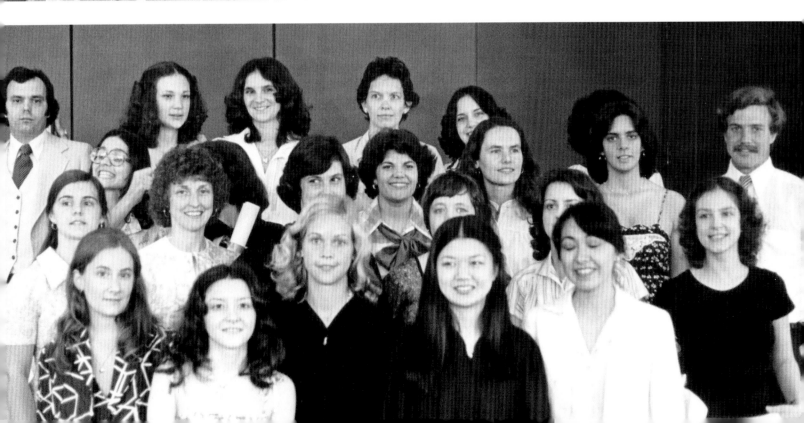

The alumni association was the glue that kept all those alumni together when the school closed. If you look at what happened to other alumni associations of schools that closed, they disintegrated. But the force of these women was so strong that they continued to hold reunions, they continued to keep that Nutting Fund strong, and they continued to work toward having university status.

Paula Einaudi

Everybody was very sad but we realized that the time had come. Then they wanted to train nurses and physicians' assistants in the same program. We could have told them it wouldn't work but nobody listened.

Betsy Mumaw McGeady, 1955

I was active in the alumni association. We felt it was incumbent on us to try to keep ourselves together as a unit in the hopes that there would be a new school. The School of Health Services came to be but didn't last long. After it closed, there were rumblings that we would make efforts to try to get the school started in another, more positive, direction. The alumni association always felt that there was a purpose other than just being: to be there, to keep things going, and to keep people involved so that when the school was reestablished, they'd have a base from which to draw support— not just monetarily, but the support of knowing that nurses before support the school now.

Sue Appling, 1973

With the closing of the Johns Hopkins Hospital School of Nursing, the alumni association faced an extraordinary reality: their reason for being no longer existed and their numbers would steadily decrease over the years. Jean S. Roberts, president of the association, spoke to these problems at the annual business meeting held just before commencement on June 16, 1973.

With this graduation, our organization's object[tive], as stated in our by-laws, ends. We can no longer "promote the interest of the Johns Hopkins Hospital School of Nursing." Therefore, we face the need for redefining our reason for being. With this graduating class, we cease to have an annual influx of new members. Our major source of income—dues—will steadily decline. Another factor which is pressing us to action is that we must vacate our office space when the Main Residence is razed for the new Cancer Institute. We must relocate before January 1, 1974.

Options for the future included dissolving the organization, remaining in the present form as long as economically possible, redefining the organization's area of support to include a project within the hospital and redefining the membership, or joining the Johns Hopkins University Alumni Association but retaining integrity as a professional group.[46] The eventual outcome, after much discussion by the leadership and membership of the association, would be to join the Johns Hopkins University Alumni Association while retaining its identity as a strong professional group within that association.

Integral to the alumni association and its relationship with the hospital and the university was the M. Adelaide Nutting Endowment Fund. The original purpose of the fund as set forth in 1915 was "to raise endowment for the school and in favor of provision for adequate financial support as necessary basis for all training work." In 1929 the alumnae association had voted that $100,000 of the Endowment Fund collected by the nurses be dedicated to Miss Nutting and be called the M. Adelaide Nutting Fund of the Johns Hopkins Hospital Nurses' Alumnae Association. Although minutes are vague as to the fund's purpose, a history of the fund appearing in the alumnae magazine in 1933 clearly demonstrated the desire of the association to provide more academic and scholastic opportunities for student nurses by providing an adequately funded school to accomplish this aim.[47]

With the closing of the School of Nursing in 1973, the dissolution of the Advisory Board of the Johns Hopkins Hospital School of Nursing, which approved expenditures from the Nutting Fund, and the possible dissolution of the alumni association, the M. Adelaide Nutting Endowment Fund became an issue of paramount importance to the alumni association, the hospital, and the university. By March 1973 the book value of the fund had increased to $466,000, with a market value of $821,000. In addition, a small sum retained by the alumni association

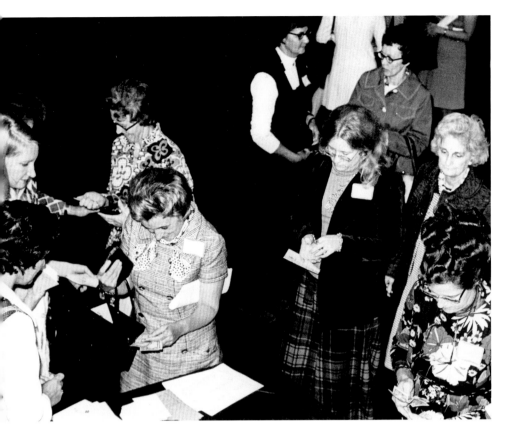

Betty Cuthbert and Joan Sutton were working so hard to have a university school, just to keep the idea of it going. They were real movers and shakers in guarding the Nutting Fund. We had this money that the alumni association had grown over many, many years of contributions. It was held by the alumni association with the hope that someday there would be a university school of nursing. The hospital really, really wanted to have access to those funds. Betty and Joan were the ones who just kept on top of it with lawyers and with the blessing of the alumni board to make sure that those funds stayed within the alumni association.

Sandra Stine Angell, 1969, BSN 1977

Nutting Endowment Fund Committee for the purpose of raising additional funds had grown to approximately $40,000. The initial goal of $1 million to be applied solely to the "educational works of the School" was clearly within reach, but now there was no school. The alumni association was eager to see its original financial goal met and the aims of the fund maintained; the hospital wanted to preserve the fund as part of its portfolio; and the university desired the monies as funding for a university-based program.

The Advisory Board of the School of Nursing continued beyond the closing of the diploma program, with the handling of the Endowment Fund as its primary purpose. No expenditures could be made from the fund without the approval of the advisory board. In addition, Michael Ventura, attorney for the hospital, determined that "after a review of the history, minutes and intention of the Nursing Association, the manner and restrictions placed on the use of the funds in its offer to the Hospital and the acceptance of the gift acknowledging this restriction to its use, it is my opinion that the *income* from the M. Adelaide Nutting Fund may only be used for such purposes as are approved by the Nursing Association Endowment Committee." Interpretations of the letter at alumni association meetings concluded that Ventura had confused the committee with the advisory board in his letter; nonetheless, the letter clarified the original intent of the fund and made evident that this money had been raised *by* nursing alumni *for* nursing education. Even

The association was looking to have funds available, if and when the nursing school became a part of the university, so that we could have our own professor. I was writing letters encouraging people to give money to the annual fund. We came to find out that our funds partially were helping to support the School of Health Services. The money wasn't being used as we had directed it. They were using the funds to pay for secretaries and paper and pencils, which is not where the money was intended to go. The funds were intended for education.

I decided that I could not ask people to support something that I did not believe in myself. I wrote a letter that said, "I cannot, in good conscience, ask you support a cause that I cannot support myself." They did send it and our contributions went way down. People said they would not give us another cent until we had our school.

Betsy Mumaw McGeady, 1955

Joan Sutton was the perfect nurse. Joan wore this beautiful starched old-fashioned uniform with the bib. She was very professional. I would work so hard to make sure I did a good job so I would get her appreciation. She was always very fair. She treated you almost like a peer.

Sue Appling, 1973

People think of Hopkins as an elitist institution. But I am impressed with Hopkins' willingness to look at problems and say, "This is a problem and we have to fix it" and not accept second best. If something's not right, nobody's going to sweep it under the carpet and say it didn't happen. That is what I feel is really great about it.

People are very aware of things that have happened, like the Nursing Education Program in the School of Health Services. There are places that would let those things just go on and wouldn't say, "This is not good enough. We need to do something different." Being able to look at something and say, "This has to be better" is a characteristic of an elite institution. I think that's good. That's what I've learned by being associated with Hopkins. That's an expectation that you are going to try to really do your best.

Susan Carroll Immelt, 1977, PhD 2000

If they had done nothing, in my opinion, in the '70s, I think the inertia for starting a school of nursing would have been too great. But because they had this School of Health Services, they had access to some faculty members and some nurse leaders so there was a nursing presence and people they could talk to. Now, imagine that that didn't exist. But because they were getting reports and they knew nursing was doing fine, that's what allowed them to flip it over into a proposal for a new school of nursing. My perception is if that failed school hadn't occurred and hadn't involved nursing, they wouldn't have gotten a new school of nursing.

Sue Donaldson

without the authority to approve expenditures directly, the alumni association, through its representative to the advisory board and through the Nutting Endowment Fund Committee, remained embroiled in discussions about the future of the fund for years.

On May 11, 1974, the alumni association voted to reaffirm the intent of the fund, namely, to advance education in nursing. In addition, the membership made a list of recommendations to the Advisory Board of the Johns Hopkins Hospital School of Nursing. The specificity of these recommendations indicates the depth of the membership's concern about the future of nursing education at Hopkins and the institution's management of the fund. The recommendations adopted were that:

—a Professorship in Nursing be established in the Johns Hopkins University for the purpose of promoting nursing practice, scholarship, and research;

—the endowed Professorial Chair be named the M. Adelaide Nutting Chair of nursing;

—the M. Adelaide Nutting Endowment Fund be used to endow the Professorship;

—the principal and interest of the M. Adelaide Nutting Endowment Fund now held by the Johns Hopkins Hospital be transferred to the Johns Hopkins University and be given the right to select the individual to fill the chair within the following guidelines:

—that the recipient demonstrate clinical competence in nursing commensurate with Professional status (i.e., in nursing practice, scholarship, and research);

—that the chair not be used for a faculty position in which the major responsibility is administration;

—the Professorship be established within five (5) years from the date of acceptance of this agreement;

—within five (5) years (prior to the selection of the recipient of the chair) the M. Adelaide Nutting Endowment Fund may be used for support of temporary nursing professorships;

—the Trustees of the Johns Hopkins University report annually to the Alumni Association of the Johns Hopkins Hospital School of Nursing, Inc., on the uses made of the M. Adelaide Nutting Endowment Fund, giving sufficient detail so that the Alumni Association will be able to determine if the Fund is being used in accordance with the above designated purposes....

—should the Professorial Chair in Nursing not be established in the Johns Hopkins University within the period of five (5) years from the date of acceptance of this agreement, then a representative of the Trustees of the Johns Hopkins University and a representative of the Alumni Association of the Johns Hopkins Hospital School of Nursing, Inc., shall meet to consider the matter and attempt to resolve it.[48]

The Johns Hopkins Hospital School of Nursing Advisory Board unanimously approved the recommendations on June 25, 1975.[49] The end result was that the fund's principal was maintained in the portfolio of the hospital, while the earned income was transferred to the university. Any new gifts to the fund would go to the university, and the eventual goal would be to transfer all funds from the hospital to the university.

In September 1976, one year after the admission of the first class of students to the Nursing Education Program of the School of Health Services, Dr. Kay Partridge, director of the program, sent a letter to the alumni association concerning the status of the M. Adelaide Nutting Chair in Nursing. A search committee had been formed to develop guidelines and review applications for the chair. The committee envisioned the work of the Nutting Professor as 50 percent research, 25 percent teaching and formal courses or seminars, and 25 percent faculty development. Applicants would be doctorally prepared and have given evidence of productivity in research and teaching. Of interest and concern to the alumni was the omission of any mention of *clinical* expertise, *clinical* practice, or *clinical* research, hallmarks of Hopkins nursing.

At the eighty-fourth annual meeting of the alumni association, in 1976, the membership directed the association to establish the M. Adelaide Nutting Ad Hoc Committee, with Joan Masek Sutton, 1963, as chair; Betty Cuthbert, 1943, and Betty Scher, 1950, as members; and Constance Waxter, 1944, Nancy Boykin, 1953, and Linda Norris as ex-officio members. In March 1977 the committee met with Dr. Partridge and Dr. Peterson to express concerns about the major emphasis on research as opposed to education, the emphasis on a joint appointment, and the status of the Nutting Professor compared to other professors in the university, particularly with regard to eligibility for tenure. The committee was also concerned that the university had not provided annual expenditure reports to the alumni association, as originally agreed upon.

However, with the resignation of Dr. Partridge in June 1977 and the announcement of the closing of the School of Health Services in February 1978, the M. Adelaide Nutting Chair of Nursing in the School of Health Services was never filled. By June 1978, the portion of the Nutting Fund held by the alumni association had increased to $62,000 and the portion held by the hospital and university had increased to $665,000, with income from the fund amounting to $105,000, for a total of nearly $770,000 to be applied to a future university school of nursing.[50] Through a time of unprecedented and unimaginable difficulty, the alumni association had persevered and triumphed in maintaining the integrity of its organization and its monies as it aimed to continue to foster nursing education within the Hopkins institutions.

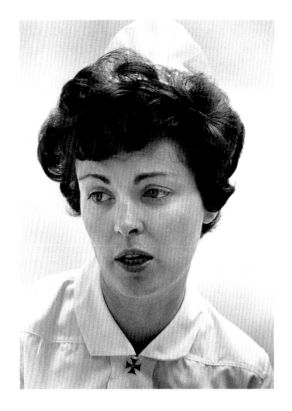

When nursing alumni voted to join the university's alumni association, Joan Masek Sutton, 1963, a favorite instructor with many students, became the nurses' alumni association representative on the executive committee. She was a stalwart protector of the Nutting Fund.

More than anyone else, Betty Liggett Cuthbert, 1943, was credited with protecting the material legacy of nursing history at Johns Hopkins. When the nurses' library closed, she hauled much of its contents to her home for safekeeping. Ultimately, university and hospital authorities recognized that establishing a university school of nursing, Cuthbert's fondest wish, was in the best interest of all.

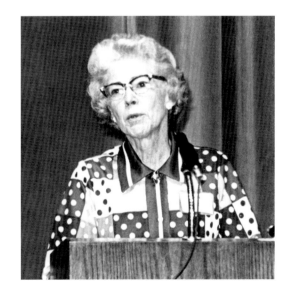

"Beyond the Bedside"

In the last few years the whole field of nursing work has been expanding and developing in an extraordinary degree. The service of nurses today reaches very far beyond the bedside care for the sick in hospitals and homes. It extends into public schools, shops and factories, into crowded city blocks, and scattered rural districts, and into every branch of city, state, and national health service. It concerns itself with education for the prevention of disease as well as with the care of the sick.

Elsie Lawler, 1899, speaking at commencement in 1921

I was immediately impressed with the architecture and the history of Hopkins. I was fascinated by the neighborhood and the cultural differences in the community. It was unlike anything I had ever seen or experienced before. It was obvious that there was a great deal of poverty and a great deal of need, and I found the juxtaposition of that community mix to this high-tech intensive tertiary care center an interesting contrast.

The Eastern Health District was one of the premier health departments and health districts in the country. In the 1920s, '30s, and '40s, there was a very strong nursing presence with Ruth Freeman and then people like Anna Scholl and others who were on the faculty of the School of Hygiene and Public Health.

Martha Norton Hill, 1964, BSN 1966

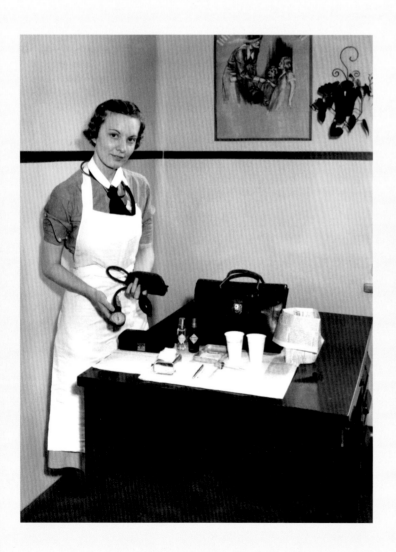

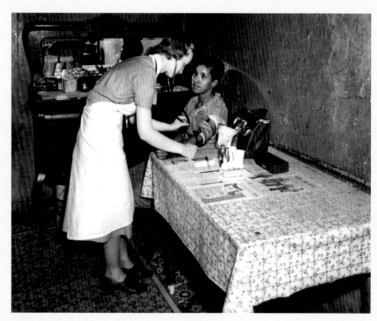

From 1934 to 1952 students explored the field of public-health nursing through the Dispensary Visiting Nurse Service. *At left*: A student gathered the equipment she would need for a prenatal exam. *Above*: She made use of her skills in the home of an expectant mother, probably in a tenement not far from the hospital.

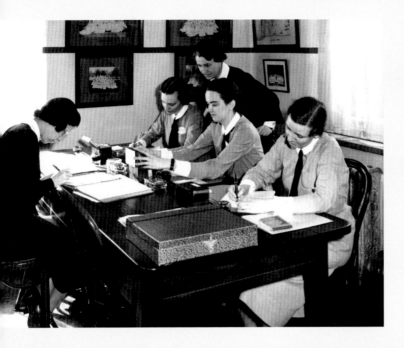

We went to the Eastern Health District, which was the public-health office for East Baltimore. It was pretty amazing. They just gave us twelve charts and said, "Go see these people." Lots of times they were well-baby visits so you'd check the baby, you'd check the mom. Other times it was general health visits. It was probably the toughest thing we ever did because you were out there on your own.

Occasionally, your instructors would come with you to watch you. I remember the first case my instructor had with me. We were going to a family that I'd gone to two or three times and I'd never gotten an answer. We walked up the steps and banged on the door and this lady started screaming through the door at me. I calmed her down. I did what I needed to do and left. Then the next family was much calmer and quieter. Then the instructor said, "You did a good job. You were able to vary your approach to different people depending on their reactions."

I never really liked community health because it was so hard. You were out there all by yourself, making decisions and having to take in many, many other factors and putting it all together and trying to synthesize things. It was very challenging. They would just keep piling cases on to us. We would see these patients, hand the records back in, and they'd give us more.

Sue Appling, 1973

In the community right around Hopkins hospital and the School of Nursing we went to visit a family and provide them with some very basic services and a support system. It would be an aunt who was raising her sister's children because her sister's a drug addict. Some of the kids end up having HIV and they have no medical insurance. They're older row houses with paint peeling off the walls and you see roaches crawling by. There were signs on the walls because they had people boarding in the house to help pay the rent. It wasn't a "There is no drug use in my house." It was "There is no f-ing drug use in my house." Kids can certainly read. It was like, "Oh, my goodness. What are they learning?" We were paired up with another nursing student. You can see open air drug deals going on all the time. My patient was an elderly woman who wasn't literate and just needed support to make sure she knew what her blood pressure medications were. We'd go in every week and check her blood pressure and make sure everything was fine and help teach her how to cook without dousing everything with salt.

Kate Knott, 2002

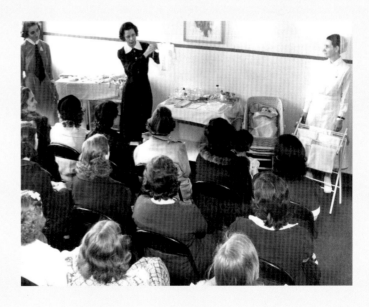

When Loretta Long and Mary Farr, both 1941, left the Woman's Clinic for an obstetrics appointment, they removed their aprons and put on a tie, transforming themselves into Dispensary Visiting Nurses. After 1952 students gained public-health experience through assignments in the Eastern Health District, a subdivision of the Baltimore City Health Department.

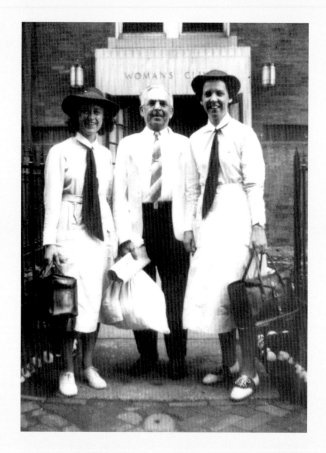

I've always thought that Wolfe Street was one of the widest streets in the world. If you were a nursing student in the hospital's School of Nursing, you knew very little about the School of Public Health. You knew it was there, but you didn't know much about what happened or what they did, what they were teaching, what their programs were. They were all graduate level. You might hear about some of the nurse faculty in the School of Public Health, and they might come and give a lecture, but there was no formal connection or relationship.

Now we have an MSN/MPH dual-degree program. It's for students who are interested in nursing and in community and public health, and with those two degrees and those credentials, they can go anywhere in the world and do just about anything. In terms of training and preparation to go out and to analyze communities, to identify problems, to design, develop, implement, and evaluate programs—whether it's an immunization program or a clinic or a maternal–child health program—they are well prepared to deliver direct care and services. Some of our MSN/MPH students are even going through the nurse practitioner program, so they will be prepared both to give direct patient care to individual patients as well as to give community and public-health nursing to groups, be they groups of families or neighborhoods or communities.

With the dual-degree programs, the walls of the three schools—nursing, medicine, and public health—are very permeable for students, and people can cross over and take courses in different schools, and some of the courses are coregistered or conumbered and co-offered by several divisions. It's a very positive environment.

Martha Norton Hill, 1964, BSN 1966

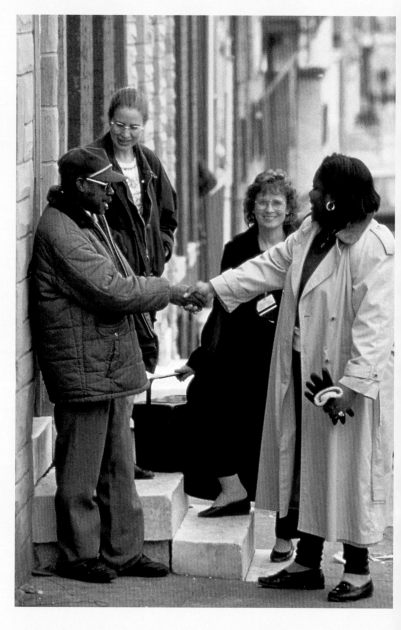

The Johns Hopkins University School of Nursing continued the long tradition of serving the community. As resources permitted, faculty and students explored new and varied techniques to bring health care to the school's neighbors. Mary Roary (right), a community health worker, greeted an East Baltimore resident and introduced him to clinical instructor Sue Hall and one of her students.

Right now I have a K Award from the National Institute of Drug Abuse, looking at substance abuse and intimate partner violence in women. I was able to integrate both my research and my practice, which was important to me. The faculty practice is probably the best thing about working here. I don't have to juggle. In one faculty role I work in clinics and my salary and benefits are paid directly to the School of Nursing, so that's not something that I ever see but it's part of my role here.

What struck me when I would do the health interviews with the women was how much violence was an integral part of their lives. There's this huge literature on violence and women, this huge literature on substance abuse, but very little that talked about substance abuse and violence. Many times women are introduced to drugs through their partners so that got me to thinking. "Okay, you have a large group of women who are introduced to drugs through their partners and at the same time, either before or after, are in an abusive relationship. How do they address that? How do you help them?" I wanted to combine the two and contribute something that helps these women.

Benita Walton-Moss, 1978

This year I have helped bring babies into the world, and I have learned to comfort those whose life will not last. But the Johns Hopkins School of Nursing goes beyond just teaching its students the skills to work in a hospital. I spent one rotation working in the Baltimore shelters, and wondering that our American health system does not, in fact, provide for all. An act as simple as arranging an appointment for a homeless woman at a free dental clinic became a source of profound gratitude.

Marni Sommer, 1999, MSN/MPH 2001

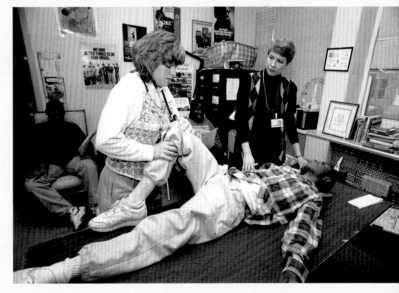

The first Lillian D. Wald Community Nursing Center, named to honor the founder of American community nursing, opened at the Rutland Center, in 1994. Founded and directed by Assistant Professor Marion Isaacs D'Lugoff, the clinic offered a place where neighborhood residents could get complete physical examinations and routine preventive pediatric services, immunizations, and lead screening for uninsured children. *Above:* Assistant Professor Sue Appling, 1973, helped a student conduct a physical examination at a Wald Clinic. *Left:* Students led a workshop with young children about the importance of hand washing.

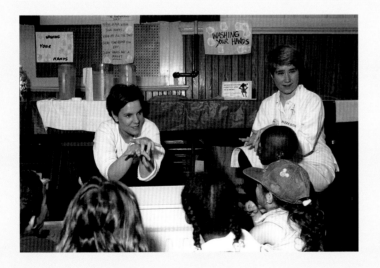

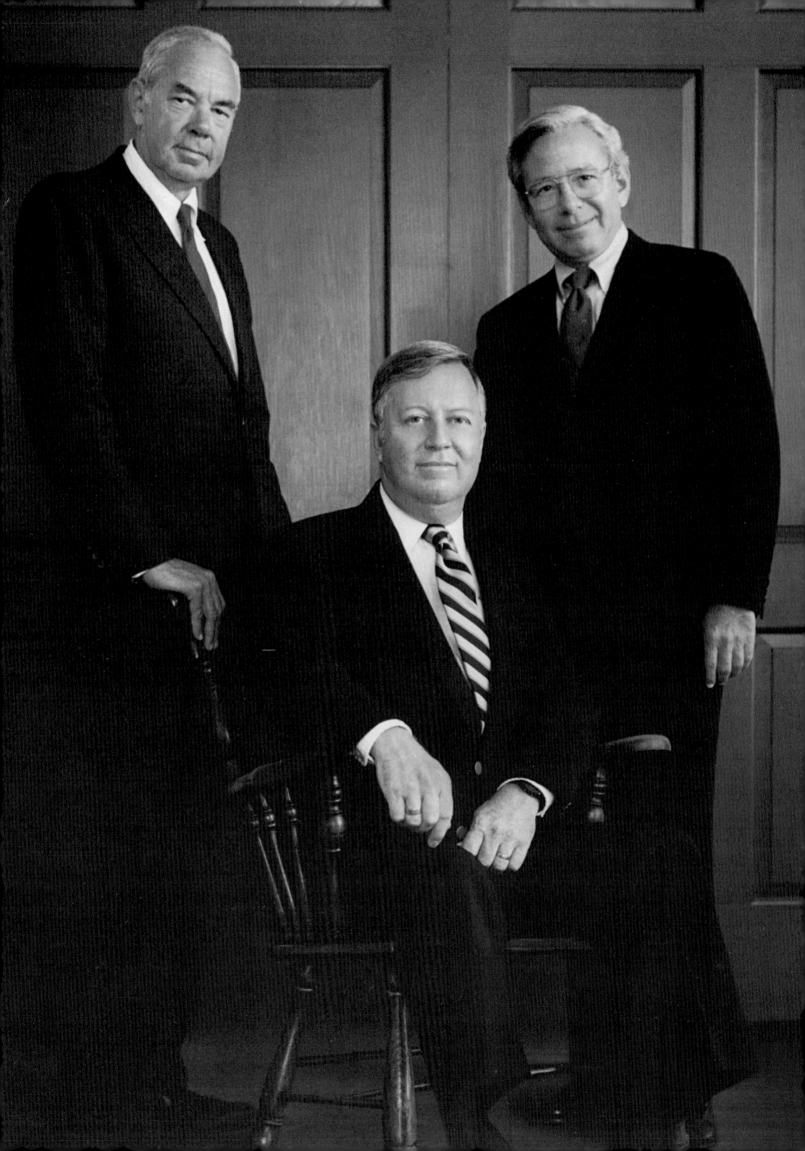

All Eyes on Hopkins, 1980–1994 · MAME WARREN

6

The Consortium for Nursing Education was founded
in 1982 as a means of creating the Johns Hopkins
University School of Nursing. Dean Carol Gray praised
the three hospital presidents who championed the idea:
Robert M. Heyssel of Johns Hopkins (left), Thomas
Gillam Whedbee Jr. of Church Home (center), and
Spencer Foreman of Sinai. "It is well to recall and
recognize those in administration at the time the new
school was established," Gray said. Those visionaries
"made a bold leap to commit to the new school.
There were many who questioned the level of Hopkins
commitment to nursing at that time."

They had the gift shop in the little house by the gate to the hospital. They sold things and put that money away, saving it for the day when they were going to have this baccalaureate school of nursing. The money grew and grew. School of Health Services had gotten a little bit of it, but primarily Joan Sutton was able to get that money back. She and Betty Cuthbert had to be convinced that this new school was in fact for real and that it was safe for the alumni to hand over that money.

Stella Shiber

What needed to be done for the nursing alumni board was to tap into the younger alumni and get them to assume offices, and interested in things happening at the school. As soon as the new nursing school started up, there was so much going on. They were easy to snag once we got some excitement going. They wanted to be on the board and do projects.

Susan Carroll Immelt, 1977, PhD 2000

Devoted alumni kept a watchful eye on the formation of the university school, then vigorously supported it. Valerie Simmons Harrison (seated left), 1965, Donna Dittberner (seated center), 1966, and Betsy Mumaw McGeady (standing right), 1955, are pictured here in 1989 discussing the alumni association and its work with other graduates of the diploma school.

AFTER DECADES *of frustration, the Johns Hopkins University established its School of Nursing in 1984. Creative thinking yielded an innovative solution to the dilemma of how to fund the new division. Many of those who helped to create the school are still with us. Their reflections offer insights into how the school became a reality, struggled through its early development, and soon soared to the top stratum of American schools of nursing. Here, their memories blend with those of alumni from the first twenty years.*

Paula Einaudi, *former director of development for the Johns Hopkins University School of Nursing:* Betty Cuthbert, class of '43, was a wonderful historian and a fabulous steward of the Nutting Fund. Every year or two, she would get a call from either Steve Muller or Bob Heyssel or someone else at the hospital and they would say, "We have a good idea for how you might want to use the Nutting Fund." It would be a nice idea, but it would be to help with nursing research on some unit in the hospital.

Betty and Joan Sutton would smile. They would listen quietly and say, "A wonderful idea, Dr. Heyssel, but we need you to know that we will be delighted to give this money, in its entirety, when the School of Nursing opens as a division of the university." That had been a goal of the alumni association for decades. The hospital trustees got to know that these women were pretty darn feisty and tenacious. About the third time they went, Betty Cuthbert told me, "Suddenly, I saw the lightbulb go on over Dr. Heyssel's head." He realized that these women were serious. He also realized that he had a serious problem on his hands because there was a severe nursing shortage. In previous decades there had always been this fresh group of young nursing students ready to take over for nurses who were leaving either temporarily or for good. With the school closed, this situation was really very tough.

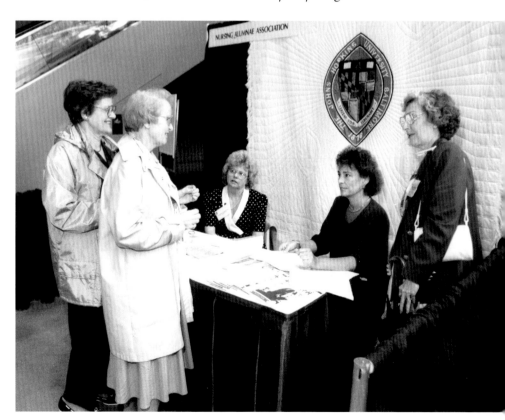

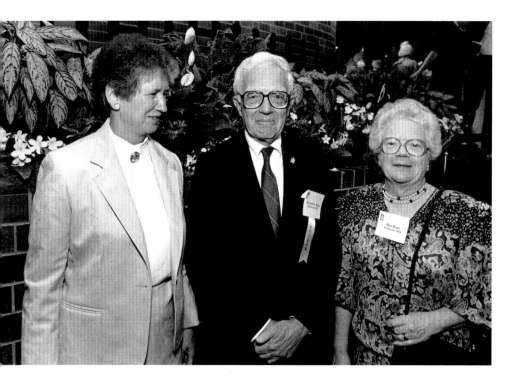

Sandra Stine Angell, 1969, BSN 1977 from the Evening College, *former president of the alumni association, and associate dean of the Johns Hopkins University School of Nursing:* I was president of the alumni association the fall that the school was dedicated. I remember sitting in the provost's office over at the university with Carol Gray my first day as president still arguing, still fighting, about the Nutting Fund money. The university had a very paternalistic attitude about the School of Nursing and the alumni association. There was always an attempt, you know, "Come on, girls. This is really going to be okay. Let us handle the finances and you worry about taking care of patients." Dr. Heyssel was persuaded, in large part, by some of the women he met in that alumni group. I think he was very influenced by them.

Robert Heyssel, *former president of the Johns Hopkins Hospital:* We were without a school of nursing. Then we had this big nursing shortage, I guess in the late '70s, early '80s. And Hal Cohen, who was then still director of the Health Services Cost Review Commission, announced that there would be money and rates for training nurses, in-hospital rates. So I was talking to Spike Foreman, who ran Sinai Hospital, and said, "You know, we ought to take advantage of that somehow. If we spread the costs of those rates over a bunch of hospitals, none of us would know the difference, whereas if they were all in one hospital's rate, it'd be more expensive than we want." He agreed to that, and so Sinai and Church Home and ourselves—that made two thousand beds among the three of us, each bed getting a nickel or so tacked onto the rates. So we went to Hal Cohen at the HSCRC and he said yes, he'd let us do that for planning purposes for a nursing school.

So then I went to Steve Muller and said, "Steve, you've always wanted a nursing school. Maybe this is your chance to get it." And Steve had, but it couldn't cost him anything.

The other departments come in and do their little things and they're gone. The doctor comes in and he visits a short time. The nurse is there twenty-four hours a day. So we have to make sure that those persons are qualified and try to provide an environment for them so that they feel fulfilled, so that they feel, "Hey, yes, I'm appreciated. Yes, my boss, my doctors, the administrators think I'm doing a good job." You have to make them feel needed and wanted and cared for, just as you're trying to do for the patients.

Medea Marella

Steven Muller, *former president of the Johns Hopkins University:* The hospital had lost a lot of reputation in nursing because, since it closed its nursing school, the quality of nursing was going down. So from his point of view, the best thing Heyssel could do was strongly support the university founding the School of Nursing because the university didn't need a school of nursing, the hospital did. Who would these nurses serve? Sure, it was good for the School of Medicine to have a nursing school, but it was not something they cared deeply about if it came to money.

Stephen McClain, *former vice provost for academic planning and budget of the university:* Academic nursing at Johns Hopkins University was a part-time program in the Evening College. Bob Heyssel, speaking for Johns Hopkins Hospital, was having conversations with the provost, Dick Longaker, that there was a shortage of higher level–trained nurses. Bob had also talked with Spike Foreman at Sinai and Gil Whedbee at Church Home and Hospital. They were also facing shortages of nurses and were interested in working with Hopkins in establishing the School of Nursing. I remember a very early conversation in Garland Hall, which was more a "Should we do this?" kind of thing. How would the hospital work with the university to establish a school of nursing?

Muller: Bob was able to get some support from a couple of the other hospitals because other hospitals felt the lack of Hopkins nurses graduating and staying in Baltimore and working for them. That was nice, but that was not the key. The key was the fact the hospital had the facilities, had the need, and had the money.

Martha Norton Hill, 1964, BSN 1966 from the Evening College, *faculty member of the diploma school, the School of Health Services, and the university school, now dean of the Johns Hopkins University School of Nursing:* In 1980 I took a position at what was then called the Evening College. Margaret Courtney was the only full-time faculty member in the RN to BSN completion program in the Evening College. There was a lot of interest in getting that program accredited, which meant they had to have more full-time faculty, so Margaret hired me. We were implementing a plan to receive accreditation from the National League for Nursing.

We advertised for somebody to join us as a faculty member and someone I had worked with in Philadelphia came down to interview. Part of the interview was at the hospital. She had a meeting with several people, including the director of nursing. She came back and told me that the hospital was working to get funding from the state with which they planned to start a school of nursing with several other hospitals and she asked me how that fit. I said, "What?" I had no idea. She said she understood that it was going to be a baccalaureate program. I said, "Then the degree would have to be given by the university. We better go talk to

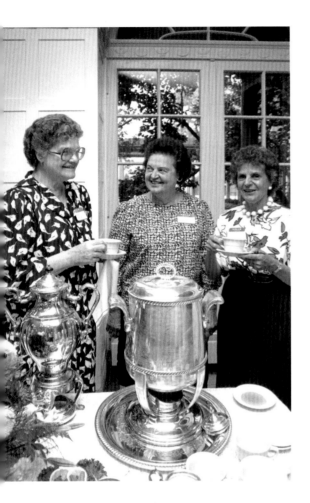

Dorothea Robertson (left) became executive secretary of the alumnae association in 1962. Here in 1987 she enjoyed tea with Anna Buchko Flatley, 1940, and Helen Peters Finney, 1954. After Robertson's death, the nurses' alumni office was dedicated in her memory and a scholarship was established in her name.

Margaret." So we repeated everything and Margaret said, "Come on," and we went downstairs to the office of Roman Verhaalen, who was the dean of the then Evening College. I said, "Roman, wait till you hear this." Roman hit the roof and started making calls because the left hand didn't know what the right hand was doing. The fact is, you cannot have two programs that are accredited awarding the same degree in the same university, which meant that the RN to BSN either had to be phased out or it had to be integrated into this new university school of nursing.

Medea Marella, *former vice president of nursing at Sinai Hospital:* The nurse shortage in late '79 and '80 perked us all up. We were all wondering, What are we going to do? It was at that time that Dr. Heyssel got this inspiration that maybe there should be a school of nursing again at Hopkins. In early 1981, he contacted Dr. Spencer Foreman, who was the president of Sinai Hospital, and Gillam Whedbee, who was the president of Church Hospital. Steven Muller became involved because if a school was going to be developed, it would be part of the university. That's how it was envisioned. Once Dr. Foreman got involved, he asked me if I thought it was a good idea and should we do it. I said, "Of course. It's the most wonderful thing I can think of."

I'm really a nurse educator from way back. The diploma nurse was a great nurse. I'm a product of a diploma school of nursing, but we needed more education. We needed to be oriented toward research, sciences, and the new technology. We needed to grow as a profession to compete and be able to converse with our physicians in an intelligent way. The most important thing is to improve the care of patients, and that would come from our being educated more. All of those things were very important to me.

Stella Shiber, *first associate dean for undergraduate education:* Dr. Heyssel saw the same thing that a lot of the physicians saw. Hopkins had to rely on somebody else to educate nurses. It got to be harder and harder to recruit, to the hospital, the kind of people that they really needed to make the whole picture complete. If you are one of the top hospitals, nursing is an extremely important part of that hospital. The odd thing was, when we opened the school in '84, there were lots of people in this country who did not know that there hadn't always been a School of Nursing at Hopkins. They just couldn't conceive that there wouldn't have been. Of course there's nursing at Hopkins.

Bernard Keenan, 1986, *member of the first class of the university school,* MSN 1993, *and part-time faculty member:* It was made very clear that this was a new program and that this was the dream of generations of nurses coming before us and that we had them to answer to in a way. I really bought into that whole aura of the history, the people who preceded

Dorothea Robertson deserves a lot of credit for keeping the alumni association as together as it was. She just loved Hopkins nurses. She had a genuine love and respect for the nursing profession. She made friends wherever she went. We called her Robbie. She was not an organized person. Her office was a disaster but she had a very good memory and could find things.

She took care of the older alumnae, even the ones who didn't live around here. She did some things for alumni that probably most alumni associations aren't supposed to do anymore. She liked older people a lot and she also loved students, so she was a natural. She always seemed to have forty-eight hours in her day.

Sandra Stine Angell, 1969, BSN 1977

Dorothea Robertson was a very motherly, perfect person for that job. Robbie really ran the alumni association. She said who was going to be elected. They had a nominating board and all that, but she did all the prephoning. I personally feel that's one of the reasons we have a hard time getting some of the older alumni to get very involved. They don't think there's anything for them to do because the alumni office is going to do it all. In fact, today it's different. Since we're attached to the university, Melinda Rose is paid from the university and she's not supposed to be doing all the extra stuff that she does. It should be the alumni.

Lois Grayshan Hoffer, 1962

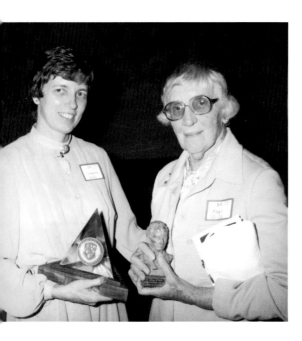

In 1981 the Johns Hopkins University honored Carolyne Davis (left), 1954, former dean of the School of Nursing at the University of Michigan, with its Distinguished Alumnus Award. Here she posed with Mary Sanders Price, 1934, who became director of the hospital nursing school the year after Davis graduated.

Nan Pinkard was on the board of the Johns Hopkins Hospital for many years, and she was upset when the hospital School of Nursing closed. Nan was very concerned about the lack of nursing education at the hospital and the university and she would frequently bring this up. She was one of the clear and persistent voices. She would say to Heyssel, "What are you going to do about this?"

Martha Norton Hill, 1964, BSN 1966

me, and having to measure up and do as well. That was something Dr. Shiber really impressed upon us. Yes, we were a new school but we just didn't come out of nowhere. We had quite a legacy to live up to.

McClain: Bob Heyssel was a very forceful person and knew what he wanted. They needed a more sophisticated, bachelor's degree–trained cadre of nurses. The university school needed to start with a bachelor's and a master's degree program. Bob was farsighted enough to realize that there was a need for nurses who were trained in management and the oversight of nurses; nurses were going to take on more and more responsibilities in the provision of health care, both within a hospital setting and in nonhospital settings, in the future.

Because this was Bob Heyssel's baby, Bob took a lot of interest and opened doors within the medical establishment to Carol Gray that probably would not have opened with ease. Everyone knew that Bob Heyssel was the godfather of the School of Nursing.

Heyssel: We got Dr. Carol Gray to come from Texas and she planned the nursing school and we renovated the third floor of the Phipps Building. She hired some faculty and they had a couple of rough years at first recruiting people, but then it took off.

Hill, 1964, BSN 1966: Carol Gray was originally hired at the Evening College to be the director of the RN to BSN program and to do the feasibility study. Carol asked me to take the day-to-day responsibility for the RN to BSN program while she worked on that report for the new university school. Several decisions were made. One was that it would be an upper-division program and that the Evening College program would be phased out. Then the decision was made to start the Johns Hopkins University School of Nursing.

Susan Carroll Immelt, *1977 graduate of the School of Health Services Nursing Education Program and one of the first PhD candidates in the new school, now a part-time faculty member:* Carol Gray was a very quiet, gentle person, sort of steely. You wouldn't picture her getting upset about something. I see her as someone who, when they hired her, they said, "We want this program," that she would just say, "Okay. We'll do this" and "We'll do that" and just move along as things needed to be done. She moved through the system. When something wasn't working out, she would just say, "Okay. Well, I'll do this then." I think people really liked her a lot.

Carol Gray, *first dean of the Johns Hopkins University School of Nursing:* I believe the mistake with the School of Health Services was putting nursing under the umbrella of another discipline, as it was then, with medicine. One of my first requirements in accepting this position was that nursing be an autonomous school within the university under the leadership of an individual with the title of dean, comparable to that of other divisions. I believe that these conditions were critical.

McClain: President Muller was kept up to date on all of this and he put his institutional blessing on it. He relied upon the discussions between Longaker and Heyssel by and large. He knew Heyssel very well and it was basically, "Bob's willing to put his money where his mouth is, he must want it badly enough to where this makes sense." Of course, it rounded out the medical complex conceptually and academically and professionally to have a school of nursing.

Donna Dittberner, 1966, *faculty member of the diploma school and former president of the alumni association:* Steve Muller was an awfully good president and respected nursing. He respected the concept. He respected Carol Gray. They had a very positive relationship. I don't think that there could have been a better choice for the first dean of the School of Nursing. Bright, warm, savvy, tenacious, her whole presence, her whole demeanor was felt on the university campus. She's engaging, good sense of humor, able to laugh at herself as well as situations. She's a "glass is half full" person, very optimistic. She'd make people feel very comfortable. She was tremendously respected by the alumni association. We felt very close to her. We felt that she was really the champion. She's a very inclusive kind of person and she included the alumni association as being critical in many ways.

Einaudi: Bob Heyssel talked to Steve Muller and the presidents of Sinai and Church Hospitals. They decided to form the Consortium for Nursing Education, Inc. Nan Pinkard was the first head of this consortium. They got the legislature to say that the State of Maryland would give the consortium one dollar per patient per day. The first year, it turned out to be $1.5 million. The idea was, "We'll give you that much this year. Next year, it will come down because, as the years go by, you need to prove yourself capable of sustaining yourself. This will be seed money."

Marella: It was an exciting time for me that we were going to establish this new school of nursing. I know that Martha Sacci at Hopkins and Joyce O'Shea from Church Hospital were very pleased to be included. Carol Gray was very easy to work with. If I disagreed I let them know. Since I was a nursing service administrator, I certainly was geared educationally because that's my preparation. But I was also clinically oriented because I had to be concerned about the patients and the quality of care they were going to be getting and seeing that the students in our program would have the necessary skills and knowledge to perform the care.

McClain: We had just finished the bad experience with the School of Health Services. That had never gotten off the ground. Heyssel and

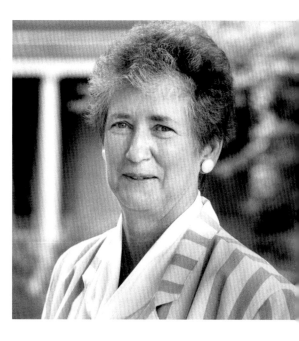

Carol J. Gray came to Baltimore in 1981 from the School of Nursing at the University of Texas Health Science Center to assume the directorship of the Evening College's Division of Nursing. The following year the Consortium for Nursing Education and the Johns Hopkins University announced her appointment as the first dean of the Johns Hopkins University School of Nursing.

Carol Gray was tall and rather statuesque, but her voice was very soft. The encounters that she had with people were always precise, efficient, and low-key. The administrators of the university liked her very much. She knew what she was about. Gradually, the curriculum developed for the baccalaureate degree, faculty members were hired, and we got under way. Carol Gray was a behind-closed-doors administrator. She was quite formal as a person but she worked very hard to see that things were done correctly, completely, and to get the school going in the direction it needed to go. As a first dean of the school, she was quite effective. She was imposing in appearance. That helped also. She was always beautifully dressed and very businesslike. When she talked with the administrators of the university or the hospital she made an impression. It was fortunate, I think, that she was where she was at the time.

Ada Davis

There were conflicting feelings in medicine. What they would like to have had back is the hospital diploma school, where they got those nice girls who were bright. They did not really think they wanted someone who was educated or someone they would need to recognize as a peer.

When we first opened the school, Dr. Muller was very clear that he wanted there to be joint use of resources. When I was putting the curriculum together, I was told, "You must find a way to use faculty from the School of Medicine." Pharmacology and pathophysiology are two things that seemed very reasonable that they could help us with. When I told the chairman about the curriculum, he interrupted me. He told me that they were the expert teachers and that they would decide what the nurses needed to be taught. I was stunned. I had my doctorate and I'd been an educator for twenty-five years. The whole time he called me Ms. Shiber. He's the only person in my whole career to whom I've ever said, "Excuse me, that's Dr. Shiber." He was absolutely typical.

He sent me to see a very young resident who, he said, would be helpful in teaching pathophysiology. I was introduced to this guy— who could have been my son—as Dr. Shiber. He came across the room and took my hand and said, "Ms. Shiber, it's so nice to meet you." He heard the word nurse and automatically went to a nurse who is a kind, hard-working person but not very well educated, not very bright. It was tough to get beyond that with a lot of them. Their sense of helping or collaborating was, "We'll tell you how it should be done."

Stella Shiber

Hospital president Robert Heyssel selected Martha Sacci as nursing director in 1977, when the hospital's administration was decentralized. "Martha Sacci understood that you pick good people, delegate authority and responsibility, and then hold them accountable," remembered Dr. Richard Gaintner, Heyssel's vice president. "She understood that her role was not to manage nursing but to be the central icon for nursing. She was a tough lady. She could run with the guys very easily. The hospital was a man's world, let's face it."

the university had put a lot of time and effort and some money into that and no one wanted to repeat that experience. It was rather obvious that the School of Health Services was in very bad financial shape, which led to its closing.

There was a move in academic and professional services and that's what the School of Health Services was designed to address, a gap between the highly trained doctors and nurses and the next level. This was right at the beginning of the push toward community-based health care. How do you provide quality health care but not at the same level of cost that the system was experiencing at that time? I think we got caught up in an academic professional fad without really understanding what the trends were. The trends only became really evident over the next five to ten years. Because the fad never took hold professionally, the federal money to sustain this kind of professional initiative quickly dried up.

Keenan, 1986, MSN 1993: At that time, there was a lot of mistrust of the university because many of the alumni were still smarting from the first attempt at a school affiliated with the university. There were funds mismanaged. Betty Cuthbert and Joan Sutton had actually threatened to sue the university to get some funds back that the alumni association had contributed to the School of Health Services. When that closed, the university just thought they'd keep the money and that was that. And that wasn't that. They didn't know who they were dealing with. Betty and Joan got the money back and held on to that money. That eventually was some of the seed money that went toward the start-up of the school.

Ada Davis, *faculty member and nurse historian:* People would say, "Did you hear? Hopkins is going to have a baccalaureate program." But they also knew about the strife within Hopkins against the program and they knew we were having back-and-forth conversations among the

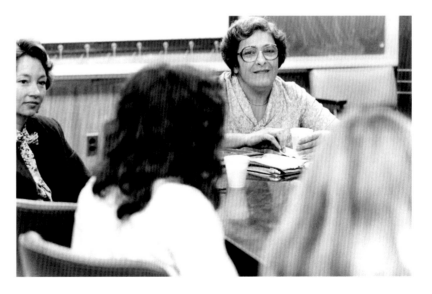

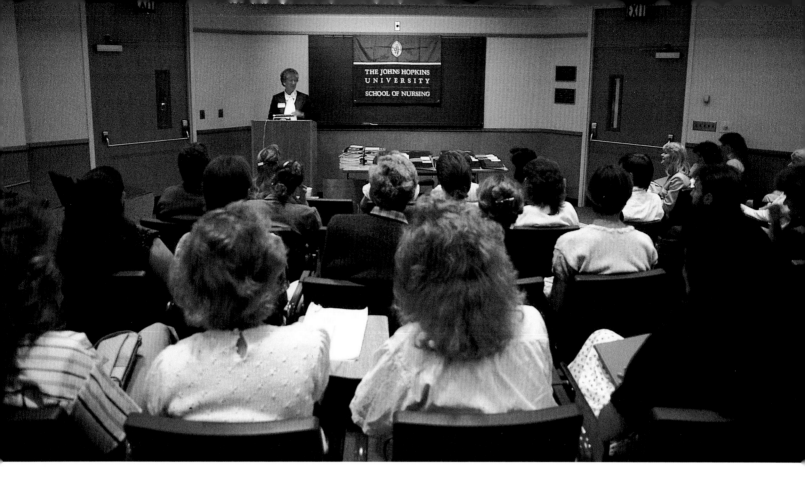

administrators of the hospital, the university, and the School of Nursing. They knew we were having a hard time making progress in the education of nurses. There was quite bit of talk because they knew our history. Some were saying, "Forget it. It will never happen." Others were saying, "Yes, it will. It has to." All eyes were on Hopkins for quite a while, not just here in Baltimore but all over the country. It's been a success story, really, but it's taken a lot of hard work, a lot of discussion, and some of the discussions were not too friendly.

Heyssel: The whole country was so suspicious because, my god, there goes Hopkins again running another hospital-dominated nursing school. And really, Carol Gray got all sorts of stuff from her colleagues around the country for letting the hospital pull the wool over her eyes. Of course, we never dictated any curricula. She put the money together and insisted on being on the governing board.

McClain: The endowment that was under the hospital's control wouldn't even have come close to providing the kind of ongoing operational support required, so you needed a major, major infusion of outside money to get this thing off the ground. Bob Heyssel had come up with the plan to convince the State of Maryland that a dedicated portion of the patient day rate for all three hospitals—Sinai, Church Home, and Johns Hopkins—would be skimmed off and dedicated to the School of Nursing.

Marella: The Health Services Cost Review Commission in Maryland was very instrumental in helping us to get this program off the board.

Classes at the School of Nursing met for the first several years in cramped quarters in the Phipps Building, which was renovated after the Department of Psychiatry moved to the Meyer Building. Here Dean Carol Gray welcomed students during orientation in 1988.

Betty Cuthbert charmed the socks off of all of us. If a Hollywood director says, "I need a bit player who's a charming, crusty old grande dame. Go over to central casting and send me someone," they would have sent Betty Cuthbert. On the surface, she was very gracious and very nice, but she had a core of steel and she knew what she wanted. She wanted a nursing school and was very suspicious of the school being within the university and not within the hospital, not because she had anything in particular against the university, but she was so attached to the hospital nursing school because that's where her memories, her experience, her institutional love was. One of the reasons some of the people like Betty were suspicious of the university being able to pull off a school of nursing was because we hadn't done a credible job with the School of Health Services and had taken and obviously misspent, at least in their eyes, a lot of their money.

Stephen McClain

Because of the terrible nurse shortage, the HSCRC came up with plans and said that hospitals and schools of nursing should try nursing education programs to staff and retain nurses. If they came up with innovative programs, the HSCRC would fund the programs.

And so the hospital presidents in the consortium met with the Health Services Cost Review Commission and the HSCRC thought it was a great idea also. They said, "Look, if you guys are a success planning this, in hiring a dean and in establishing the school, we will help pay for it." In order for each hospital to pay its share of the cost, the HSCRC raised their rates of reimbursement for hospital patients; that's how they funded the school. Initially it cost about a million and a half for one year. Sinai paid $36,000 a month, Hopkins paid $68,000 a month, and Church about $18,000 a month. That's how we got the school started because neither the hospitals nor the university had that kind of money. Once the school was established, they planned to get some funds through raising money for endowments as the university has done with all of its other programs.

We formed a steering committee that worked for about two years planning for the school. We met at least once a month. Our discussions were lively at times. Once they accepted that, yes, we're going to go ahead and do it, they really put their hearts and souls into developing this school. The committee was certainly male-dominated, and strong men. We seemed to think along the same lines so there weren't any real problems about what we decided had to be done. It was just, How are we going to do it? working out who's going to do this and how much money. Money was very important.

Bob Heyssel was very authoritative. Dr. Foreman was another strong person. We called him Spike. He was gregarious, a real happy guy. Sinai always felt a little inferior to Hopkins but he and Bob Heyssel had a great relationship, which helped a great deal. Gil Whedbee was another very nice gentleman, but the other two presidents of the hospitals were much more forceful and in control of all the goings-on.

McClain: My task was taking the academic part and figuring out how big the school could be and how big it needed to be to be financially viable. How many students did you need to bring in so much tuition income? How many faculty would you need? How many of them would be full-time faculty, part-time faculty, et cetera? You had all sorts of variables to work with. You also needed to channel some of that patient-day-rate money into establishing a long-term endowment for the school to give it the financial bedrock to be successful.

Then you had the added complication of working with two other separate corporate entities. You had to think about the governance apparatus, given the involvement of the hospital, the university, and then the two outside hospitals—how you put that together because, of course, Sinai and Church Home and Hospital had their own special needs for nursing. They were involved on both the nursing curriculum as well as on the financial side. Both wanted to attract Hopkins-trained nurses.

Marella: At Sinai and Church, we knew that we couldn't keep graduates unless they wanted to work in our hospitals. We knew from the very beginning that we couldn't get our hopes up because they had the freedom to do and go where they wanted once they graduated.

McClain: I was the one who wrote up the original consortium agreement. My academic background is as a political scientist. I've always been interested in Aristotle and Plato. Aristotle did a famous study of the constitutions of Greece. Being more interested in political theory than political science, I've always been interested in constitutional structures and how you put, in this case, political organizations together to achieve certain objectives.

When I sat down with Carol Gray in this process, it was much more on the academic side. What's the minimum that you need to make this thing viable academically but then also to make it financially viable? Then if everything broke your way, what would be the best or the optimum set of circumstances that you would want? Obviously and usually, you wind up somewhere in the middle.

Ninety percent of Carol Gray's focus was on the academic side. She left the rest pretty much to me and to Ed Meerholz, who was in the finance office. He did a lot of the number crunching. I had come out of the controller's office and therefore knew payroll and all of the nuts and bolts of what a school needed to run itself. You needed someone who looked after the payroll and an admissions person, et cetera. The school was very small when it started. In fact, we shopped out a number of the services early on to the School of Public Health. They did the payroll initially, any research accounting that was needed. It just didn't make sense to hire full-time staff for administrative responsibilities.

Dittberner, 1966: Carol Gray asked for input from the nursing alumni association. We said, "It's got to have an extremely strong clinical component." We were seeing so many nurses come from baccalaureate programs never having really had any true-life clinical experience. I think that's what makes the School of Nursing today stand out: it has an unusually strong clinical focus. That doesn't mean that undergrad-graduate isn't strong on theories and research, but the clinical skills are there.

Betsy Mumaw McGeady, 1955, BSN 1955 from McCoy College, *former president of the alumni association:* Carol Gray was in the right place at the right time. She was able to take our vision and, along with hers, get the basic structure of the university school worked out. When she came she

When they taught us breast self-examination in the diploma program, they showed a film and they asked me to leave the room so as not to embarrass my classmates. I was at a conference recently where Martha Hill was speaking and I mentioned that to her. She just shook her head. She said, "I can imagine that's probably the way it was. That was the culture at Hopkins." When we were on the floor dealing with patients, believe it or not, I never once was given a female patient. I remember walking in on one of my classmates to tell her something and the patient looked at me and said, "Who are you?" I said, "I'm a student nurse." Without missing a beat, the patient said, "Are you a sissy?" I said, "No, I have a wife and two kids." "Oh." So that was the atmosphere back then.

My program was so much on-the-job training because it was just a diploma program. With my son's program, a bachelor of science in nursing, he did spend a lot more time in classrooms and probably less time in a clinical area than I spent. But they did give him female patients. It's a different type of education. We learned through osmosis by being there all the time. He actually learned out of the textbook. There are a lot of people with PhDs in nursing, PhDs in anesthesia, who have a lot less experience than I have in terms of actual patient contact. But that's the trend now. Back then a diploma in nursing was sufficient.

Herb Zinder, 1971

Stella Shiber was the center in the early years for making sure that the academic programs were in place, that they were strong, that we got appropriate faculty, and that we met the NLN standards. She had a good feel for organizational development. She knew the importance of interacting with other schools. She was devoted to the school. She was certainly devoted to the students.

Sandra Stine Angell, 1969, BSN 1977

The research faculty has made a tremendous difference. Jackie Campbell and Jeri Allen are not only recognized but also respected among the physicians with whom they work. Jackie's well known in the area of domestic violence, which has become a huge area of concern not only here but in other countries as well. She has shed light on causes and treatments and ways to remedy the violence. She's added a lot to what we know and what we're able to do, which to me is a significant contribution.

Jeri is a quiet person. She's very competent. Despite her small size, she's like a fire engine. She just forges ahead. Everything she does is of outstanding quality. Writing, researching, teaching, whatever, she's just an extraordinary person. And we have a lot of them. Some people just give half of themselves to a job, you know, and others give their whole selves. The ones who give it all stand out. Individuals with outstanding qualities always stand out.

Ada Davis

said she would only stay for a definite period of time. We were thrilled when she decided to become the first dean.

Hill, 1964, BSN 1966: Carol Gray was offered the deanship by the provost, Richard Longaker. To my knowledge there was no search committee for the dean. Carol had done a very thoughtful and well-organized job in the feasibility study and I think she had established good working relationships with people. Heyssel, Whedbee, and Foreman were comfortable with her. She was in many, many ways the right person at the right time in the right place. She knew undergraduate education. She knew what to do and how to do it so the program would be accredited. Then Stella Shiber was hired and then Margaret Dear, who had been on the faculty at the School of Public Health, and Leah Bonovich, a maternity nurse who had taught for and worked with Stella very closely. They took the lead on developing the curriculum.

Angell, 1969, BSN 1977: Carol Gray was absolutely the right person for the opening of the school because her background certainly was in developing curriculum. That's what we needed. Not being from the area, not really knowing the Hopkins community, she needed some people who did have contacts and did know folks. I think that she relied heavily on Stella Shiber for that and then certainly Martha Hill, who is Hopkins through and through.

It was a very small faculty initially. Everybody taught multiple courses. Jeri Allen was one of the early faculty members. Leah Bonovich taught obstetrics. Maureen Maguire's been around for a long time, not from the very beginning but she was one of the earliest faculty members. Sue Appling came early on.

Elaine Larson, *faculty member:* Stella Shiber was the backbone of the curriculum. She was the pedagogical expert and the main contact for the students and she really helped to establish the undergraduate academic programs.

Marella: By 1983 all three hospitals and the university had committed themselves—they were going to go ahead. Everything had been worked out, the school was established, and we began to plan and enroll students in the type of program we wanted. It was going to be a two-year, upper-division program, which meant that the students had to have nursing education preparation courses. The faculty all had to be master's or doctorally prepared or working on their doctorates. We enrolled our first students in 1984. The name was a big attraction. They were going to be affiliated with *the* Johns Hopkins University. There was no doubt in our minds that this school was going to be fully accredited as soon as the National League for Nursing came if it met the expectations of nursing education programs. I guess we really thought a lot of ourselves.

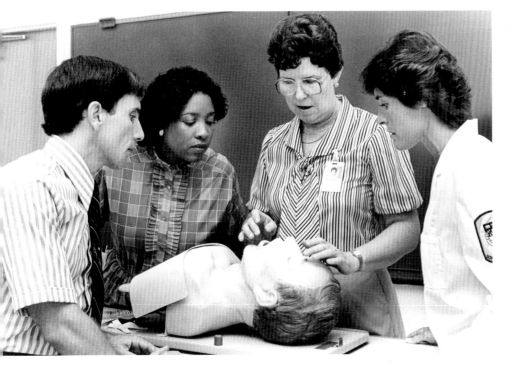

Stella Shiber was on the faculty of the hospital school and of the Nursing Education Program in the School of Health Services. Here she is pictured in 1984, teaching a lab to members of the first class of the university school, where she was responsible for developing the curriculum. Bernard Keenan recalled that Shiber had trained as a psychiatric nurse. "Many of my classmates would go to her when they had a problem. That warmth and, as we say in psychiatry, that positive self-regard, unconditional acceptance, seemed to be there and students would listen to her."

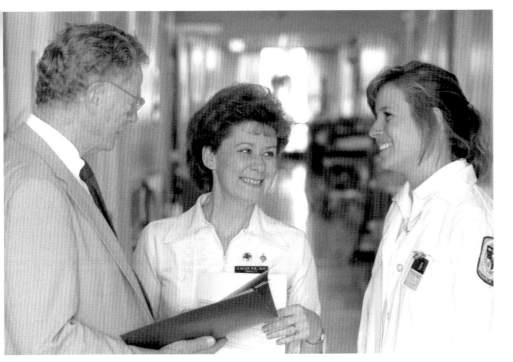

Many Johns Hopkins physicians, such as Worth Daniels (left, with Assistant Professor Jerilyn Allen, center, and senior Laurie Cerniglia, 1991) have been appreciative and influential champions of nurses. Before his death, Dr. I. Ridgeway Trimble wrote that "the longer one practices medicine the more one comes to realize the importance of the nurse's role in the care of the sick patient. The morale of the patient, of the ward, of the hospital division, is dependent on her, as indeed is the morale of the doctor. Her role in the case of a desperately ill person, through her vigilance, judgment and skill, often means the difference between triumph and disaster."

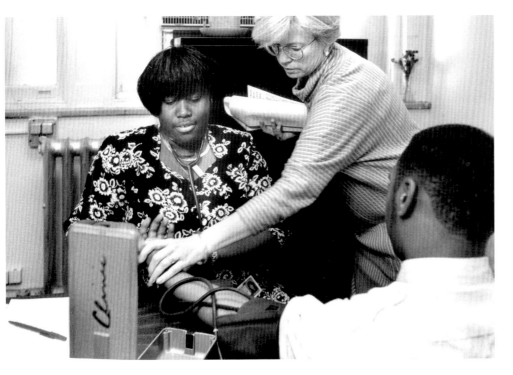

Martha Norton Hill (standing), 1964, became director of the Center for Nursing Research in 1992. Here she instructed a student, in 1993, on how to take a patient's blood pressure.

Maureen Maguire (left) joined the faculty in 1985 as coordinator of nursing for child health. "I like to share my view of what nursing can do and what nursing is,." Maguire said. "I like the whole 'aha' feeling that students get when they master a particular concept." In labs like this one in 1991, she explained, "We practice on each other. Students practice on students, on faculty, or on dummies. We have all kinds of gadgets that we use and we improvise when we don't have a gadget for real."

Angell, 1969, BSN 1977: I remember discussions with potential students. We did a lot of talking, cajoling, and pampering and gave a lot of individual attention to every single applicant. We spent a ton of time on the phone and had success with some people and not with others.

This was an upper-division nursing program so that made us different from the beginning from a school where a student would go right out of high school. We thought we'd have more students transferring to us as juniors. What we really found, pretty quickly, was that we were attracting career changers.

Keenan, 1986, MSN 1993: About half of us had been through school and were older. The other half were coming into their junior year of college. It had a very good balancing effect on the makeup of the class. The students knew all the tricks about how to study and cram and take tests and take notes. Then some of us who were coming back to school, we had the life experience to be able to maybe calm them down. If they didn't get a 98 percent, there really were bigger worries in this world than that. We were helpful to each other.

There were only three men. By then I had been working for five years at a hospital with nurses. I was used to working with a lot of women so that wasn't a new experience. I tried to keep very neutral. I never wanted to have anything perceived as me being favored because I was one of such a few men, but nor did I want to have that held against me either. I guess it helped me academically because I stood out. I was the only one with a beard in the school. I never missed a lecture except on one occasion, in the third semester, I went over to the Welch Library to finish working on a paper. When I came back for another class, Dr. Shiber said, "Oh, Bernie, I missed you in class earlier." I thought, "Wow. Here I've got classmates that have probably missed ten or fifteen days, much

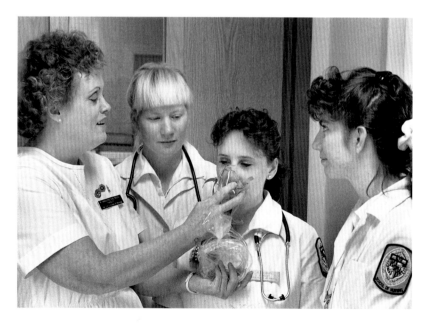

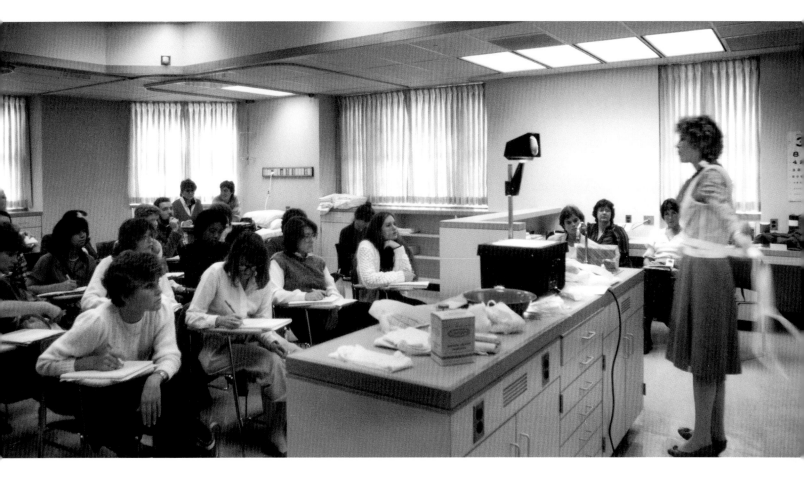

less lectures, and I miss one lecture and here it is pointed out to me." That kept me on my toes.

Sue Appling, 1973, *faculty member:* They developed the curriculum beginning with the most basic courses and building up in complexity. Students would go from just knowing information to applying information to synthesizing and analyzing information to the point where, as they graduated, they could achieve these more dynamic program objectives.

Keenan, 1986, MSN 1993: The faculty made it clear that this school was going to be based on science. It wasn't merely that we learned to do something, memorized it, and always did it that way. Health care was changing; we had to be prepared to change with it.

    The faculty all thought about what their experiences were as students. They thought about what was important and what wasn't important. They did away with things that didn't need to be done. They turned things upside down or reinvented the way nursing education could be. It was not just a matter of "This is the way we've always done it and so we're going to do it that way" or "We were miserable doing that and, by God, they're going to be miserable doing it too." Things were really very well thought out. That's the way the school is, trying to always make a better experience for the student because, then, better students make better nurses make better care for patients.

"Of one thing I am certain, you have been the singular force that made the School and the setting a reality," Dean Carol Gray wrote to Dr. Heyssel in 1984, thanking him for making space in the Phipps Building available to the school. That year Susan Appling (standing), 1973, became one of the first faculty members hired by the Johns Hopkins University School of Nursing, where she taught for twenty years.

Sue Appling was a person who knew how to do just about everything. She was very strong technically. She had been a critical care nurse. She was also a nurse practitioner. From the time we opened the school, the nursing practice lab has been Sue's area. That unquestionably has always been extremely well done. I've always felt fortunate that she was the perfect person and that she stayed with it all these years. Students see her as the model for what a nurse should be.
Stella Shiber

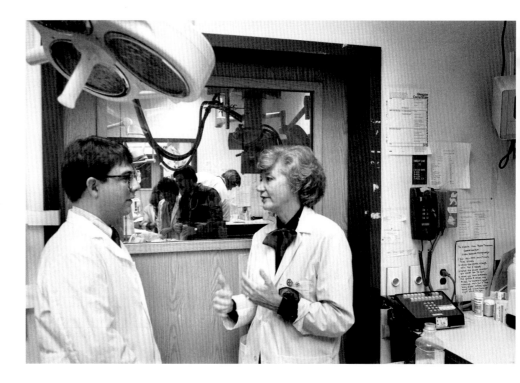

Dorothy Gordon (center) had been on the faculty since 1985, when she became, in 1989, the first person to hold the Elsie M. Lawler Professorship. Five years later Dr. Gordon was elected chairwoman of the advisory board of the National Center for Medical Rehabilitation Research.

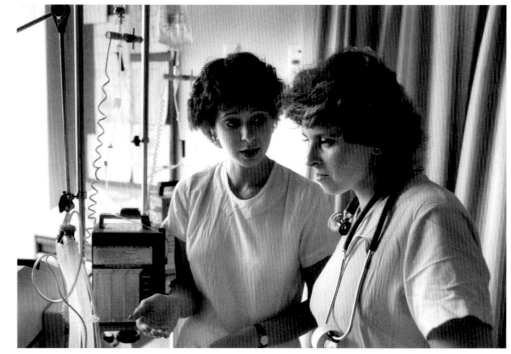

All three consortium hospitals provided clinical placements for students in the university school. Liz Packer (right), 1986, listened intently as Melinda Marchum, her staff preceptor at Sinai Hospital, explained a procedure. Medea Marella, vice president of nursing at Sinai, enjoyed hosting students, but she acknowledged that she "had to be concerned about the patients and the quality of care they were going to be getting and seeing that the students in our program would have the necessary skills and knowledge to perform the care."

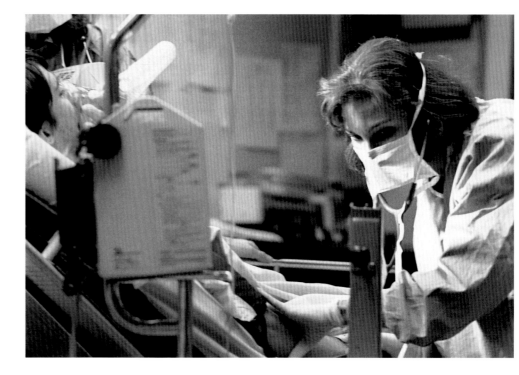

Johns Hopkins was the clinical site preferred by most students. When the first class graduated in 1986, most of its members accepted positions at hospitals participating in the consortium: two went to Church Home, three to Sinai, and twelve to Hopkins. Here, in 1990, a student monitored a patient's condition.

It was very important that we all earned a bachelor of science degree, that we didn't earn a bachelor of science in nursing. The message it sent was that, look, nurses are just as academic as all the other disciplines. You don't get a bachelor of science in biology, you major in biology. It was very clear to us that we would earn a bachelor of science and we majored in nursing.

Shiber: From the very beginning I included in the curriculum more clinical time than most baccalaureate programs had and made it clear that we were going to graduate a student who knew what to do, who was clinically competent. Philosophically we decided that we were never going to have our students observing. We were going to have them actively learning by doing, which meant two things. I'd better have faculty who know how to do it and enough of them so that students can all actively practice. We were looking for faculty who were strong clinical role models, who were not strangers to the hospitals and the clinics.

Marella: Each hospital had its own faculty that would be supervising or educating the students when they came to each respective hospital for their clinical experience. We had four nurses at Sinai who were prepared at the master's level so that they could fulfill the role of a faculty member at the Johns Hopkins School of Nursing. They were Sinai Department of Nursing employees but they had faculty appointments.

We were excited to be associated with an upper-division program in nursing. My staff, the ones who were the faculty members, really put themselves out and they loved having the students. We'd had students all along from different schools, like Towson and the University of Maryland, but they brought their own faculty to take care of their students in our hospital. This was different. These were *our* students and it was *our* hospital and *our* faculty, so it was a totally different ballgame. It was a good feeling.

Larson: One of the really exciting things was the close link between the hospital and the clinical practice at Hopkins and the School of Nursing. We really were kept honest in terms of making sure we weren't going off into a cloud or just theoretically understanding the profession, but really getting in there working, collecting data, and doing research in the community with the staff at the hospital.

Keenan, 1986, MSN 1993: Sue Appling was teaching Principles and Applications of Nursing. When you know nothing about nursing, what you think is important are these tasks. You don't have an appreciation for the critical thinking that needs to go on. Sue would show us how to do procedures. Now I am on faculty teaching that very class along with

I never wanted a student to forget that when they were dealing with equipment that there's a patient attached and not to nurse the machine. You know how frustrating that is to patients and families— to have a nurse run in and turn buttons and run out and never even recognize that there's a patient there. There are a lot of nurses who totally forget to make the patient a part of what they're doing.

Stella Shiber

Sue and I hear Sue with the same enthusiasm that I remember hearing twenty years ago. Nothing was too much trouble. Everything was very doable. Always a positive attitude.

Maureen Maguire, *faculty member:* We've always had a combination of full-time faculty and clinical faculty, whose primary job is in a clinical facility. The idea of that is to have people who are at the very cutting edge of what's happening in clinical practice because it changes so much. They teach pediatric nursing, or psychiatric nursing, or OB for the period of time those courses are being taught, and then they're back doing their regular clinical specialist job or nurse manager job in between.

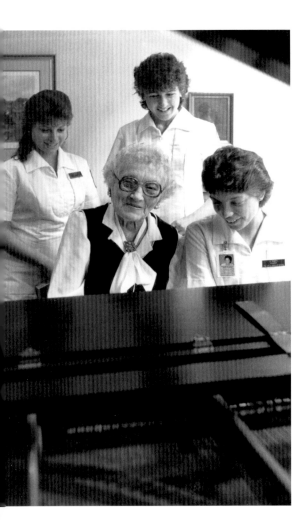

Amy Berman Heyman, Karen Weiland, and Judith Raboy, all 1987, gathered around Church Home resident Gertrude Rice to listen as she played the piano, in 1986.

McClain: There was a lot of good professional contact in using the clinical departments as sites for training nurses. The quality of the students showing up in clinical settings was good and, in some cases, quite extraordinarily good. Much of what the school was doing, at least within the hospital and medical part of the operation, began to speak for itself.

Larson: There was in the hospital a culture of nurses who were, at the very least, aware of needing to ask questions that needed research. Because it's an academic health center, a lot of nurses were part of research teams, primarily from the School of Medicine. There was a lot of research going on and many, many nurses in the hospital collected data for other studies.

Keenan, 1986, MSN 1993: They rotated us through all the hospitals. We would be two weeks out at Sinai, and then two weeks at Hopkins, and maybe two weeks at Church Hospital. That didn't go over well at all. It had good logic behind it. It forced us to think of the science of what we were doing, rather than just going and memorizing some procedures of the way this or that hospital did it. But a lot of my classmates felt that by the time they got feeling comfortable somewhere, it was time to go.

Shiber: It was an uncomfortable arrangement for the first few years because we would have to do our best to keep the consortium hospitals happy. The students came to the Johns Hopkins School of Nursing for an education at Johns Hopkins. They didn't take kindly to being shipped off to Church or Sinai to do their clinical learning. It was always a tension. We had to convince these students to at least think they were getting a quality education that included spending a significant portion of their time at facilities other than Hopkins.

Maybe 60 or 75 percent of the students in our first classes stayed at Hopkins. They came to Hopkins because they wanted to be at Hopkins and it's not a bad idea to have a few years of experience on your resume from Hopkins. Very few chose to work at Sinai or Church and that was always a real bone of contention.

Angell, 1969, BSN 1977: We got financial support from the three hospitals, Church, Sinai, and Hopkins. There was a tremendous amount of determination from other places to make sure that it did succeed. We had a consortium board that we answered to. Whenever those meetings were about to occur, that was a very tense time because they had financial oversight, they asked a lot of questions, and we had to defend everything that was done. I would describe the first couple years as very tense.

McClain: Neither Church Home nor Sinai ever got an appreciable number of our graduating students to work there. In terms of its own institutional self-interest, neither was seeing much benefit of staying in the consortium. When Church Home dropped out I think that Sinai rightly said, "This was a good thing. We're glad we did it but it's not serving our particular interest anymore since we're not getting any demonstrable benefit."

Keenan, 1986, MSN 1993: The first year there were only the twenty-some of us and we were the whole school. Then the next year it was stunning. There were thirty or forty that came after us. Now the school had doubled and suddenly it was filled halls and maybe even going to another room for a lecture. The first year it wasn't uncommon for us to be in one lecture hall for the whole day or one classroom for the greater part of a day.

Maguire: Those first couple of years, there's a real bond between the School of Nursing and those graduates. Many friendships grown out of that time have lasted over the years. They will be some of my cherished memories when I look back, being here at the beginning. There was a lot of flexibility. We could really express ourselves. There was a lot of creativity in the teaching. We had a good time. There weren't as many administrative things that take a lot of the teachers' time.

Angell, 1969, BSN 1977: Those of us who were involved in the school knew we were going to be accredited because the standards that were set were so high for the academic program and the clinical experience. Stella Shiber and the other faculty knew what acceptable standards were. The goal was just to always set our standards higher. We knew that for anybody who graduated before the accreditation was received, that it would be retroactive and they would be protected.

By the third year, when such a high percentage of students were passing the NCLEX [the national council licensing exam] and being successful and being able to say that employers were very pleased with their performance, we had more data to go on. But for the first two years, admissions were a big sales job. We would go over into the hospital. At that particular time in the school's history, it was important that I was a nurse because I was able to speak about the clinical aspects of being

For a few years the former Phipps Psychiatric Clinic became known as the Frank M. Houck Building, but then its name reverted to the Phipps Building. The university School of Nursing made its home there from its opening until 1992, when the 1913 structure was slated for a demolition that never took place.

We were learning about doing physical exams. We were practicing on each other, looking into each other's eyes and ears. Then Martha Hill and Sue Appling explained we were going to be listening to heart and lungs and even a breast exam, and that at some schools the students would wear bathing suits or keep their undergarments on. They thought that that just really was a waste of time because you weren't learning anything. You could have heard a pin drop in the class. I thought, "Well, I guess everybody's pretty okay with this." Sue Appling left the room and I got swarmed by my classmates because I was the class president. They said, "You've got to go and explain that we can't do this."

You have to understand that we were on the third floor of the Phipps Building and that's all that the school was. The whole building was being renovated and there were all these construction workers. In the practice lab, there weren't any curtains. Everyone was imagining that there would be workers pressing their noses up against the windows watching all these disrobed women. I explained the situation to Sue Appling and Sue said, "We'll fix that. We'll hang sheets up on the windows and we can hang sheets for examining areas. You let everybody know it'll be just fine."

Martha Hill and Sue Appling demonstrated how to do a breast exam. I guess my classmates felt at least that they weren't being asked to do anything that the faculty weren't willing to do. The idea of us practicing on each other was purposeful in sensitizing us to what it's like to be a patient. That was important.

Bernard Keenan, 1986, MSN 1993

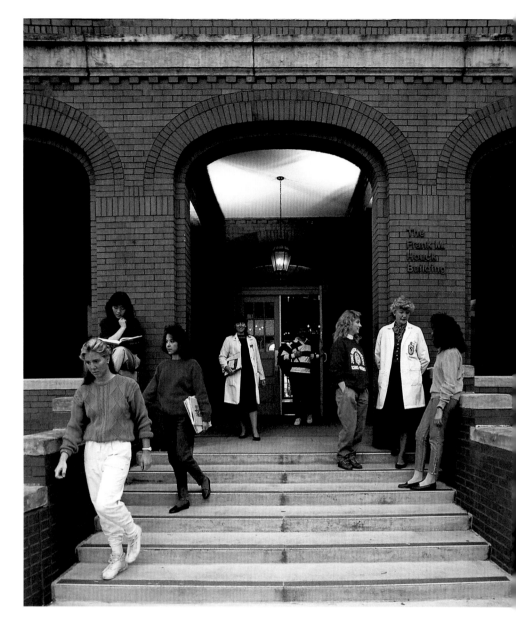

a nurse. We really used the hospital as an enticement. It's hard to come to Hopkins and walk through the hospital and not be excited about it. Even if you have no desire to be a health professional, it's a pretty impressive place.

Keenan, 1986, MSN 1993: We were attending a school that was not accredited. In order to have the program accredited you had to graduate your first class. Well, we were the first class and, quite honestly, we didn't know if we would pass the state boards because, of course, this was a new program. Did the faculty really know what they were doing?

In preparing us for that, we took what were called the National League for Nursing exams. Dr. Shiber told us the state board exam was testing to make sure that we knew enough not to kill somebody. As Hopkins nurses, we were expected to do a whole lot more than just not kill somebody. But when we took these NLN exams, our scores were much lower than any of us imagined they would be and we thought,

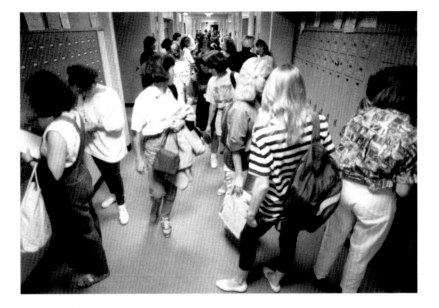

As enrollment continued to swell, conditions in the Phipps Building became increasingly crowded. Students had their own lockers but, unlike alumnae who had attended the diploma school, they had no dorm rooms in which to study or relax.

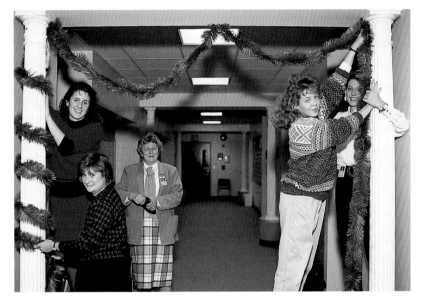

Administrator Arlowayne Swort (wearing a plaid skirt) joined students as they decorated for the holidays in 1989. As director of admissions for the fledgling university school, Sandy Angell, 1969, BSN 1977, knew firsthand how austere things were in the early years. "We were on a very, very tight budget. There were no frills. We'd have a Christmas party and we'd all bake cookies."

"Oh, my God." It was a whole new way of testing and we were pretty stunned. It made clear to us that we had better study so that we could bring those scores up because we weren't going to be allowed to sit for the board. We weren't going anywhere unless we were going to pass this exam and do well. We weren't going to be out there embarrassing the alumni, the faculty, and for some, their parents, and in my case, my wife, by not being able to pass.

Maguire: There was no question Dr. Shiber was the titular head of the baccalaureate program. With her leadership we passed the NLN accreditation the first time out. We got full accreditation for eight years without any recommendations for change.

Shiber: Early on, it didn't seem to me that we were entirely meeting the needs of the occasional young person who already had a degree. We treated her or him just like the person who had two years of college.

We should have known they were different. They are much more sophisticated learners. That's how the second-degree program came about. I thought there would be a small group of people but what happened, of course, was they overran the whole school. We announced the accelerated, second-degree program in February and that June we had sixteen. The next year we had sixty. And then it went to seventy-two, then eighty-four, and then it went over a hundred. It stayed over a hundred.

Then applicants to the two-year program shifted in large part from people who had two years and sixty credits from someplace to people who had finished a degree and were going to do nursing as a second undergraduate degree. The decision got to be, do I want to do this in thirteen months or two years? When I designed that curriculum, I didn't really expect that it was going to impact the school the way it did. It is probably the single biggest thing that happened to the school.

Appling, 1973: That accelerated program was the salvation. They started in the summer and ended in the summer, so our summers were filled with accelerated students paying full-time tuition at the same time as we had regular two-year traditional students paying full-time tuition during the spring and the fall semesters.

The accelerated program was about getting people through in thirteen months and giving them, essentially, the same number of hours of education and of clinic, just compressed. The idea was to get very strong students. All they had to do was come in with anatomy and physiology and microbiology. They were very motivated. Many of them had other types of jobs, other types of careers, and were changing for whatever reason. They could get their nursing education done quickly and they could get back out in the work force. Even though it was a big hunk of change, it meant that they only had to take thirteen months out of their lives to do it.

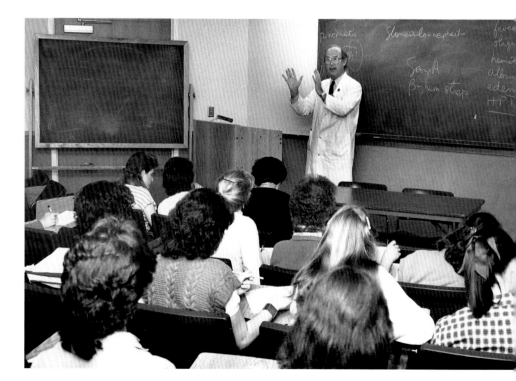

Following a longstanding tradition in nursing education at Johns Hopkins, members of the faculties of both the School of Medicine and the School of Public Health often taught classes to nursing students. Here Dr. Langford Kidd focused on the complexities of pathophysiology.

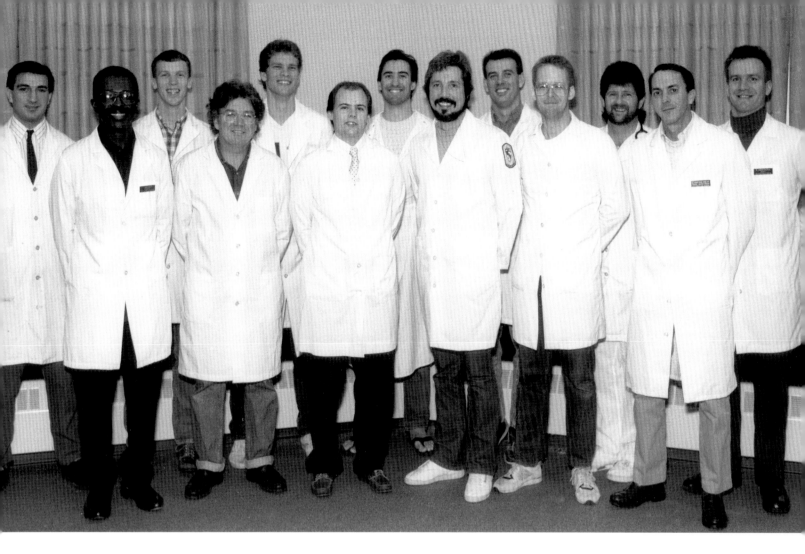

Maguire: The accelerated class comes in the first week of June and takes two semesters of the skills course and the one-semester dimensions course in a ten-week period. Everything's speeded up, doing double time. Instead of one day a week or a half-day a week of skills lab, they're doing a whole day a week of skills lab. Instead of one lab, they're doing two labs for assessment. They get the same education; it's just at an accelerated pace, particularly that first semester. After that, they're on the same kind of timetable except they have shorter vacations in between.

Accelerated students already have a baccalaureate degree, at least, in some field other than nursing. It can be in anything. It can be in music, biology, anything at all. We've had people with business backgrounds. We've had people with artistic backgrounds. We've had performers.

This program is thirteen and a half months long. The accelerated students are mostly people who have seen something of the world, made a decision to become nurses, and are very anxious to get out there and be nurses. They're all very bright. They come with very high GPAs. Our idea was that if these people have been successful in another educational program and have gotten a degree, that counts as most of the prerequisites. They don't have to take so many credits in chemistry and so many credits in history or humanities. The only prerequisites are six to eight credits in human anatomy and physiology and at least three credits in microbiology.

As the profession expanded and nursing began to attract a greater number of men, the ranks of male nursing students and alumni at Johns Hopkins also grew. By 1991 the school boasted thirteen male students.

You talk to my son and it was like just another college program. He didn't have a minute's trouble with anything. His classmates all wore short white lab coats. He blended in with his classmates, which I think is good because I stuck out like a sore thumb. His experience was totally different. He keeps telling me how hard it was. I got a diploma, he got a degree, and I remind him that I had a wife and two kids.

Herb Zinder, 1971

Elaine Larson brought a very steady enthusiasm and commitment to the profession of nursing. She brought a sense of excellence. It was the first time within the school that we had a faculty appointment that people there could say, "This is what we should be doing." She was very, very good. She was the personification of what the school could be in terms of the quality of its faculty. We were lucky to have her as long as we did.

Stephen McClain

Johnson & Johnson expressed an interest in funding something with the School of Nursing. I put together a proposal for a postdoctoral program to train nurses to do research in the field of infectious diseases and infection control. Now, the astounding thing about this was that we didn't have a doctoral program then. It didn't deter us for a minute. We thought, "It will enhance the school's research so that when we're ready to start the doctoral program, we'll already have a good track record of training postdocs and having funded research."

Johnson & Johnson really liked the idea. They decided to fund nine postdocs. Senior, highly educated nurses applied. Every year we had many more applications than we could take. The nurses who were recruited to this postdoc program had to do original research and write grants for funding. The stipend was better than you could get as an NIH-funded postdoc. It wasn't comparable to a nurse's salary, but it was certainly a livable wage, which was unusual.

Elaine Larson

Kate Knott, 2002: For your first semester of the traditional program, the hardest class that you take is pharmacology. The second semester, the hardest class you take is pathophysiology. The accelerated students have the delightful pleasure of taking in their fall term pathophysiology and pharmacology at the same time. They all look like zombies by the time January rolls around because nobody's slept and everybody's completely stressed out.

The real difference between the accelerated program and the traditional program is really more personality than anything. I would say it's more a type A personality who might be the one to go for the accelerated program. I knew that I didn't retain information as well when it was so jammed down my throat. I wanted to do traditional because I thought, "This is information that you need for the rest of your career" so I wanted to be able to digest it.

Maguire: We have done some follow-up studies and have found some interesting things. After six months, you cannot tell the difference between the one who took it in thirteen months versus the one who took two years. It didn't make a difference what their previous major was. We all thought the ones with science and biology backgrounds would do better than the liberal arts or business backgrounds. It makes no difference in six months.

Angell, 1969, BSN 1977: Stella Shiber has a creative mind when it comes to being a little bit ahead in designing curriculum that other schools hadn't thought of yet. To say you have an accelerated program doesn't mean much anymore because everybody has one. But at the time that ours was put in place, it was one of the first and it's been widely imitated. She was generous with that information if people asked her about it.

I hold Stella in very high regard. She's a psychiatric nurse by background and that's a wonderful asset in management. I give her all the credit for those early years, the real putting-us-on-the-map years, for our educational programs. She has a wonderful breadth and depth of knowledge about nursing and about historical trends. I don't think we'd be where we are if she hadn't been so central for so many years.

Marella: Steve Muller knew exactly what the university was going to do and how they were going to help to implement this school and how the university was going to control certain aspects of the educational program. The curriculum for our School of Nursing had to match other programs at the university.

McClain: If this School of Nursing was going to survive in the Hopkins context, it had to have a research component from the very beginning. Even if it was modest it needed to be there. Even though it didn't get going until the school was well established, the idea was that it would eventually have a doctoral program. If nursing was a profession coming into its own academically and if it was going to be within a Hopkins context, then it had to have the full array of what Hopkins is about on both the educational and the research side. That was one of the reasons for the master's degree program being an integral part of the thinking early on. That would be the first entrée into at least a modest research program with the School of Nursing.

Larson: The admissions policies brought us extremely mature and bright students who knew what they wanted. We were able to have a student body motivated toward a more scholarly career, not necessarily an academic career, but scholarly in the sense that whatever you do, whether it's clinical practice or whatever, you ask questions, you think about how to solve things.

Shiber: Because of the money that we got from the alumni to endow a chair, Elaine Larson became the first Nutting professor. That was quite unusual to have an endowed chair for a new school with just a baccalaureate program. Elaine was very well known in infection control prevention research, and because of her research she was able to attract Johnson & Johnson funding that brought postdoc fellows to the school. It was unusual that we had a school of nursing with no doctoral program that had postdocs. From a very early time, Elaine was able to bring some credibility and national attention to the school.

Larson: Nursing research at Hopkins was on the fast track compared with other schools that had had university degrees and baccalaureate programs for several decades longer. The focus from the beginning was really very clear: that it was a scholarly place, that it was also clinically based, and that what mattered was patient outcomes. There was also a very strong commitment to the community. I think that was very important. And having all the schools physically close—the School of Medicine, the School of Nursing, the School of Public Health—meant that we would have collaborative research. That was just a gold mine for high productivity and for really being able to not feel limited.

We thought of a lot of innovative teaching strategies. For example, for the research course for the undergraduates, the traditional way to teach it would be to have them write a draft of a research proposal. We didn't do that. We had them go out in teams. We found a bunch of clinical mentors, like head nurses or staff nurses, who had a clinical problem they were interested in. They were assigned a group of students and the students' job was to review the literature in that area and figure out ways the literature might be applied to the problem area. We called it STUR, Student Teams Using Research. As far as I know, nobody had ever done anything like that. Being new was nice. I didn't think about

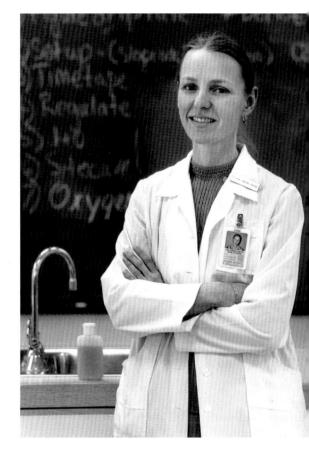

Elaine Larson was the first occupant of the M. Adelaide Nutting Chair in Clinical Nursing. During 1986, her first year on campus, Larson initiated or consulted on twenty research and program studies at Hopkins, Sinai, and Church Home. Under Larson's guidance, the postdoctoral program got under way in 1987, and two years later she established the school's first laboratory, which enabled students and faculty to accomplish basic scientific research that could be applied to clinical practice.

"How is it normally done?" I thought more "How *should* it be done?"

Shiber: Elaine was the director for the Center for Nursing Research, so she was known as someone who could be very helpful and had some solid thinking about research and nursing. Georgetown asked her to come down there as a consultant about how they might be able to bring more research to the nursing program at Georgetown. After being a consultant, as sometimes will happen, they asked her to be the dean.

Einaudi: The Center for Nursing Research furthers nursing research and encourages faculty members. They help faculty members to write grant proposals and when the money comes in, it all gets funneled through the center. Graduate students are learning right from the start about good nursing research and how to get it done. For a young nurse researcher, that's the place to get nurtured and mentored.

In 1987 Arlene Butz (pictured showing a toddler to Senator Paul Sarbanes) and Denise Korniewicz became the first postdoctoral fellows. Dr. Butz later joined the faculty of the Department of Pediatrics in the School of Medicine.

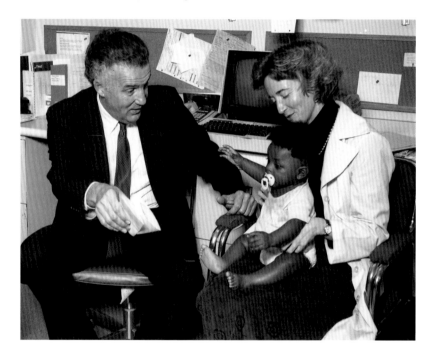

The first graduates in the Johns Hopkins University School of Nursing's master's program gathered in July 1989 to receive their degrees.

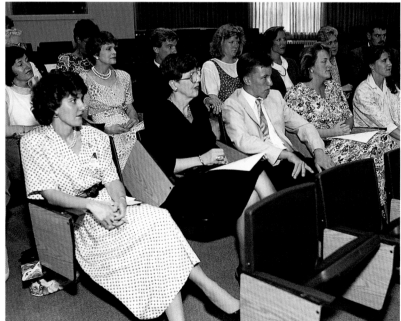

McClain: Bob Heyssel and Carol Gray did have a good relationship. Carol understood very well on which side of the bread her butter was. Because Bob had invested so much of his time, energy, and his personal and professional prestige and money into it, he took a rather benevolent view of the School of Nursing. Some of the most vicious battles I've seen fought anywhere within this university, particularly in East Baltimore, are about space. That land where the new building sits was Bob Heyssel's gift to the School of Nursing. That was prime, prime space and you know that he had at least half a dozen department heads coming in and saying, "Bob, *what* are you doing?" Even in the school's early years, Bob did pretty well making sure they had good space within the East Baltimore complex. The School of Nursing could have wound up three miles from East Baltimore in some rented second-rate space. Bob did things for the School of Nursing that were quite significant.

The public is not clear about just how important nurses are. They have this concept of the ever-present, caring angel, which is a nice concept, but at Hopkins, the nurses were outspoken. They were educated. They were knowledgeable. They were assertive. They acted. They didn't just sit at the bedside and mop your brow. They were looking at your med charts and analyzing your laboratory data and plotting the next step for what you, as a patient, needed in your care. They were the organizers of the care. I saw that over and over again. The nurses were outspoken, but not in a disrespectful way. When they thought something needed to be done, they stood up. You followed the chain of command but you went to the intern or the resident or whomever you needed to go to explain your concern. I'm always trying to explain to anybody who will listen about how important nurses are. I am convinced they are the glue in the health care system.

Cathy Novak, 1973

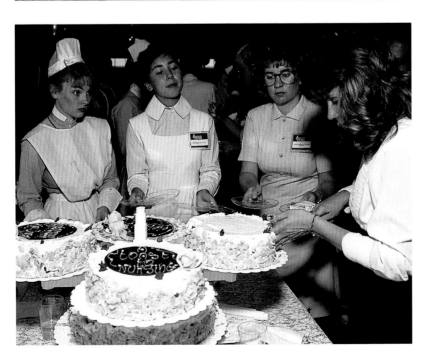

Friends assembled in the Turner Concourse in 1989 to listen as Dr. Robert M. Heyssel (holding a microphone) offered a toast to nursing as a highlight of the centennial celebration both of the hospital and of nursing education at Johns Hopkins. After the testimonials, students wearing uniforms of their predecessors waited eagerly for a slice of celebratory cake.

MAME WARREN

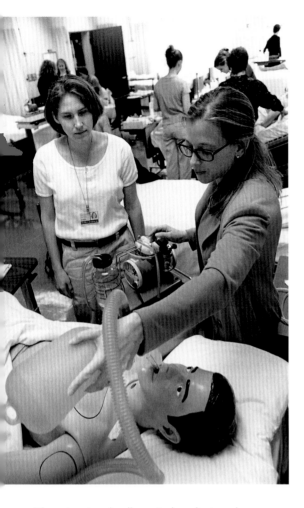

The university school's curriculum eliminated many hours of clinical time in the hospital and instead made provision for students to learn in practice labs using mannequins to simulate patients. Here Rene Rubenstein Shumate, 1991, demonstrated the use of defibrillator paddles to shock a "patient" whose heart had stopped beating.

Shiber: At Hopkins, space is a tremendously important asset. Everybody fights over every little closet that becomes available. If you're going to control your own destiny, you'd better control your own space. We're right in front of the hospital. I think that makes a statement in and of itself. We've got Dr. Heyssel to thank for that space.

Einaudi: The hospital trustees gave the land to the school for a dollar a year and said, "You can have it and you build the School of Nursing there." Suddenly, everybody's outlook changed. This was an unbelievable vote of confidence. It energized all of us to know that we were really going to be given a presence right across the street from the main entrance to the hospital. You could not do better than that.

McGeady, 1955, BSN 1955: When I heard that we were going to get it on *the* prime piece of real estate left in East Baltimore, I could not believe it. I did not really believe that I would see the nursing school in its own building in my lifetime. The idea of being able to have a home on the Hopkins medical campus in a prominent place encouraged me that perhaps the medical community was saying, "We value nursing."

Einaudi: The School of Nursing was in the Phipps Building. We were on the third floor and half of the fourth floor. Within a year and a half or two, we were in six different buildings. We had no real identity.

The accelerated program got started with sixteen students. The following year, they had sixty. Well, you can imagine how many more faculty members you've got to hire, how many more lab spaces, how many more classroom spaces you've got to have. It was very clear that something had to be done. How do you get any sense of identity if you're all spread out like that?

Marella: Once the school was established, one of the first things they tried to do was get a fund-raising person and start raising money for an endowment. They've been very, very successful. The very first two or three months they raised $200,000 just like that! It was going to take off and it has. Money comes to Hopkins because it's a fine institution; it's a great university, and so people are drawn to good schools, good hospitals.

Davis: Many alumni from the RN program married physicians and came into wealth. In their positions as physicians' wives, they have been very influential in raising money among themselves or with associations or businesses that their husbands are involved in. They have been a great boon and have contributed so much to the school. It's made it a showplace, really. The state has been helpful in many ways, but private donors have made a big difference to this school because of their position in society and their influence with corporations and organizations.

Shiber: Carol Gray had a very heavy job in raising funds and interacting with alumni. She was more an outside person and I was the inside person. I never felt I had anything but her complete trust. Before the National League of Nursing came for their visit to accredit us, she had me come into her office and said, "Now explain to me what a typical day and week might be like in the School of Nursing for students and faculty." She really didn't know.

Carol seemed incapable of just sitting down and chatting. She was always very prim and proper and very formal. She never hung out with us. She was not a person that you could easily get to know. Students would see her at graduation and that would be the first time. They didn't know who she was. She was always in the dean's office behind closed doors. She was not the kind of person who was visible.

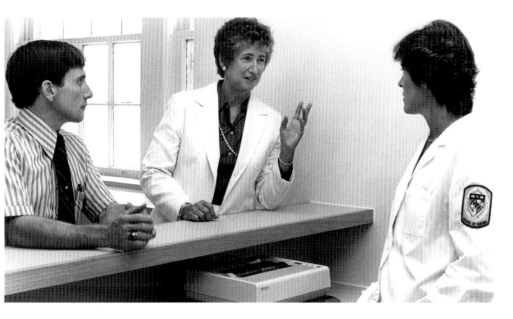

Dean Carol Gray elicited mixed reactions from colleagues and students. Some found her aloof while others considered her warm and welcoming. All agreed that she was an effective leader who established an innovative school firmly based on Hopkins' tradition of excellence.

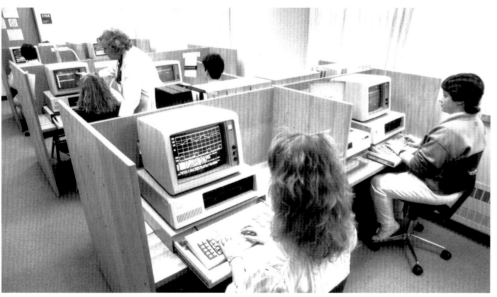

In 1985 the Women's Board of the Johns Hopkins Hospital provided $30,000 for the purchase of computer equipment for the school. A computer lab was essential for courses required in the new curriculum, which made the school one of the first to provide the skills nurses would need to work with information technology systems.

Keenan, 1986, MSN 1993: Dean Gray made a substantial impact on me personally and professionally. She presented me with opportunities and unquestioning support that was, Well, of course we would succeed. There was never any doubt in her mind that the things we were being asked to do could be done. She did a great job of knowing what was going on.

Dean Gray would come to meetings to be helpful to us. She was very interested in knowing how things were, what the student experience was like for us, and she helped us fix things or at least listened to our concerns. She had such a gracious way about herself, very unassuming. I just wanted to do all I could to please her and to rise to whatever her expectation was.

Shiber: As faculty, one of the things that we have the responsibility of doing is to recruit and educate people for our profession. We have certain values and there are certain responsibilities that are going to come with being a member of that profession. One of those responsibilities is to the professional organization. I feel strongly that nurses should be members of the American Nurses Association and, for me, as an educator, the National League for Nursing. Isabel Hampton Robb founded what is now both the ANA and the National League for Nursing. The only requirement to be a member of the ANA is to be a nurse.

Keenan, 1986, MSN 1993: Dean Gray said that it's important for students to have a mechanism of being able to know what's going on in the school and have an impact. Then she told us, "It's important as a professional that you belong to your professional organization, the National Association of Student Nurses, so you all ought to join." We got eighteen people that joined. Then it was, "There's a state affiliate to the organization and, you know, Hopkins nurses are meant to be leaders. All through the history of the school, Hopkins nurses have been leaders. You've got to learn how to be leaders." So I got involved on the board of directors there. Then I got other of my classmates involved with that as well.

Einaudi: Carol Gray resigned the very semester that the PhD program was approved at the state level. She stayed from 1984 to 1994. It was a perfect end of her deanship. She could say, "I came to lay the academic foundation and I did it. The school is on really strong footing and now I can hand it over to someone else."

McClain: Was Carol Gray an effective dean? The answer has many dimensions. She got the school started so she did quite a few things right. She did communicate particularly well with the older alumni from Hopkins hospital, and she did bring in some good people like Elaine Larson, for example, and Martha Hill. She got on famously

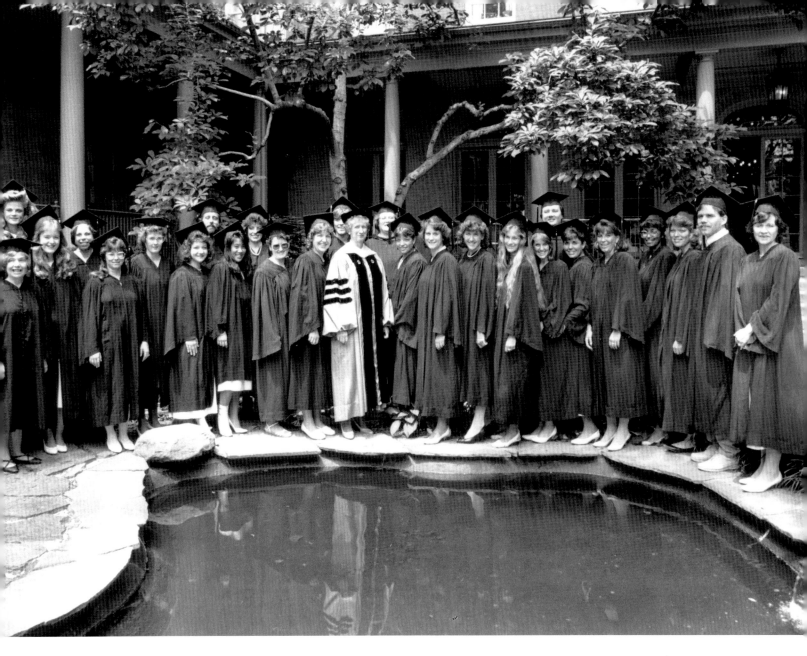

with donors, especially Nan Pinkard. By the time she left, though, it was well time for her to leave. She was beginning to take the school in certain directions that, for the longer-term future of the school, would not have been particularly good for the school.

Carol Gray was asked to step down, not because she'd done anything wrong or not because the school was in such bad shape. It became obvious to the provost and to the president—certainly it was obvious to me—that we had gone considerably beyond phase one and Carol was simply not the dean to move the school forward. She had accomplished what she had set out to accomplish. She became less open to thinking strategically about the school, whether she was simply tired, whether she had become complacent, or whether she was resistant to thinking about new ideas. The faculty was getting restless and wanted the school to move in certain directions. It was just obvious that as long as Carol was there the school was not going to move much. At Hopkins five, six, eight deans over the years have been asked to leave and not because they did anything wrong. Their time had passed.

Like generations of nursing alumni before them, the class of 1987 gathered in the garden behind the Phipps Building for a formal portrait. Unlike most of their predecessors, these graduates were about to receive baccalaureate degrees. Their dean, Dr. Carol Gray, stood proudly at the center of the group.

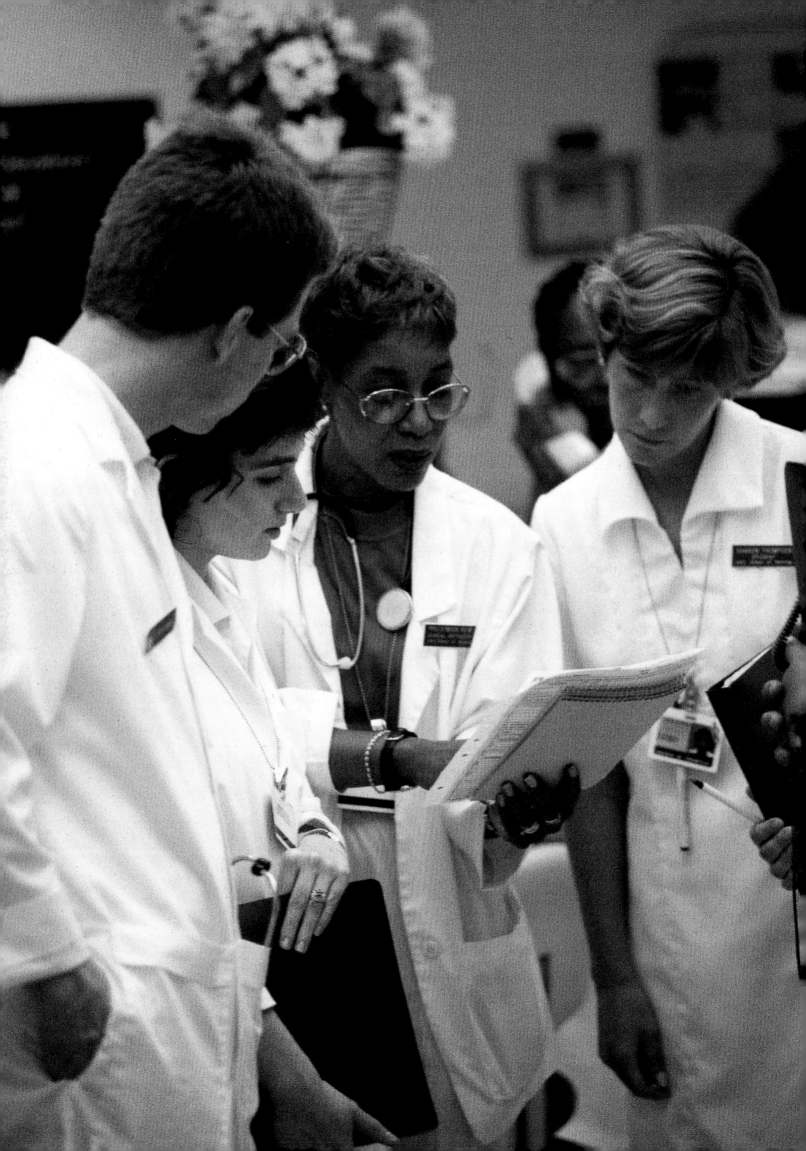

7

A Different Vision, 1995–2005 · MAME WARREN

Peter Connors, Nelli Bogdanovskaia Zafman,
and Sharon Thompson, all of the traditional
class of 1995, listened intently to their clinical
instructor, Phyllis Mason, as she reviewed a
patient's chart in a busy hospital setting.

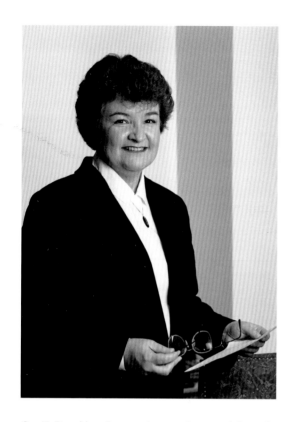

Sue K. Donaldson became, in 1994, the second dean of the Johns Hopkins School of Nursing. Dr. Donaldson arrived from the University of Minnesota Schools of Nursing and Medicine, where she had been a professor since 1983. A fellow of the National Academy of Nursing and the Institute of Medicine, National Academy of Sciences, Donaldson quickly set to work encouraging research among faculty and students.

Opposite: The Johns Hopkins *Gazette* highlighted the school's continuing success with a cover story in 1996. Dean Sue Donaldson posed front and center with her "dream team." From left: Karen Haller, vice president for nursing and patient services at Johns Hopkins Hospital, and faculty members Jacquelyn Campbell, Fannie Gaston-Johansson, Marion D'Lugoff, Kathy Sabatier, and Martha Norton Hill, 1964.

This is a very exciting place to be because it keeps changing. We keep adding programs. For a while, we just had a baccalaureate program. Then we added a master's program; that was very exciting. Now we have a doctoral program. There's no opportunity to get bored. There's always something new and different, moving into this building, planning for the next building. It's not possible to be stagnant around here.

Sandra Stine Angell, 1969, BSN 1977

William C. Richardson, *former president of the Johns Hopkins University:* It was clear, when Carol Gray was ready to retire, that we needed somebody who had the academic credentials that would go with Hopkins and the energy to fund-raise, build a building, and really be a model for those students and faculty, especially the graduate students. We looked high and low because there are a limited number of people who would feel comfortable at Hopkins working with the rest of the medical center as a dean. They are a very bright, aggressive group of people. In Sue Donaldson we got a good scientist with a very good track record and certainly with no problem at all in standing up to other people; perhaps, in some instances, more standing up than the system could handle. She just had so much energy and was so driven to get things done.

Immelt, 1977, PhD 2000: One of the very first things that we read in our PhD program was an article that Sue Donaldson collaborated on in the early '80s. It was called "What Is the Discipline of Nursing?" The PhD in nursing is relatively recent. Nursing PhD programs were developed because strong nursing scholars who wanted to get PhDs and were needed to teach in academic settings had to get PhDs in different disciplines, like Sue Donaldson's was physiology or Martha Hill's was public health. This article was about What is nursing? What is the essence of nursing? What is the discipline of nursing? It was a very good article that I go back to: that nursing is about human responses to health; that the profession of nursing is there to serve the public and to be aware of what public needs are; and that we need to really listen and assess what health needs are and be responsive to them.

Sue Donaldson, *second dean of the Johns Hopkins University School of Nursing:* The school had done a fine job of putting in all of the infrastructure and initiating all of the programs, from baccalaureate degree through master's to PhD, but it was still not established as a research division of the university. That doesn't mean there weren't very fine faculty members conducting research and even funded research from the National Institutes of Health. It meant that the sum total was not visible enough to warrant listing the school as a research division. That's in contrast to medicine and public health. If nursing did not become a research division, its long-term survival at Hopkins was questionable.

Maguire: Dr. Gray's background was education. We reached a juncture where the university, now that we had a bachelor's program and a master's program in place and were beginning a doctoral program, wanted to see a stronger research emphasis in the school. Sue Donaldson was hired because of her background as a researcher. She had headed up a big lab and had administrative experience. Sue brought excitement

The Gazette

July 22, 1996   The newspaper of The Johns Hopkins University   Volume 25 No. 39

In This Issue

2   Two JHU alumni were on board TWA flight 800. In-Brief

5   Four faculty are promoted to professor. For the Record

6   *Gimme Shelter, Wattstax* on screen as "Movies Rock." Calendar

Employment Opportunities 4

Notices 6

Classifieds 7

Hopkins is online with InteliHealth

Steve Libowitz
Editor

Scott Sherman says that recently he has has been sleeping at night like a baby. He wakes every two hours.

It's not crying, though, that stirs him. It's more like tossing and turning, of a good sort. Sherman, an assistant dean at the School of Medicine, oversees the Johns

Photo by Louis Rosenstock

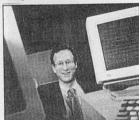

Scott Sherman heads the medical institutions' consumer health information efforts.

Hopkins Office of Consumer Health Information. Last week, he was among those who announced the formation of InteliHealth, a company created to produce and distribute consumer health information through myriad electronic channels, including the World Wide Web.

U.S. Healthcare is the funding partner, extending up to a $25 million line of credit to InteliHealth in exchange for a majority stock position in the company.

The Hopkins schools of Medicine, Nursing and Public Health, along with the health system, will be responsible for the informational content, lending their names and prestige to the venture. In return, they will be minority stockholders and earn royalties. Faculty will be compensated for their time spent reviewing and editing content.

Continued on page 8

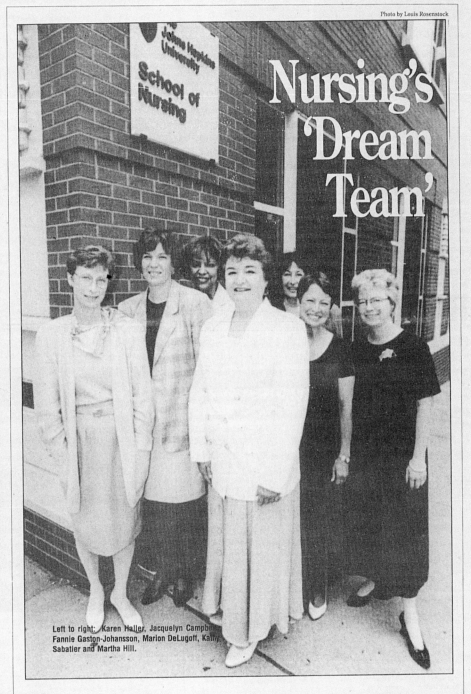

Photo by Louis Rosenstock

Nursing's 'Dream Team'

Left to right: Karen Haller, Jacquelyn Campbell, Fannie Gaston-Johansson, Marion DeLugoff, Kathy Sabatier and Martha Hill.

I n its first decade, the School of Nursing focused on attracting the best faculty and students while creating a complete curriculum, from baccalaureate to doctorate. Now, with a new building in the works and a new institute that melds academic research to clinical practice, Hopkins Nursing prepares to take on the world, led by a group of academicians and practitioners who are Nursing's own Dream Team.

See story on page 3.

I think that nurses have and had many opportunities that they were just unaware of. There was no reason in the world why a nurse couldn't hang a shingle and go into business for herself or himself. I did it and I couldn't see why nurses felt compelled to work in a hospital or a doctor's office. You need grounding in business. I told everyone who would listen that I thought that nursing schools, and medical schools for that matter, should teach the business of medicine and nursing. You get a newly minted doctor who opens up an office and has no clue how to bill or what to pay a secretary. They know medicine but they don't know the business of medicine. And it's the same with nurses.

Herb Zinder, 1971

Caring for children with asthma was a particular interest of faculty member Kathy Kushto-Reese (left). Here she worked with a student, in 1996, showing her how a gentle touch and a confident manner can reassure a young patient.

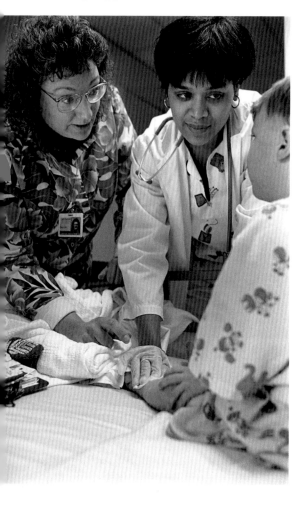

about research and hired a number of faculty. We now have two different pathways here for faculty with the educator clinician and the educator research tracks.

Einaudi: Sue Donaldson had an entirely different style from Carol Gray. They were probably as different as Elsie Lawler was from Anna D. Wolf. Sue Donaldson went to nursing school after she got her baccalaureate degree. She's a scientist first and a nurse second. She had absolutely stellar research credentials.

Sue Donaldson's mandate was to increase the prestige of the school. Well, the way to do that is to increase the amount of research that's done by the faculty members. She made it her business to encourage faculty to apply for grants and to champion them for doing it.

Maguire: Initially, the master's program was a combined nursing administration and clinical degree. You had to do both and you had to do a thesis. That was burdensome because it was a long program. That was the dream and the brainchild of the associate dean for the master's program, Arlowayne Swort. She thought that there were not enough programs preparing nursing administrators.

Under Sue, we broke out into many more majors in the master's program. We have several kinds of nurse practitioner programs. We have a clinical specialist program. We have the combined MSN/MPH program with the School of Public Health. Elaine Larson did the initial negotiations with the School of Public Health to get that off the ground. Under Sue, we got the combined MSN/MBA program with the School of Professional Studies in Business and Education. We really cover a lot of areas now.

Keenan, 1986, MSN 1993: I came back for my master's degree. I did it part-time because I was working full-time. Some of the courses were here at the School of Nursing but some were over at the School of Public Health. I really enjoyed that a lot, being mixed in with not only other nurses but also doctors and the business people. It was a real eye-opener and it was exciting.

Immelt, 1977, PhD 2000: In the PhD program, we started out with the history of philosophy: how do you know what you know? We studied in the first semester the received view, which is you can prove things, and how that whole view gradually loosened up. This was very new to us. We thought it was all about controlled clinical trials and proving that this treatment works and this one doesn't. We learned about how to do state-of-the-art literature reviews, how to investigate interventions and how you know whether they work or not. There was a big focus on health promotion, what that means working with sick people and helping them to be as healthy as they can.

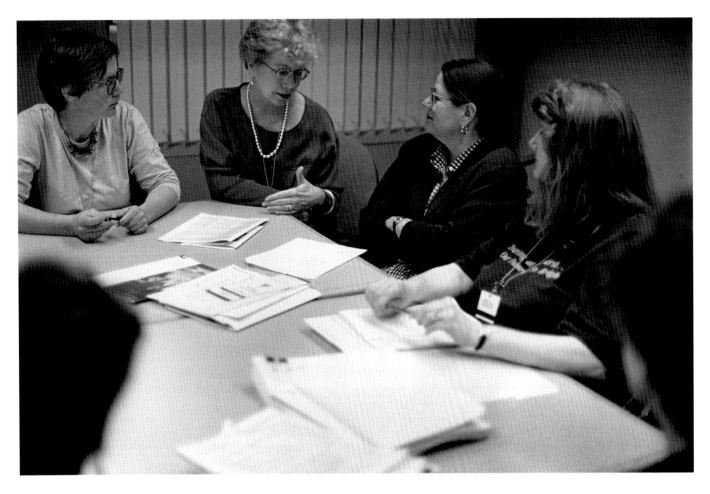

Then we had Charles Rohde from the School of Public Health and we learned very complex, multivariate statistics. We were there all weekend. The class was Wednesday afternoon and then we had a lab with this teaching assistant and we would get home at ten-thirty or eleven at night. We were all people with families and were overwhelmed. We'd sit in our computer lab and try to do these statistics. Someone always was crying because they couldn't figure it out, but we were trying to help each other. That was the research that semester.

McClain: Sue Donaldson had a very strong research background. Very few deans come into the position with extensive administrative background. They may have served as a department head and she had. Particularly at a place like Hopkins, where the deans have much more authority and control and responsibilities than you would find in many, many other universities, she was not out of the ordinary. It was mainly her research credentials that the school thought it needed to move into its second and third phases.

Sue was a very bubbly, very enthusiastic person compared to Carol Gray. Here was someone who was such a different personality type and she seemed genuine. The committee not only thought well of her on the academic side but most of them liked her. Sue Donaldson, in public,

Susan Carroll Immelt (left), 1977, PhD 2000, explained her incentive for becoming, in 1993, one of the school's first doctoral candidates: "You can't really teach in an academic setting if you don't have a PhD." Here Immelt listened while Professor Martha Norton Hill, 1964, explained her perspective to Jane Fall-Dickson, who completed the program in 2000.

I stopped working in 1986, because that's when my children were born. Then I said, "I'm not going to start working again until I get my PhD and I really want to get my PhD at Johns Hopkins." You knew it was a new program, but they knew what they were doing. It was exciting—nice, supportive people—and great scholars. The students were really bright and the faculty was really great. It was small but it was very rigorous and I enjoyed it a lot.

Susan Carroll Immelt, 1977, PhD 2000

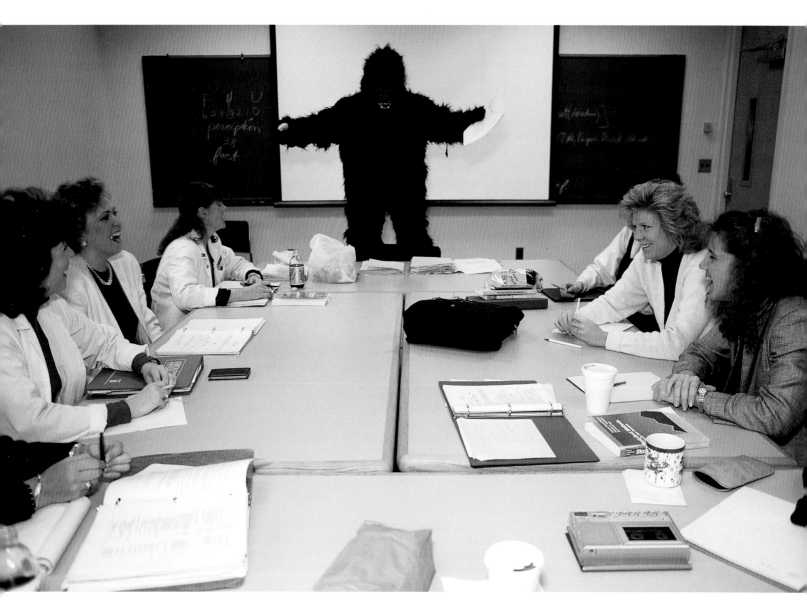

Professor Ron Berk delighted students in 1988 by dressing as a gorilla on Halloween. Colleague Ada Davis appreciated Berk's antics, "He has a wild sense of humor. He has studied the effect of humor on students. He says it's positive and most of his students love it."

Statistics might be more boring than learning how to change a bed. Ron Berk teaches the best statistics class ever. That man is a nutball. He's crazy. He's so funny. Every year he dressed up for Halloween. He added music and every lecture had some theme. He changed the words and would make us sing along. He has written books about how to bring humor into the classroom. He's legendary for his antics.

Kate Knott, 2002

always had such enthusiasm for what she was doing and for the school and that got communicated to people. On the public occasions, she was enthusiastic, exuberant, and at times, which could be effective, a little bit wacky.

Donaldson: Within the first week of my arriving, the faculty had a party to welcome me and each person had found some clever thing to signify my becoming a dean. There were little red beaded slippers with a note that said, "You're not in Kansas anymore." There was a top hat for fund-raising. One of the gifts came from Sue Appling, who's an alumna of the hospital diploma school of nursing. She had taken a red cape and then used yellow felt and made it into a Superman cape.

Davis: Sue Donaldson was a totally different person altogether from Carol. She was very outgoing, very friendly, liked jokes and laughter. She was like a breath of fresh air, in a way, but did not have the administrative experience, really, that Carol had had. I remember one meeting soon after she came here. I was involved in the meeting at the university. Sue came with a superman cape. She came into this room with prominent people in the university and flaunted the superman cape. That made an impression. People were impressed with Sue's bravery. She didn't flinch. Sue, when she came with her personality and her abilities, changed the whole school, really. Things became a little lighter.

Donaldson: When I came here, the School of Nursing had gotten all of its accreditations from the National League for Nursing and other accrediting bodies. The graduate programs were new and they hadn't existed long enough with enough graduates to be eligible for the rankings. So at the point I came, it had never been ranked. There were over two hundred schools they would be compared to in the ranking. Then they said to me, "Well guess what, we're eligible this time around and it will come out in the spring." And I thought, what if it doesn't come out in the top twenty? Top fifty, maybe that could be done. But you know Hopkins. How do you think Hopkins would view a ranking less than top twenty? It's done on the quality of the graduate programs and the leadership. The deans vote.

I have never been so grateful in my whole life. When the first rankings came out we came up fourteenth. I breathed a sigh of relief. Next time we were in a tie with five other schools for eighth place. You live and die by the rankings. Students choose the school based on the rankings.

Einaudi: The school, under Sue, went to fifth in the rankings and that's remarkable. Here's a school that opened up in 1984. Its graduate program opened up in '88 and by 1998, they're fifth in the country. Sue was well known in the field and loved to go out and talk about the quality of research being done at Johns Hopkins. If she had been quiet about it, I'm not so sure that we would have gotten the recognition.

Immelt, 1977, PhD 2000: Sue Donaldson could talk about anything. I'd run into her in the hallway and she would start talking about something and I'd say, "Oh, yes, that reminds me of this, this, and this." "Yes, that's right," she'd say, "but what about this?" She had a brain that just really rolled. She really had a wonderful capacity to just take whatever this issue was that you were talking about and really think about it and come up with a way to discuss it and make it meaningful.

Benita Walton-Moss, 1978, *faculty member:* Sue Donaldson was very encouraging. It took me two tries to get this K Award, which apparently is not very unusual, and she was very helpful in terms of "How are things going? Think about this." When she was no longer dean, just bumping into her in the halls, she gave me lots of ideas. You know, typical Sue. "Call up so-and-so and tell them I told you to call." She's been

You get your bachelor's and you get your master's and you get your nurse practitioner and, by God, we've got to have a lot of doctorates too. That's what I'm seeing. I think that's too bad. Research is all well and good but what about the people who take care of people? Maybe they just don't fit in at the Hopkins School of Nursing, but that's something we were good at and something we were known for. I fear that people will go off with the Hopkins name and different things will be expected of them than they're capable of.

Lois Grayshan Hoffer, 1962

Associate Professor Miyong T. Kim (right) met often with Korean women at the Greenmount Senior Center (pictured here) and at other facilities as part of her grant-funded research on the prevalence, treatment, and prevention of coronary heart disease among Korean-American immigrants.

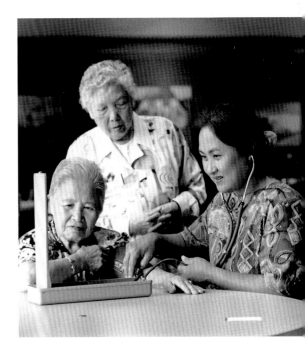

Instructor Diane Aschenbrenner (left) demonstrated for her student how to assess proper functioning of a wound drain. Aschenbrenner also stressed her areas of expertise: pain management, preventing errors in administering medication, and effecting medical procedures.

very supportive. "We are here to support you as a developing researcher. That's our goal here."

Sue's always liked the idea of having a teaching and a practice track. I don't think Sue ever blinked an eye in terms of a practice-track person who's also trying to go down the research road. It made sense to her. This is Hopkins and it is a research university so it only makes sense that everyone should be going down this road to some extent. I cannot imagine coming here and not becoming involved with the research.

McClain: I give Sue much more credit than I think a lot of people did. She walked into a rather tough situation. The school hit some financial bad times pretty early on. There was something professionally immature and unself-assertive about nurses who still thought that the sun shone out of the doctor's backside. Sue Donaldson, whether she was fully accepted or not by her colleagues, had operated in schools of medicine, rubbing elbows with the prominent doctors. She wasn't particularly intimidated by them. On the academic value side, she gave the school some oomph in the first couple of years of her tenure; I think she did a good job.

Donaldson: Maryann Fralic had come a year before I arrived. She is an absolutely fabulous leader with a national and international reputation. The hospital and school, under her leadership and Carol Gray's, were already in the process of determining how you could create a center bridging the hospital and the school.

The Institute for Johns Hopkins Nursing does continuing ed, patent rights, and copyright. As long as that exists, it's going to keep us very close to those nurse leaders in the Johns Hopkins Hospital. This institute has positioned us nationally and internationally. It's very visible and it's given us the power to do continuing education in a way that is

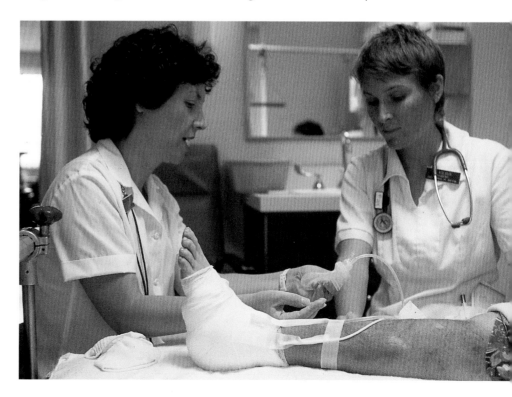

significant. The certificates issued are signed by the dean and the vice president for nursing. We quickly gained a reputation across the nation and even internationally.

Einaudi: The Institute for Hopkins Nursing got an enormous boost when Sue Donaldson came along. The institute has forged a strong relationship between the nurses at the hospital and the nurses at the School of Nursing. The idea was to come up with an entity that would allow the nurses within the university and the nurses at the hospital to market their services in an effective way. Among the things that they have done is to put on certification series. It gives you a leg up in terms of administration. It's a nice way to market what Johns Hopkins nursing is all about.

Davis: Maryann Fralic was head of the Institute for Hopkins Nursing. The idea was to provide education to nurses from around the country on topics that were current at any given time. They present three- or four-day conferences, or sometimes weeklong conferences, on a particular area that is developing. We're in the forefront of trying to disseminate information about new things, which is helpful for the school. It's in conjunction with the nursing department in the hospital, and many of their nurses teach in the conferences or conduct groups around the hospital. It's a learning center, really.

Hill, 1964, BSN 1966: The School of Nursing was evicted from the Phipps Building. Then we had space in the 1830 Building and we had to go up to Monument Street to 2024 for classes. That was the last straw. If you don't own your own building you're always on the potential eviction list, because he who owns the space makes the rules. That's when we realized we really had to raise the money to build the building. This was absolutely intolerable. And we really needed to be on this campus because out of sight, out of mind.

Donaldson: When the board looked at the cost of renovating 1830 Monument Street versus building a new building they said, "Well, if it's cheaper to build the new building, we'll build the new building." Pulling out walls to put in fiber optic cabling is extremely expensive.

Einaudi: Barbara Donaho was class of '56, a tremendous leader as a student, and really one of the illustrious alumni. She went on to become one of the few nurses to be a hospital president and she was on the board of trustees. Barbara Donaho was the obvious person to lead the campaign for a building for the School of Nursing. She said, "I'll do that on one condition: that we will no longer talk about renovating a building. The School of Nursing deserves its own building." That was absolutely pivotal.

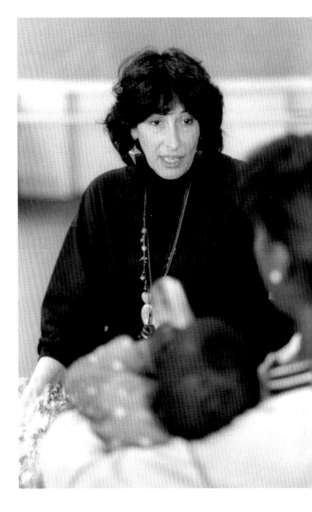

Assistant Professor Marion D'Lugoff concentrated her efforts on vulnerable populations throughout Baltimore City. She founded a network of outreach sites through the Lillian D. Wald Community Nursing Center, where students and faculty gave physicals and counseled families, such as this young mother, on caring for their children.

This is the only school of nursing I've been at in my career where there are such warm, cordial, truly collaborative relationships among professional nurses who are leaders in a business that medicine's running. When you interact with the nurses from the hospital it's very collaborative. It kept us in touch with the real world of health care. There's always been linkage between the Johns Hopkins Hospital, which had the original School of Nursing, and the new school. There is a unique passion here for the hospital.

Sue Donaldson

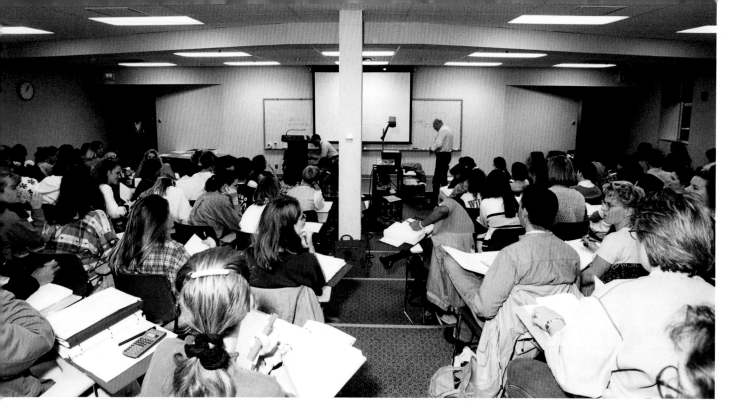

Administrators in the School of Nursing learned in 1992 that it would have to abandon its home in the Phipps Building. At first the school occupied temporary quarters on the third and fourth floors of the 1830 Building, on Monument Street, and when that space proved inadequate as enrollment continued to increase, classes were also held two blocks away, at 2024 Monument Street. There a vertical support in the middle of this classroom made it a challenge to view projected images on the screen in the front of the room.

Angell, 1969, BSN 1977: That was a very exciting time. Alumni really came together to help in many ways. They gave lots of money. Reunion classes for a number of years went all out. There was a school, yes, but this was tangible. This was the culmination of all the years that the alumni had fought to have a separate school and they really came through.

Donaldson: The hospital president, Jim Block, said, "I think there's going to be a concern on the part of the hospital that you don't have any red brick on this building." The first proposal for the school looked very much like the School of Public Health. I said to the architects, Ayers Saint Gross, "You'd better come to that meeting with another rendition of the building with some red brick," which was a total design change. Dan Nathans, who was the interim president of the university then, and I looked at it together and there were some things he didn't like about it. He actually used the word—and for a geneticist I considered this very significant—he said it looked like a hybrid and that was not a good thing. He said, "I hope the architects are paying attention. This is a significant building." I thought, "All right, I'm sure I could go in there and fight, but do I really dislike this red brick?" I went and stood on the site. I realized that the red brick would be the height of the base of the building. There were row homes just across the street. So much to everyone's surprise, I said, "I like this red brick because of how it blends into the neighborhood."

Einaudi: There was an unwritten rule that hospital buildings are in red brick, university buildings are not. What's brilliant about the building's design is that it says, "We're part hospital, part university. We're the bridge." It gave it a unique quality.

Shiber: The fact that the building was designed just for the functions that the School of Nursing performs was very important. The architects who worked with us were just terrific. They were very responsive. They included us in on everything. We put together our wish list, our dream of what the school would be, and then the harsh reality of how much money we had and what we could have sort of hit us in the face. We lost a lot of things that would have been nice. We had to give up a lot of conference rooms, the size of some of the classrooms, things that now are significant problems.

Hill, 1964, BSN 1966: The mandate Sue Donaldson had was to build the building and build the research program. Sue devoted an enormous amount of her time and talent to literally thinking through every aspect of the significance of this building: the meaning of it for people; what kind of community were we trying to establish? and how did the architecture reflect that? She was very involved in everything from choosing paint colors and furniture.

The Pinkard family, through the France-Merrick Foundation, has given millions to Hopkins. Every part of the campus has been touched. Nan Pinkard was involved with the Consortium for Nursing Education, which really provided a lot of money at the inception of the school. Nan became a mentor to Carol Gray. She served as a mentor to me. Nan is a very modest, gracious person. It took quite a bit of convincing, probably mostly by her family, to allow her name to be on the building. I think she's now pleased. We are thrilled because she has been so wonderful to the school.

Sue Donaldson

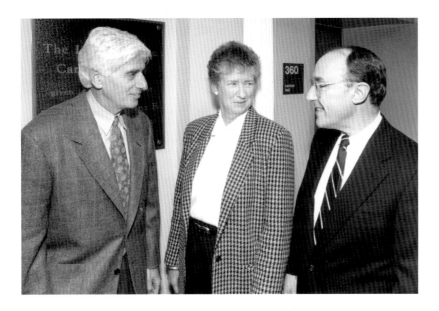

Hospital president James A. Block (left) and university president William C. Richardson (right) met with Dean Carol Gray and her faculty on November 17, 1992, just after the school moved from the Phipps Building. "I am feeling more committed than ever to nursing education at Hopkins," President Richardson said as he and Dr. Block announced the site for the first building to be constructed specifically for the School of Nursing. "There is a sense of cooperation among the schools on the East Baltimore campus that is unparalleled in the country. We intend to capitalize on that."

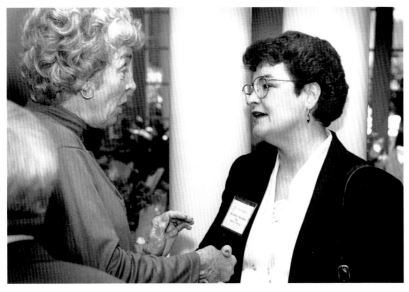

In 1994 the Jacob and Annita France and the Robert G. and Anne M. Merrick Foundations announced a gift of $3 million to the School of Nursing, which enabled plans for the new building to move forward. Here Dean Sue Donaldson expressed her gratitude to Nan Merrick Pinkard (left), who chaired the foundations' boards and who had served on the nursing consortium's board from its outset. William C. Richardson recalled how essential Nan Pinkard and her family were. "The wonderful support of the Pinkards was really the lynchpin of the success of getting that building. Theirs was a deep and abiding commitment to nursing. As the years went by and it was clear that we needed new space, they stepped forward, in their quiet but very potent way, and said, 'This is something we want to take on.'"

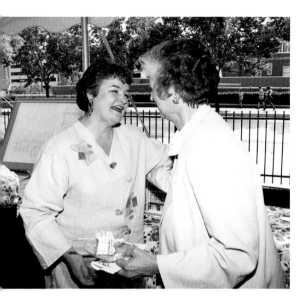

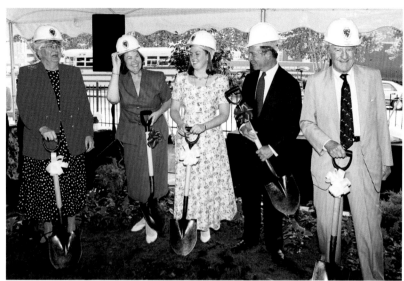

After she retired, Carol Gray rarely returned to Baltimore, but on June 6, 1996, Dean Sue Donaldson (left) warmly welcomed her predecessor to the groundbreaking ceremony for the new School of Nursing building. Hospital trustees had voted in 1992 to lease land across from the hospital's main entrance to the School of Nursing as a site for its permanent home "at a token rate such as $1 per year with provision for a reversion to the Hospital and/or renewal at the end of the lease."

Above right: Hard hats were the order of the day for Barbara Donaho, 1956, Patti Wilcox, 1967, Holly Villepique, 1997, and university trustees Michael Bloomberg and Steve Peck as they prepared to heft their shovels for the ceremonial groundbreaking.

It's really great to finally have a school because we never had but a few classrooms and we got shifted around depending on what the hospital and the medical school were doing. We had nutrition classes in the School of Hygiene. We had our anatomy classes in the medical school. We had pathology in the pathology building. Just to see everything all under one roof, it was just, "Finally, we made it." Kind of unbelievable but it's happened and I'm glad.

Constance Cole Heard Waxter, 1944

Angell, 1969, BSN 1977: Sue enjoyed the process thoroughly, from being involved with the legislature to talking to donors. She really worked very hard to develop friends of Hopkins who were non-nurses but who had the potential to be donors to the school. She was good at that. She went to the alumni. She got the students involved. She got the faculty involved. She got the hospital involved.

Donaldson: I practically lived down at the legislature. I would speak to each of them in terms of the needs of their constituents and how nursing met them. They would say, "I know you're here about that building." I said, "I want to talk to you about your constituents because I'm preparing the nurses who are going to take care of them." I like legislators. They want facts. They want you to be honest but tell them what they're going to miss. Don't get emotional over it; don't get angry; just let them know. I made many good friends in the legislature and I continue to stay in touch. They came through and gave us $2.5 million.

Angell, 1969, BSN 1977: Sue really insisted on a building that was going to be functional but attractive at the same time and that also had some oases, like the courtyard. That was important to her. She didn't want it to be a totally utilitarian-looking building. When Paula Einaudi was here as our development director, she really listened to Paula about the importance of incorporating the past into this building and I think the results are quite good.

Einaudi: Sue Donaldson wanted that building to be elegant. She knew that it was going to be her legacy and she wanted to make it beautiful. The donors were generous and so we were able to do it. The older alumni were so thrilled that the school was in the strong position it was in and that it was going to have its own home, they were really ready to give very generously.

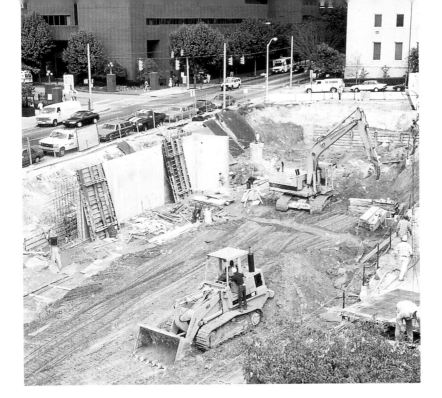

Associate Dean Stella Shiber recalled the planning of the building as a stimulating, cooperative experience. "Our architects were wonderful. They tried really hard to get to know us, to watch how we taught and how people moved around in the building." The structure they designed rose quickly from a deep hole in the ground to a handsome home for the School of Nursing.

On December 20, 1997, a gleeful Dean Sue Donaldson cut the ribbon and presented her faculty, students, and staff with the completed Anne M. Pinkard Building. Paula Einaudi, who as director and associate dean for development worked closely with Donaldson to raise funds for the building, beamed just inside the door.

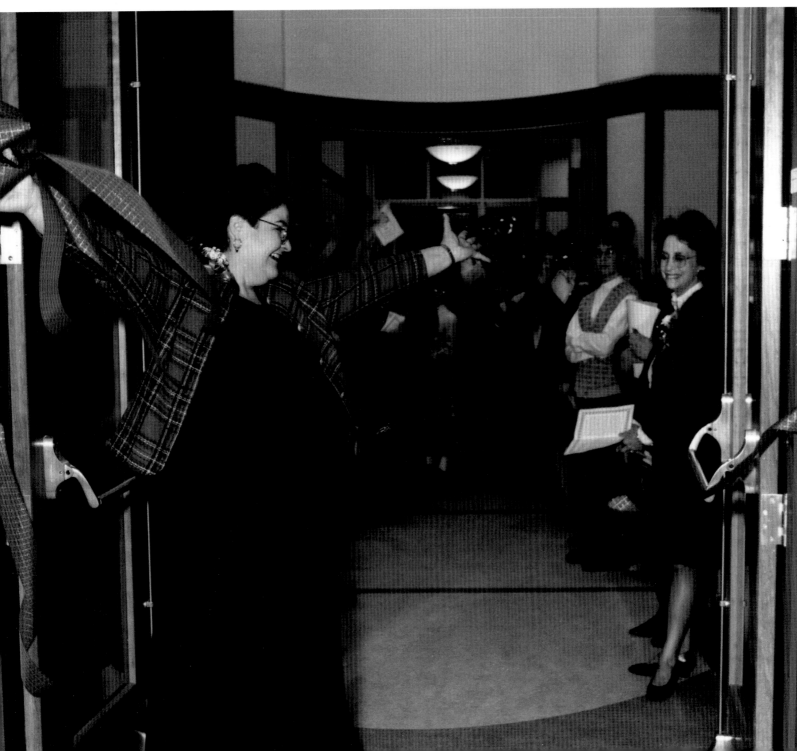

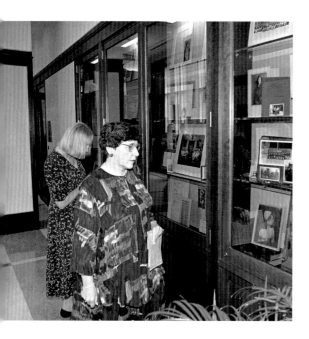

Alumni took great pride in the new home for their school. In particular, they enjoyed viewing exhibits, which featured treasures from their historical collections, in the large display cases on the first floor.

The torch gets passed. Individuals like Betty Cuthbert and some others before her have always been aware that these things should be preserved. For a long, long while, many things were kept in Betty's basement. Then Sue Appling took a great interest in making sure things were preserved. Then individual nurses keep everything. I know that one of my classmates has her original student uniform.

Betty Borenstein Scher, 1950

We have a home of our own now. This identifies us and we're centralized. Everybody who passes by the hospital always sees the School of Nursing. It's been a great boon to our morale here, and others recognize that the school is here to stay.

Ada Davis

McGeady, 1955, BSN 1955: Our older alumni have been *very, very* generous. I'm sure that this building in many ways would not be what it is without the support of the alumni. We were given a goal of $500,000 in order to have the auditorium called the alumni auditorium. It didn't take long to get that. Now it is our gathering space. We have our meetings there. We can have lunches there. Now, it's like this is our space and we come home to celebrate.

Shiber: Having a School of Nursing where there are classrooms and offices gives permanence to nursing's presence as part of the Hopkins community. That the building had NURSING chiseled in the stone was recognition that nursing was on the campus and that it was part of the community. It gave us a permanent home.

Keenan, 1986, MSN 1993: Betty Cuthbert was dying at the time they were finishing the new building. I would give her updates. I told her about how the name SCHOOL OF NURSING slid in at the very top and she said, "Well, if they can slide it in that easily they can always slide it out and turn the building into something else." For some of the older alumni who had had relations with the university that were not as cordial, it really was taking a lot for them to come over and take this chance. I was pleased that I was able to finally get a picture of the building to Betty and give it to her before she died.

Donaldson: Our goal with the building was to honor the very wise, intelligent, compassionate, and elegant women who had preceded us and to carry it forward. The alumni were passionate about the building. You get a different perspective of the School of Nursing talking to the alumni than you do from the current faculty, some of whom are alumni, but it's a different vision and a different view. It's truly a privilege to have been here. I'm not a Hopkins alumna. I'm glad they trusted me enough to do it and it's just been great. Alumni are very, very special in their trust and their commitment.

After we hit our campaign goal, Paula Einaudi and I were at a trustee dinner. Michael Bloomberg had done this wonderful thing with a big silver bowl. When your division hit its goal, your name was engraved on it and you got to keep this big silver bowl in your possession until the next school did. They called Paula and me to come forward. I slipped on the superman cape. There was a ripple of laughter and applause. Michael Bloomberg's up at the podium looking at me over his glasses and he said, "Donaldson, what's going on here?" This gave me the rare opportunity to thank everybody in that room for their support of the school and for their campaign donations. I said, "I wore this tonight to thank all of you because now you've given me a building to leap over." People had tears in their eyes. It was emotional for me but it was emotional for them, too.

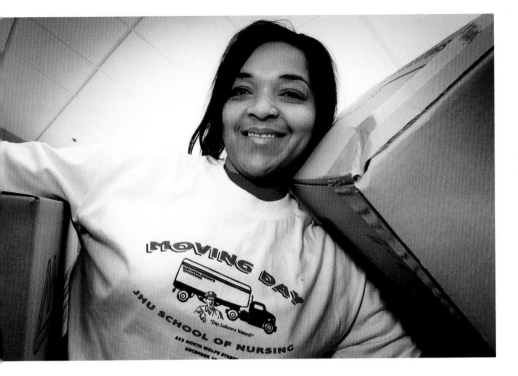

It was all smiles on moving day and everyone got involved. Furniture, books, and equipment were delivered from the six different sites where the school had been conducting business. Administrative assistants, such as Sheila Saunderlin, wore commemorative T-shirts as they hauled boxes from room to room, making sure everything arrived at its proper destination.

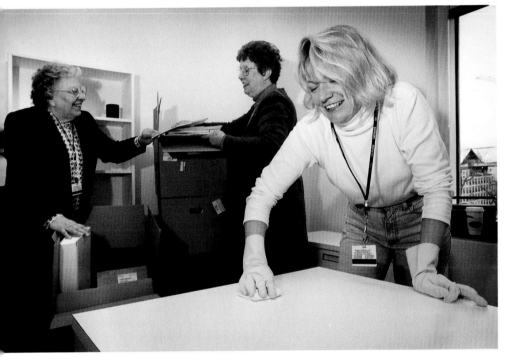

Professor Ada Davis (left) passed files to Associate Dean Stella Shiber while Assistant Professor Rosemarie Brager wiped off a work table. By the time students returned the next semester, the school was ready to resume business.

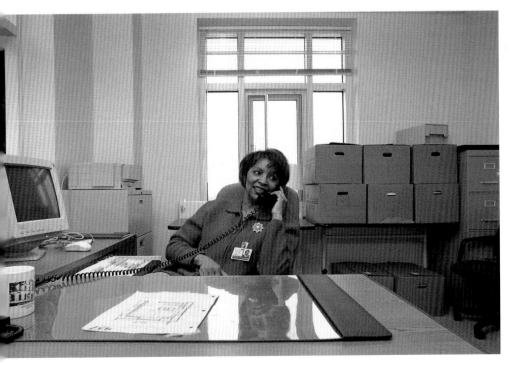

Setting up her computer came before unloading boxes for Fannie Gaston-Johansson. She was already making calls on moving day, continuing her responsibilities as director of international nursing programs and director of the Center for Health Disparities Research. In 1998 Dr. Gaston-Johansson became the first African-American woman with both tenure and a full professorship at the Johns Hopkins University.

Nan Pinkard and Carol Gray genuinely liked each other. I think each appreciated the other's soft-spoken tenaciousness. They were both very gracious. That was the seed that ultimately made for the largest gift that the school had ever received, the largest gift that the France-Merrick Foundation had ever made.

Paula Einaudi

In 1991 Paul D. Coverdell (left), director of the Peace Corps, Interim Provost M. Gordon "Reds" Wolman, and Dean Carol Gray signed an agreement creating a program for returning Peace Corps volunteers to study nursing at Johns Hopkins. The first such program in nursing in the United States, it brought lasting benefits to everyone in the classroom since Peace Corps veterans often introduced new perspectives on how to approach challenges.

Nurses returning to school for additional degrees came with a practiced eye and touch for their work. Dennis Kuzmikis (left) was pursuing a master's degree when he examined a young patient at St. Bernadine's School with Assistant Professor Beth Sloand. School-based health centers and pediatric primary care were the focus of much of Sloand's work.

Angell, 1969, BSN 1977: Sue Donaldson knew that even as it was going up it was already too small. We all knew that. That was the one sadness about this building. We were limited in the amount of money that we could borrow and so we have a building that was already at capacity when we moved into it. We gave up some things that we needed and that we miss, seminar rooms and some additional faculty offices. We're going to have to build another building to get those, so that's the next step.

McClain: When Martha Hill became dean, one of her major tasks was finding more space. Well, that didn't surprise me at all. Whatever's the time horizon that you think a building will suffice, cut that in half, because that building's going to be filled up in some way twice as fast as you had imagined. Where they thought the building would hold them for let's say ten years, after five years they said, "We need more space." Okay. I just shrug when I hear that and I say, "So what else is new?"

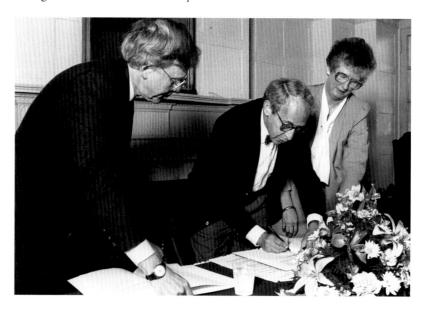

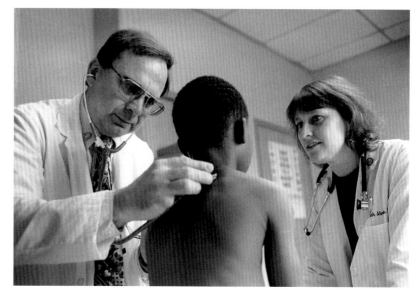

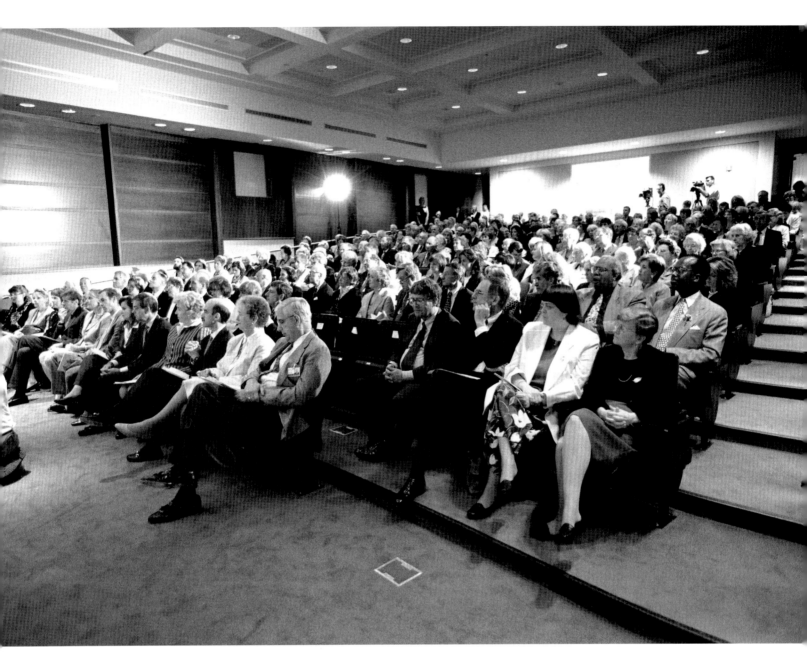

Maguire: We had the first partnership with the Peace Corps. Many of the people who were in the Peace Corps were in developing nations. They were there teaching agriculture or English. Then they realized that one of the primary needs in this country is health care and that nursing offers a holistic approach. It looks at nutrition, child development, sanitation, and all those kinds of things. We have a large cadre of people who are return Peace Corps volunteers who are part of our overall program here.

Einaudi: The Peace Corps program came about because of Jackie Baldick, the director of development, and Stella Shiber. They saw this as a terrific opportunity to recruit students who had dedicated themselves to increasing the quality of life in other countries. Wouldn't they

On June 11, 1998, a host of devoted alumni and friends gathered in the alumni auditorium for the dedication of the Anne M. Pinkard Building. Members of the Pinkard family filled most of the seats on the front row, but former dean Carol Gray and Edward Miller, dean of the School of Medicine, also found seats there.

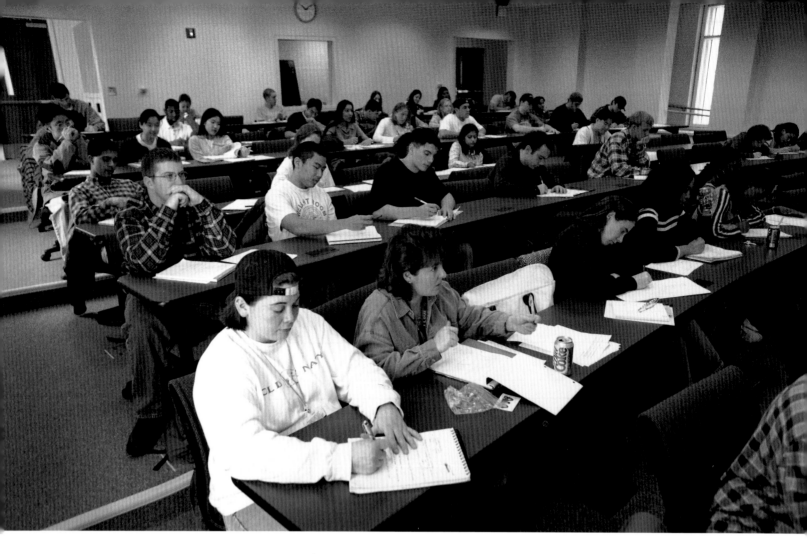

Classrooms in the new building were a huge improvement over the makeshift quarters of the past decade. Other changes were also apparent as recruitment efforts attracted a more diverse student body and men began to fill more seats in lectures and seminars.

A lot of the students coming in now in the accelerated program are already graduates of other universities. I've heard it said that, in fund-raising, your first university or college is the one that you'll usually give your money to, and I think we are running up against that problem. I am concerned about this group of alumni not being able to help us to maintain this alumni association. They get demands all the time from lots of places. Their focus is, more or less, "Hopkins is one of the things I've done." We have to convince them that this is one of the things that they need to continue to support. We need to find some way to have them value the history of Hopkins as nursing education.

Betsy Mumaw McGeady, 1955

be interested in coming back and learning nursing so that they could increase the quality of life in the United States? We were the first nursing school in the country to have a program with the Peace Corps.

These students changed the tenor of what went on in the classroom. Many of them came so that they could do community health nursing. That totally changes the conversation. These returning Peace Corps students learn about the high-tech stuff that goes on in the hospital. But the other students who have come in primarily to learn all that high-tech stuff also learn about low-tech nursing, which, in terms of cost per dollar, really provides an enormous amount of fabulous health care.

Davis: It was such a pleasure when so many ex–Peace Corps students came into the school. They brought a global perspective. Many of them had been in countries that were underdeveloped. They saw conditions they had never expected to see. Many of them were very successful on their own as agents of change among these groups of people. The experience gave them a whole new perspective on life. Many of them who went into the Peace Corps never dreamed of becoming nurses, but after their experience in these poor countries, they said, "Gee, nursing would have been so helpful if I'd had that education." Both men and women from the Peace Corps came to medical school or nursing school. That had become their goal and, of course, Hopkins is the best.

Knott, 2002: Twenty-six was the average age of a student in my class. There were about ninety people in my class, some of them married coming back for a second degree, some of them straight out of their first two years of college and coming to complete their first bachelor's degree. The men in my class did very well. I think three got married to other people in my class. There was a large contingent of people, maybe ten to fifteen, who had finished a stint in the Peace Corps. There were some women coming back for second degrees who had children. They were probably in their forties. I was twenty-nine, so I was just over the average age.

Hill, 1964, BSN 1966: The majority of our students now have at least one bachelor's degree before they come to us. We have people with master's degrees, we have lawyers, we have engineers, we have two PhDs in one of the classes. It's an extraordinary student body.

More and more of them now are going directly into the master's program. That's where they can get nurse practitioner credentials or a joint degree with an MPH or an MBA. We have several degree programs with other divisions of the university. Since they're such exceptional students, they're very quick and they move forward rapidly. They are stimulating, and very appreciative because they are so eager to learn and maximize every opportunity.

Keenan, 1986, MSN 1993: I was the first president of the alumni association who had graduated from the university School of Nursing. Now, not only had the alumni done all this for the school, but now there were alumni from the school who were actively participating in the alumni association. It was shortly after I graduated that I became active on the board of directors. Fran Keen was the first woman who was president of the alumni council at the university. I guess Fran and I broke both of the barriers at a similar time.

Hill, 1964, BSN 1966: When the dean, Sue Donaldson, announced in April 2001 that she would be stepping down July 1 to teach and do research, the provost and the president announced that they would appoint an interim dean and then form a search committee for a dean. I was asked by the president to take the interim deanship. I was very reluctant to do it but also very willing because I saw it, literally, as an interim situation. It was a difficult year because I had all my other roles and responsibilities, being the director of the Center for Nursing Research. I had all my grants. I had students. I had a full load because my expectation was that I would return to those roles, which I found fully satisfying and very stimulating. I had no intention of staying as the dean but I did feel an obligation to step in as a form of university service. There were urgent needs in regard to development and some administrative

Melinda Rose has brown-bag lunches. For example, this winter students came and we talked about what it's like to be in academic nursing, what it's like to teach in a university, because that is the big need. She also does lunches with the clinical nurses at the hospital so the students get to know people who are already in nursing and get an idea that this is what alumni do. She does things like that so that the students start to get connections with alumni, particularly alumni who are already involved in the alumni association, and they see it's a good thing to do. Members of the alumni association are generally enthusiastic, very high-functioning people.

Susan Carroll Immelt, 1977, PhD 2000

In 2002, after serving for a year as interim dean, Martha Norton Hill, 1964, became the first alumna dean of the School of Nursing. Suspending her research career, Hill accepted the charge with enthusiasm. "The challenges are huge in the delivery of health care today," she declared. "I believe that nurses are critically important and essential."

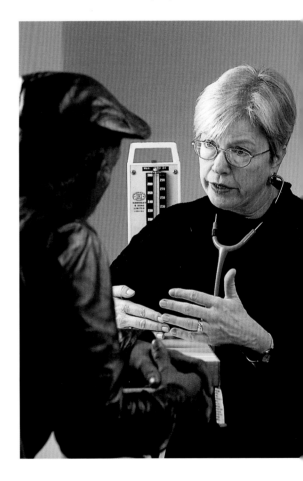

The profession and academic nature of nursing from the late '60s into the '80s and perhaps even up until today was going through a tremendous change in terms of its professional status of switching from a vocation to a profession, reflected in the greater proliferation of bachelor's and master's and in doctoral programs in nursing. One of the big indications of that was when Martha Hill was elected president of the American Heart Association several years ago. She's a nurse. That's indicative that attitudes about that profession have changed.

Stephen McClain

At East Baltimore you have the Schools of Medicine, Nursing, and Public Health, and then we have the Johns Hopkins Medical Institutions. This is a collective term that refers to the East Baltimore campus. Faculty can move effortlessly to find others who share the same intellectual interests and to collaborate. The walls of these buildings and these institutions are very, very permeable, which is one of the things that makes this place so special. Students have considerable flexibility.

Martha Norton Hill, 1964, BSN 1966

Students made frequent use of their library, which featured current journals and books as well as an extraordinary wealth of early nursing publications.

issues. Then Dr. Stella Shiber announced that she would be retiring. She had been here eighteen years, the whole history of the school, the head of the academic program. These were major matters to deal with.

Immelt, 1977, PhD 2000: I was really happy that Martha was first appointed interim dean and then became the dean. She taught in my PhD program. All through the time that we were in the program, she had a big research program. She would involve us in different things that she was doing because it wasn't just research. She was a very strong public figure. Then she moved on to the American Heart Association for a while. She has a huge amount of energy, a fun person, a really interesting person, a great leader, a great mentor, able to zero in on what's important. I'm thrilled that she's dean. Everybody seems very happy about it. Of course she's a Hopkins alum, which makes it really nice too.

McGeady, 1955, BSN 1955: I remember when Sue was introduced to the alumni at an event at Peabody Library. She had on a brilliant red cape and everybody knew that things were going to be different. She was very good for the school in a way different from Carol but yet I think, in our heart of hearts, all of us wanted a Hopkins nurse to be our dean.

Hill, 1964, BSN 1966: I was a graduate of the hospital diploma school. I got my bachelor's from what was then called the Evening College. I then was a student in the first nurse practitioner cohort in the School of Health Services. And then I got my PhD at the School of Hygiene and Public Health. I was on the faculty in the hospital diploma school, the School of Health Services, and the university school.

McGeady, 1955, BSN 1955: I've known Martha Hill since she graduated. I tracked her career and I thought, "She has to be the one. She's going to be the one to do it." I was thrilled when Martha became the dean because

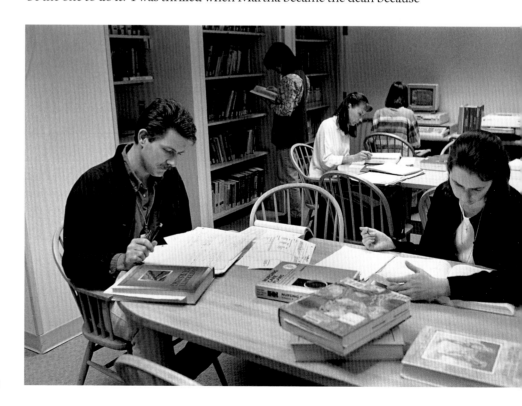

she carries the Hopkins message far and wide. Certainly her personal accomplishments are incredible and to have her be *the* Hopkins nurse for the world to see, we are thrilled. I don't know anybody I'd rather see in that chair than Martha Hill. She has the institutional memory. She has the experience of working at Hopkins not only in the highest levels but at the very basic level of a nurse on the floor. She's able to be comfortable with any nurse at any level and, of course, various and sundry other people. I can't say enough for her. She's the perfect dean.

Einaudi: Everybody gets bowled over by Martha Hill because she's brilliant, she's personable, she's clever, she can teach, she does fabulous research, and she's so likeable and so funny. She made us all so proud when she became head of the American Heart Association because she was the first nonphysician. We weren't really surprised because Martha is a strategic thinker. She's big picture, she's long term, she knows how to network, and so she had been garnering support from lots of different places for a lot of years.

Martha headed the subcommittee for interdivisional collaboration for the Committee for the 21st Century at Hopkins. What she brought to that was looking at the entire university and trying to build on the strengths and forge collaborative efforts among the different schools. She brings a sense of collaboration but also an enormous sense of vision to the school.

Hill, 1964, BSN 1966: When President Brody approached me about becoming the dean, I was extremely reluctant. I found the faculty role very rewarding and stimulating. I knew that if I took the deanship I would not be able to continue to be a leader of a major research program because the deanship requires too much of one's time and attention. The roles, I believe, are incompatible. President Brody was extremely persuasive. I was impressed by his understanding of the importance of having a top-ranked school of nursing in this university, of his understanding that to have a major academic health center you can't have a school of medicine and a hospital without having a school of nursing. I felt his vision was compatible with what my vision had always been as a student and as a faculty member throughout the history of the university school. It was out of my sense of loyalty to the institution that I was persuaded.

Davis: Martha Hill is much more a businesswoman than Sue Donaldson was, or even Carol Gray. She's looking at ways that the school can make money. Our student numbers have increased. She has a good sense of humor but she's also on the formal side. She knows where to be at the right time, meeting the right people, or inviting them here. She's been at Hopkins forever and she knows the people here. She

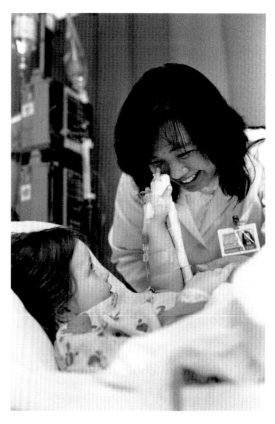

Like their predecessors who enjoyed working in the Harriet Lane Home, nursing students in the university school vied for clinical placements in the Children's Medical and Surgical Center. This young patient seemed to benefit from the attentions of a student who stopped by to chat.

It was usually about eight students in a clinical group for one faculty member. The first rotation was with the elderly. You really didn't do anything clinical other than take their blood pressure. That was just to teach you how to form a relationship with a patient and get comfortable talking to a patient. From there we went to the emergency room. The whole purpose of that was, again, to get you more familiar with being in an actual hospital situation. You weren't starting IVs or anything like that. It was to gain more experience being able to take a good patient history. We were scattered everywhere, Sinai, Good Samaritan, Union Memorial. There were some at Hopkins emergency room, maybe at Howard County.

Kate Knott, 2002

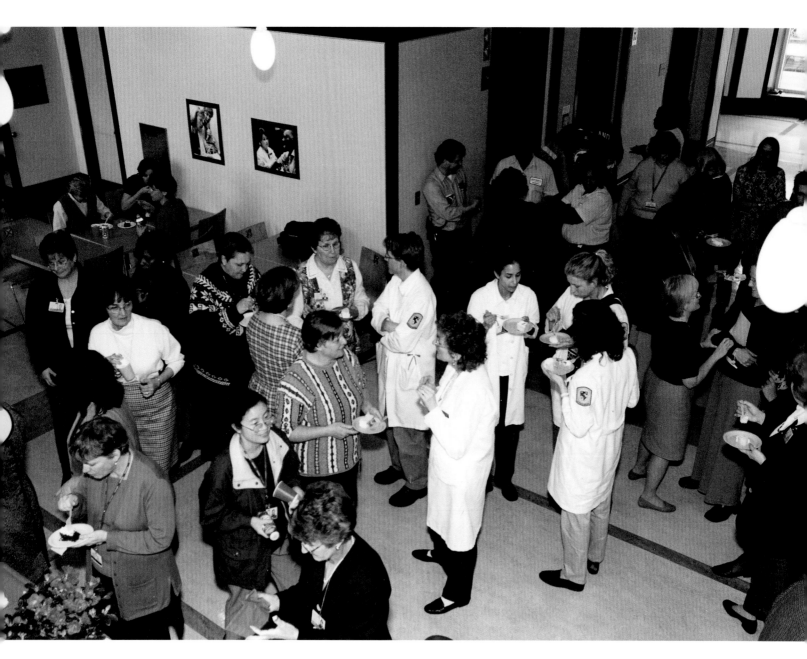

On March 30, 2000, the School of Nursing received word that it had tied for the number five position in the rankings of graduate schools in *U.S. News & World Report*. The announcement sparked a celebration as faculty, students, and staff gathered in the café to enjoy cake and beverages. Associate Dean Sandra Stine Angell (left), 1969, BSN 1977, cut slices with help from alumni director Melinda Rose and communications director Kate Pipkin.

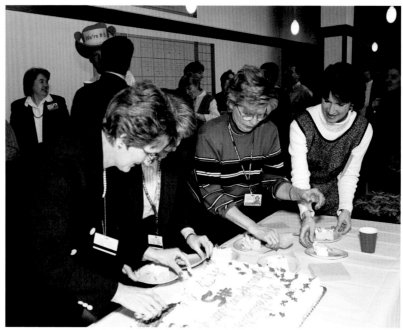

knows what the needs of the school are and she goes about filling the positions that are needed. She's very good at sizing people up.

Hill, 1964, BSN 1966: One of the hardest things about becoming the dean was to realize that my relationship with some people that I had known and worked with, who were personal friends, needed to change because no longer were we peers in the sense of being fellow faculty. They now reported to me directly or indirectly. To avoid even the perception that those relationships involved favoritism or bias it was necessary for me to have to say to several people, no matter how reluctant I felt, that we needed to readjust the personal relationship because the primary relationship was the work relationship. That was very, very hard.

McClain: Martha has done and will continue to do a good job. She has very good basic academic grounding. She knows what quality is. She's been associated with Hopkins nursing for such a long time that she knows where the bodies are buried. She knows the university very well. She knows how to try to manipulate the university to her advantage and that's something a dean should know.

Einaudi: For the older alums, it must be so heartwarming to know that it's an alum who's the dean. She has spent most of her adult life as part of this institution. She's connected to all three medical divisions, so she embodies collaboration. She embodies what Hopkins nursing is all about. Good nursing is really about relationships and making things happen and forging the future.

Maguire: The leadership course is the final course. You work thirty-two hours with a preceptor in a clinical area. Then you have a faculty mentor

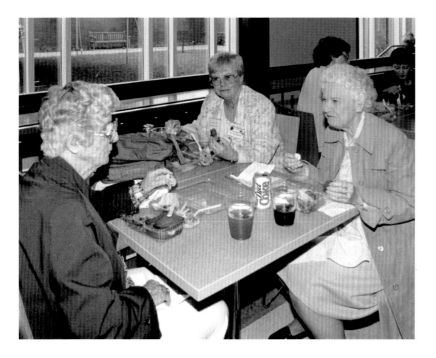

Alumni also enjoyed gathering in the café area during homecoming events at the school. Most marveled at the quality of the facilities in the new building, and found satisfaction knowing that their devotion through the years to the concept of nursing education at Johns Hopkins had made possible much of what they saw during their visit.

in your specialty area at school whom you meet with every week. I had two of my pediatric students working in the pediatric emergency room at Hopkins. I had one working in the pediatric intensive care unit at Sinai. I had two working on the infant floor over at Hopkins Hospital, which is like an ICU anyplace else. I had one in inpatient pediatric oncology and one in outpatient and one over at Kennedy Krieger. They all did the same role as a staff nurse would do. They carry a staff load. Even though they had a preceptor, they're carrying a regular load of patients. It's a transition course and they are doing a fabulous job. A lot of them get hired by the units where they do their leadership.

Knott, 2002: Your rotations are, to a certain extent, based on specialties. You start with geriatrics. You get to see a little bit of what it's like in an emergency room. You go through labor and delivery. You do a

This student working a clinical rotation in the emergency department brought a firm hold as well as a soothing touch to a child receiving sutures in his head.

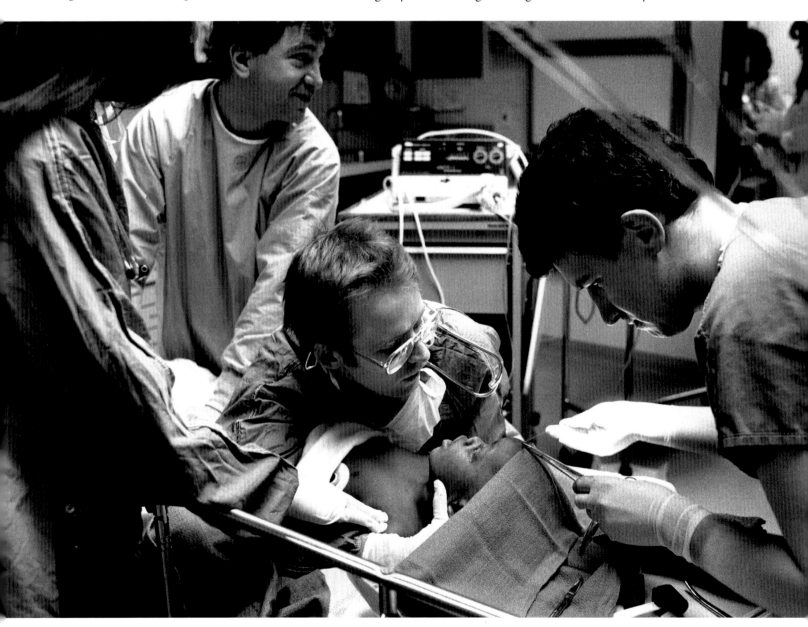

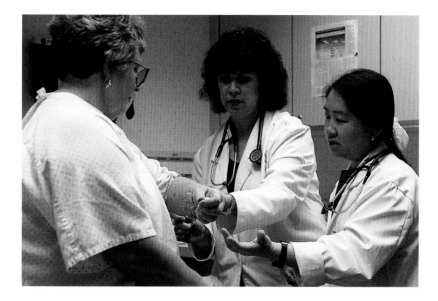

Nurse practitioner Janet Selway (center) demonstrated a procedure for student Anna Sam as they examined a patient in 1998.

pediatrics rotation. The medical surgical rotation is adult so you certainly see what adult hospital medicine is about. From there you got to do a psych rotation, a community health rotation.

The leadership course, to me, hands down, makes the tuition to Hopkins all worthwhile because you do one-on-one with a nurse. You pick whatever specialty you want to do. You work seven weeks, one-on-one, with a nurse in whatever field you choose, whether in a hospital setting or an outpatient setting. I thought I wanted to do pediatrics but I thought, "This will be my testing ground. If I really like it, then that's what I'm going to do when I graduate." They said, "We have a slot open on the adolescent floor." I talked to some people who had done their pediatrics rotation on that floor and they said, "Oh, the nurses are great." I did it and loved it. I applied for a job right after I finished and that's where I still am today, two years later.

Hill, 1964, BSN 1966: We are continually looking at the curriculum. We meet with Karen Haller and the directors of nursing at the hospital and ask about the needs and requirements in the practice setting today so that our curriculum is relevant. Our graduates don't have trouble getting jobs. They are in great demand and they do very, very well when they're hired. They move up the ladder very quickly.

Heyssel: I think a medical center like Hopkins needs a nursing school for very straightforward reasons. You can't run a hospital without good nurses, and you can't run a good hospital without very good nurses. They're the only thing there that makes it bearable for the patient. Damn few of the doctors do.

Marella: The bedside nurse has the toughest job in the whole world. They get these seriously ill patients. Sometimes it's even frightening. The patients are so sick that you're afraid to take care of them. I think

The Hopkins nursing education exposed us to many challenges. We have developed the courage to be leaders, the flexibility to adjust and grow from change, and the courage to pursue our dreams. Today, our dreams come true as bachelor's and master's degrees are earned, finally. Our courage has grown through the many career avenues the School of Nursing has offered us: from a nurse practitioner and specialty cares to a master's in public health and nursing, and the dual degree of a master's in business and nursing. Hopkins nursing graduates are executives, running their own clinics, conducting and publishing their own research, and using today's technology strategically. The School of Nursing has expanded our courage, taught us not to give up when obstacles are stacked high, and we, as Hopkins alumni, will pass this courage on.

Dara Lawrence Geiser, 1991, MSN 1998, graduation address, May 21, 1998

This building was designed with three dedicated big rooms for teaching both nursing skills and physical assessment. The same spaces are used for both courses but on different days. We have all the up-to-date equipment that they'll be using out in the real world of nursing. We have two teaching computer labs on the third floor for the growing informatics part of nursing now. Thursdays and Fridays for major specialty courses, they're all out at clinics someplace. Classrooms those days are used primarily for graduate students.

Maureen Maguire

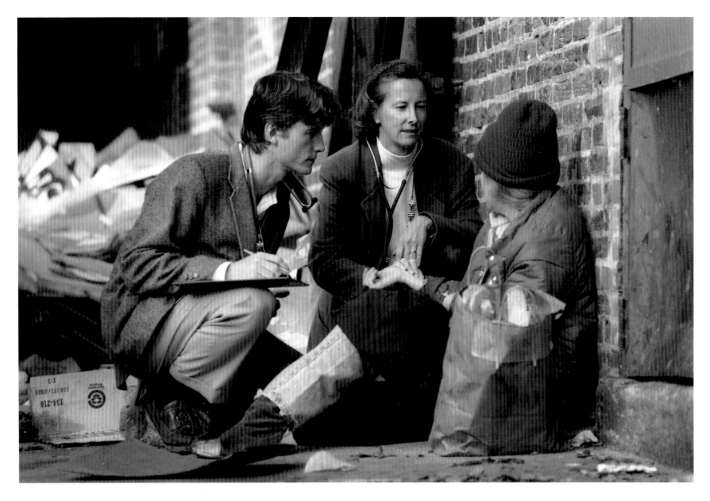

Continuing in the tradition of dispensary visiting nurses and students serving the Eastern Health District, Robin Evans-Agnew, 1994, took careful notes as he and Assistant Professor Kathleen Becker interviewed a homeless person in East Baltimore.

today, most of the people at the bedside are older women because these young people have so many more opportunities. At one time you could work in a hospital, you could work at a doctor's office, or you could do private duty. Those were the three options for nurses. Today, graduate nurses can work completely away from a hospital and not have to take care of patients who are ill, I mean really ill. It takes a certain person and there are, thank goodness, still a lot of young men and women who do want to care for people and do go into a hospital. Not enough of them but, thank God, we're still graduating some of those that say, "Yes, I'm just going to work in a hospital. I want to work in the ICU. I want to work in critical care. I want to work in the coronary care unit. I want to work in labor and delivery." They have so many different areas and they're highly specialized and their patients in those areas are really a challenge to care for. It takes a good, intelligent person to put it all together and render the quality of care that these sick patients need. Those patients would not survive if it weren't for good nursing care.

Today, the hospitals are almost entirely intensive care units. Patients stay so little so they're in there when they're acutely ill. The school has its own intensive care–unit laboratory. They prepare the students for all the latest equipment and different technologies that are being implemented for better patient care. They had to be very visionary in developing the curriculum that would meet those needs.

Shiber: We really are truly blessed with the quality of student who applies to us. Some of the best people around are choosing to be nurses and to come to Hopkins. My job was made so much easier because we had such outstanding people who wanted to come to Hopkins. It was a significant strength. That carries with it a huge responsibility. These very bright, talented people have to be given an opportunity to develop and not just do what everybody else is doing. These unusual people are bringing so much that you don't want to force them into a mold that would accommodate a much less stellar group of people. For a new school, we were extremely lucky.

Keenan, 1986, MSN 1993: The School of Nursing has really been for me the best thing in my whole professional life, bar none. I treat the students I teach much like I remember the faculty treating me, with respect and as a colleague. In the very beginning, the faculty tried to socialize us into this role of being colleagues because that's what nurses are supposed to learn to be, professional colleagues. And so I try to promote that with the students.

Angell, 1969, BSN 1977: We've had now three deans, all very different but all very appropriate for the stage of the development of the school. Carol Gray's charge was to get the school up and running, get the programs in place; not necessarily that she did that herself, but that she got the right people to do that.

Sue Donaldson's charge was to get this building built, get the doctoral program and research to be a more important part of education here. If we were going to be part of Hopkins on the same par as everybody else, we had to have a research faculty; we had to be getting grants. Sue Donaldson developed the Center for Nursing Research and she brought on some faculty who were researchers. She brought in Jackie Campbell. She brought in Fannie Gaston-Johansson. She supported Martha Hill's development in the American Heart Association in the years before she became president and certainly while she was president of the association.

Martha Hill's charge, as I see it, is certainly going to be development; also to take the research program to the next higher level; and probably to develop more of an international thrust.

Larson: Johns Hopkins went, in fifteen years, from nothing to one of the top schools in the country; that's just amazing. Some of the things we did, like the postdoc program, the new courses, the joint-degree programs, and the joint courses, we did partly out of commitment to quality and partly out of naiveté. We didn't know you couldn't or shouldn't, and we did.

I like to have my options open. I never like to be anywhere where I feel like I'm stuck. I can always go someplace else but whether I really would, probably not, because I'm still having a good time. It's not just about the money. I'm a perpetual student and I could never take advantage of everything that's available here to keep learning. That, for me, is first and foremost, to be in an environment where I'm never bored. I would never be bored here, ever.

Benita Walton-Moss, 1978

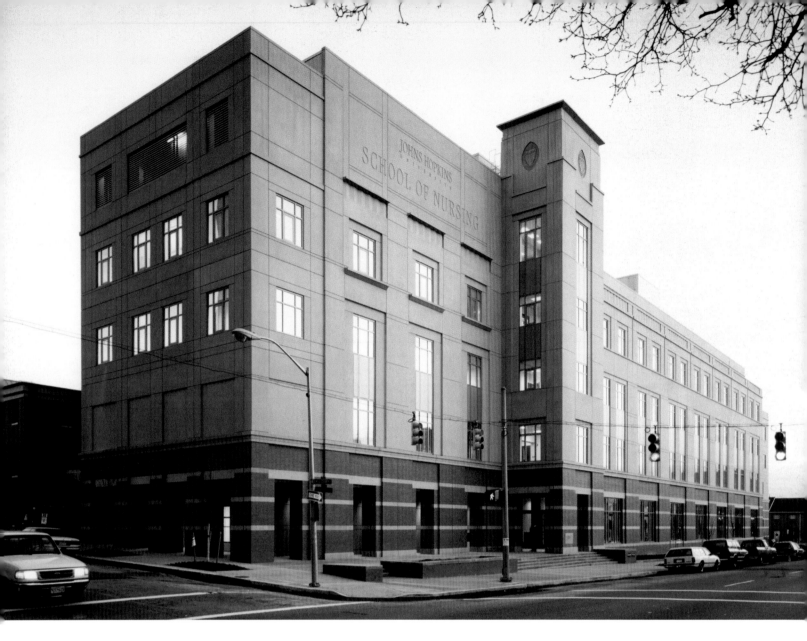

Adjacent to the Bloomberg School of Public Health and across Wolfe Street from the hospital, the Johns Hopkins School of Nursing occupies a prominent position on the East Baltimore campus. Its success brought new challenges: in less than ten years the Anne M. Pinkard Building was already filled beyond its capacity and plans were under way for its expansion.

Marella: To know that school today and what it has achieved and is still achieving, it's just wonderful. I think it's the biggest asset of that hospital and of the university. It's given the School of Nursing at the University of Maryland a real run for its money although it was well established and a fine school of nursing. But in the short time that the Hopkins School of Nursing has been in existence, it has far exceeded expectations.

McClain: The school has come of age within the Hopkins family. What Martha Hill will have to do, if she does her job well—and I think she will—is really begin to define niches. What are you going to be distinctive for? Because you can't be distinctive in everything. No one can. Harvard can't. Stanford can't. Hopkins can't. You've got to say, "How is it we're going to make our mark?" I am quite satisfied with the way things turned out. The kid's come out of adolescence quite well and I think it will grow up to be a pretty fine adult school.

Hill, 1964, BSN 1966: Finding ways to stay innovative and maintain the high quality of education, to continue to build the research program,

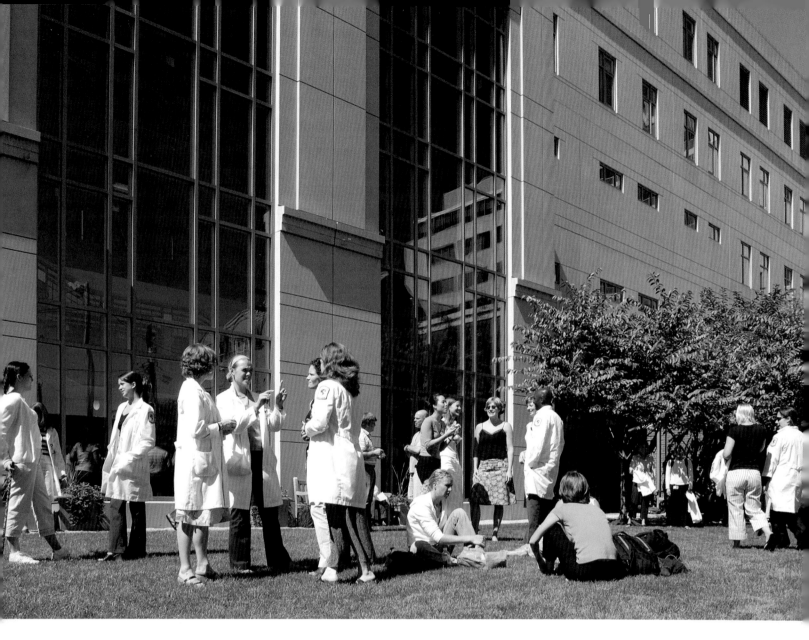

which is now ranked among the top in the country, and to attract the best and brightest students and support the faculty in their development and career progression, those elements of the mission have not changed. Being able to be flexible and innovative while you're still small and in very constrained quarters is challenging. We're going to have to really focus. Our four major goals are maintaining excellence, developing a community and a culture that's based on values, building our activities to position Johns Hopkins nursing as a leader globally in health care, and planning growth that is both innovative yet financially sound. Everything we do needs to fit with this.

You've got to have a very strong team internally and have the leadership and the management of the school be absolutely seamless. Whether I'm here or not, the daily operations need to be first-rate. It's about building teams. It's about having people understand the roles and responsibilities of the dean, the associate deans, the various administrators, the faculty, staff, and our students—it's about all of us sharing a full understanding of the mission and why we're here and what we're trying to do and how very important it is that it be done and done well.

Associate Dean Stella Shiber recalled that the architects wanted the building and its courtyard "to be an oasis from the harried world of the clinical arena, where there's a lot of stress and a lot of activity. The garden and the large open stairway and all the light accomplished that."

Dean Carol Gray selected the design for the school's pin, which incorporated the university seal. In 2005 the board of the alumni association voted to make the pin a gift to each new alumnus.

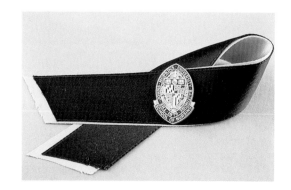

Chronology

MAME WARREN

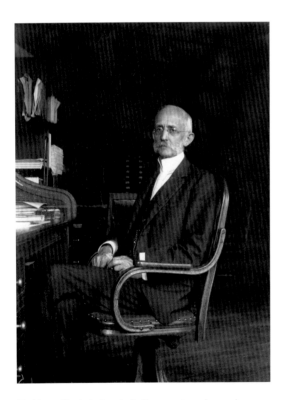

Dr. Henry Hurd, the hospital's first superintendent and an enthusiastic advocate of the nursing school, spoke at its opening. In 1906 he wrote an article entitled "Shall Training Schools Be Endowed?" for the *American Journal of Nursing*, in which he argued for endowments for both medical and nursing schools because hospitals were subject to financial liability.

1867

August 24: Johns Hopkins, a wealthy Baltimore merchant, incorporates both his university and his hospital.

1873

March 10: In his letter to the trustees of the Johns Hopkins Hospital setting forth the principles they are to follow, Hopkins states that the hospital must provide for "the indigent sick of this city and its environs, without regard to sex, age, or color, who may require surgical or medical treatment, and who can be received into the Hospital without peril to other inmates." His letter also directs that the hospital accommodate four hundred patients and that a school of nursing and a school of medicine be established in conjunction with the hospital.

December 24: Johns Hopkins dies at his residence at 81 Saratoga St. in Baltimore at the age of 78. The *Baltimore Sun* estimates his estate at $8 million. In an editorial, the *Sun* says of Hopkins, "It is gratifying to see a man who had thus successfully labored turning his attention ere life's close to great schemes of beneficence, by which an undoubted good is to result which cannot be interred with his bones. The good which such men do lives after them, blossoming and bearing fruit for the improvement and happiness of future generations."

1889

April 9: Isabel Hampton accepts an offer from the Board of Trustees of the Johns Hopkins Hospital to serve as the first superintendent of nurses at the hospital and principal of the Johns Hopkins Hospital Training School for Nurses. Later, Dr. William Osler recalled the initial interview with Miss Hampton. "She entered the room looking like an animated Greek statue. Mr. Gilman looked at Mr. King and smiled; then he looked at Dr. Billings and smiled again; then he threw a glance at Dr. Welch and he had no time to smile before he looked at me with a yet wider smile, and we knew it was all settled. It did not require anything further. Her certificates were looked at in a very perfunctory manner and the appointment was made in a very few minutes." Hampton's salary is set at $1,000 a year, her work to begin when the school opens.

May 15: First patient is admitted to the Johns Hopkins Hospital, where Louisa Parsons serves as acting superintendent of nurses.

October 9: Dr. Henry Hurd, the first superintendent of the hospital, tells those assembled for the inaugural ceremony for the training school that "in the eyes of the Trustees, nursing the sick is not to be considered a trade but a learned profession. When it is realized that here practical work is but a part of the nurses' training, and that carefully devised courses of study and systematic mental training will accompany it, the work of the school at once enters upon a higher plane of excellence. Its course of study should be more thorough and systematic than that of any other school in the land, as it must inevitably feel the influence of the great University to which the Hospital is so nearly allied."

On this same occasion Isabel Hampton expresses her own vision: "It is not so much the great amount of work that she can accomplish practically that is desired, but the kind of work, and to render unto each patient under her care nursing in its best and truest sense."

1890

Lavinia Dock joins the faculty as assistant supervisor and instructor of first-year students.

1891

January 28: Miss Hampton convenes the first meeting of the Nurses' Journal Club, "to promote a feeling of *esprit de corps* among the members of the school, to keep in touch with what is being done in other schools and hospitals by means of reports and discussions drawn chiefly from English and American weekly and monthly magazines, and to ensure a reading of such papers by all."

June 5: Dr. William Osler, physician-in-chief of the hospital, addresses the first class to graduate from the School of Nursing. The ceremony takes place under the dome of the hospital. He tells the new alumnae, "Practically, there should be for each of you a busy, useful, and happy life; more you cannot expect; a greater blessing the world cannot bestow. Busy you will certainly be, as the demand is great, both in private and public, for women with your training. Useful your lives must be, as you will care for those who cannot care for themselves, and who need about them, in the day of tribulation, gentle hands and tender hearts. And happy lives shall be yours, because busy and useful; having been initiated into the great secret—that happiness lies in the absorption in some vocation which satisfies the soul; that we are here to add what we can *to*, not to get what we can *from*, life." The class of 1891 includes M. Adelaide Nutting.

1892

June 3: Alumnae meet to form the Alumnae Association of the Johns Hopkins Hospital Training School for Nurses of Baltimore City and elect Helena Barnard, 1892, as the first president. This is the third nursing-school alumnae association organized in the United States. A constitution and bylaws are drafted and the association is incorporated under the General Laws of the State of Maryland. The object is "the promotion of unity and good feeling among the Alumnae, and the advancement of the interest of the profession of Nursing, and also of providing a home for its members, and making provision for them if ill or disabled." During its first year, a building fund and a sick benefit fund are established. The Sick Benefit Fund provides interest-free loans for members. The motto "Vigilando" and a badge, a Maltese cross in blue and black enamel on a background of gold with the letters *JHH*, are adopted.

1893

June: Isabel Hampton attends the International Congress of Charities, Corrections, and Philanthropy in Chicago and serves as chairman of the subsection on nursing. She addresses a symposium concerning "Standards for Nursing."

George W. Grafflin offers a vacant house at 219½ E. North Ave. as a home for alumnae who practice as private duty nurses or are disabled and in need after learning from Charlotte Ewell, 1893, who cares for Mr. Grafflin's daughter, about the new alumnae association and its need for a home. Mr. Grafflin proposes to give the house to the association after five years if the property is being successfully managed and promises to aid in the purchase of the ground rent "in order that both land and building should be the property of the association." The association accepts the offer in 1895.

1894

June 12: Isabel Hampton resigns in order to marry Dr. Hunter Robb in London.

November 14: M. Adelaide Nutting, 1891, becomes superintendent of nurses and principal of the training school at age thirty-five.

1895

July 4: The alumnae association's clubhouse opens for occupancy at 219½ E. North Ave. with Ethel Barwick, 1893, as registrar and housekeeper. Mr. Grafflin dies in 1896 and leaves $5,000 "for further development." By 1898 the house is too small for the number of nurses who want to live there and Grafflin's son William offers to pay half the cost of an addition. Work is completed in 1899 at a cost of more than $7,000. Additional improvements over the years bring new furnishings, a furnace, and electricity.

Josephine "Teeny" Waldhauser begins work as a waitress in the dining room of the Nurses' Home. Her career with the school continues for fifty-five years.

1896

February: Miss Nutting presents her research and recommendations for improving nursing clinical education to the American Association of Superintendents of Training Schools for Nurses, the forerunner of the National League for Nursing.

April 14: A special committee of the hospital trustees approves a three-year course of training and study. The program, designed by Adelaide Nutting, recommends eight-hour workdays, ending student allowances, and establishing scholarships.

June 4: The alumnae association adopts a code of ethics written by Isabel Hampton Robb, assisted by Katherine De Long, Mary Heriot, and Alice B. Conover, all members of the class of 1894. The code's first article, "The Duty of the Nurse to the Physician," states that "a nurse should always accord to a physician the proper amount of respect and consideration due to his higher professional position." Other topics include the nurse's duty to the patient, the school, the public, and her fellow nurses; the duty of the physician to the nurse; and the duty of the public to the nurse. For fifty-six years this code serves as "an unfailing guide to Johns Hopkins Hospital nurses."

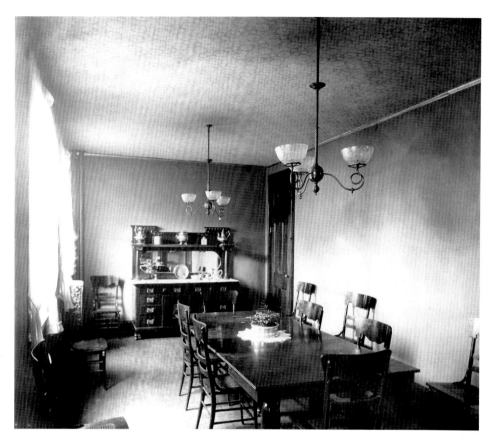

For almost a half century, many alumnae private duty nurses lived in the alumnae association's clubhouse, the gift of a grateful father in 1893.

June: The alumnae association's Registry Committee establishes a registry for private duty nurses practicing in Baltimore.

The Associated Alumnae of Trained Nurses of the United States and Canada organizes with Isabel Hampton Robb as its first president and Helena Barnard, 1892, as secretary. The alumnae association votes to become a part of this national association, which later becomes the American Nurses Association.

Nursing students begin accompanying interns and medical students into the homes of women in the neighborhood who are about to give birth. The student usually remains in the home for up to eighteen hours after the delivery. This outside obstetrical service is supplemented when the hospital creates an obstetrical ward for cases that require special attention.

1897

A separate registry exclusively for Johns Hopkins alumnae is created.

A senior student oversees the newly established children's ward at the hospital.

1899

As the hospital celebrates its tenth anniversary, staff nurses' salaries are $30 per month. Miss Nutting earns $100 per month.

The first class completing the three-year curriculum graduates.

Isabel Hampton Robb chairs a committee working to establish the first-ever postgraduate program for nurses at Teachers College, Columbia University.

1900

When she accepts Mary Bartlett Dixon, 1903, as a student, Miss Nutting tells her candidly, "I cannot develop our school unless I have the understanding and active support of the Board of Trustees. Your father is President of the Board and through you, as a student of this school, I believe I can demonstrate the reasonableness of one of my most important plans." Nutting is referring to the need to establish a probationary period for new students before they are thrown into patient care. Nutting tells Dixon, "You are about to enter the School of Nursing of a very great hospital. We are all of us here working together day and night, year after year, to give our patients the best possible care and service. You will be a small cog in this great wheel, but always remember a cog, however small, is of vital importance. I shall trust you to give us the best that is in you."

1901

Requests for information about the school increase from 320 the previous year to 1,223. According to the first circular of information, "applicants must not be under twenty-three years of age and not over thirty-five and of at least average height and physique. They must

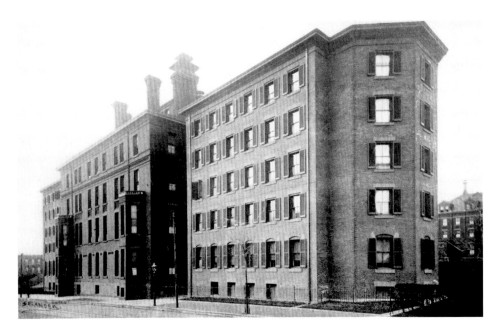

Helen Wilmer, 1905, funded a much-needed addition to the Nurses' Home as a memorial to her father in 1906. A second addition was built the following year.

give evidence of having had a good general English education and ability to undertake this course of study, and while it is indispensable, applicants are reminded that women of superior education and cultivation will be preferred, provided they meet the requirements in other particulars."

Georgina Ross, 1894, takes charge of the school's first six-month training for probationers (similar to what already existed in English schools) in housekeeping; selecting, cooking, and serving foods; preparations of bandages and surgical supplies; sterilizing; anatomy; physiology; hygiene; materia medica; and the elements of practical nursing.

December: Ada Carr, 1893, edits volume one, number one of the *Johns Hopkins Nurses Alumnae Magazine* and continues as editor of the quarterly publication for two years. Subscription price is 50¢ per year.

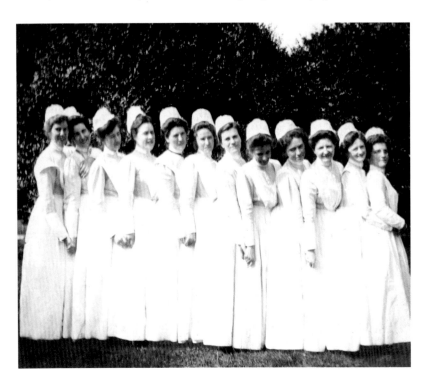

Members of the class of 1906 formed fond friendships during their rigorous training under the directorship of M. Adelaide Nutting.

1903

The alumnae magazine reports that the Nurses' Home and its annex are so crowded that for the past year "most of those on special duty have had rooms in some of the houses nearby on Broadway."

The board establishes a tuition fee and sets it at $50 per year.

1904

April: The Great Fire in February, which destroyed much of downtown Baltimore, including many buildings owned as investments by the hospital, prompts John D. Rockefeller's son to write to the trustees: "In view of the high character of work which the hospital and medical school are doing in medical instruction and research, including the training of nurses, which work he understands will otherwise be materially curtailed because of the losses, my father will give five hundred thousand dollars ($500,000) to Johns Hopkins Hospital."

Summer: At the same time the State of Maryland is drawing up its first guidelines for registration of nurses, M. Adelaide Nutting reads a paper entitled "Suggestions for Educational Standards for State Registration" at the International Council of Nurses in Berlin, Germany. Nutting emphasizes the importance of preliminary training: "It is well known that many people, among them doctors, and even the heads of some training-schools, still honestly believe that it is not only not necessary, but undesirable that nurses should be educated women." She recommends that practical work should occupy about six hours a day, leaving three to four hours for theoretical instruction.

1905

Adelaide Nutting becomes the first nurse licensed in Maryland and helps to establish the Maryland State Association of Graduate Nurses.

December 13: Miss Nutting assembles all head nurses and the entire senior class to discuss the advisability of forming a group devoted to the study of nursing history. They name themselves the Society of Teresians to honor St. Teresa. The alumnae magazine later reported that the group met for many years to discuss "the origin of sisterhoods, the development of hospitals, the lives of saints," and other topics.

1906

Helen Wilmer, 1905, gives an addition to the Nurses' Home as a memorial to her father, a noted Baltimore attorney.

The alumnae association commissions Cecilia Beaux to paint a portrait of M. Adelaide Nutting. Susan Read Thayer, a classmate of Nutting's who married Dr. William Thayer, speaks at the unveiling.

1907

Miss Georgina Ross, 1894, succeeds M. Adelaide Nutting as the director of the School of Nursing when Nutting goes to the

Department of Home and Institutional Economics at Teachers College, Columbia University, where she later becomes the first professor of nursing in the world.

Student vacations increase to seven weeks with three weeks off at the end of the first year and four after the second.

1908

Dr. William Welch addresses the nurses' alumnae association on "Public Health with Especial Reference to the Work of the Trained Nurse."

Ada Carr becomes the first full-time instructor for nursing.

December: An editorial in the alumnae magazine declines to involve the publication in the widespread discussion of women's suffrage, even though the previous issue included a fascinating article on the subject. "Our Constitution's first expressed object, 'the promotion of unity and good feeling among the Alumnae,' demands, it seems to us, in view of the divergent views entertained by our members, at least a fair degree of reticence as to our suffrage proclivities in print in the *Magazine*." Later in this same issue, however, a talk on the subject by Dr. Florence Sabin is reproduced. In subsequent years some alumnae and members of the faculty become deeply involved in the suffrage movement.

1910

March 15: Elsie Mildred Lawler, 1899, returns to Johns Hopkins to become the superintendent of nurses and principal of the School of Nursing after Georgina Ross resigns because of ill health.

April 15: Isabel Hampton Robb, 49 years old, dies when she is struck by a streetcar in Cleveland, Ohio.

1912

September: Announcement is made that a new building named for Charles L. Marburg (whose heirs had given the hospital $100,000 in 1907) will be constructed for the use of private patients. The building opens the following year.

October 9: James Buchanan "Diamond Jim" Brady makes a surprise visit to East Baltimore to inspect the new urological building for which he provided funds. He is so pleased with the nearly completed building that he draws up a new will to provide money for its maintenance and improvements. The *Baltimore American* reports that, "as usual, Mr. Brady wore a princely array of diamonds."

The Harriet Lane Home for Invalid Children admits its first patient.

1913

The Phipps Clinic, America's first clinic for the treatment of mental illness, opens, thanks to a generous gift to the hospital in 1908 from iron and steel magnate Henry Phipps. The philanthropist also endows a professorship of psychiatry at the university.

1914

On the occasion of the school's twenty-fifth anniversary, Adelaide Nutting calls for the establishment of a committee to work toward creating an endowment for the school.

1915

Elsie Lawler's annual report notes that "in the first annual report of the training school read in June, 1891, the staff all told was 57. In 1910, the staff was 142; and now in 1915, the staff is 272, not including the 84 special nurses." She makes the point that the size of the Nurses' Home has not kept pace with the growth of the school.

October 9: Eight members of the staff of the Instructive Visiting Nurse Association take advantage of courses offered to teachers and social workers by a new division of the Johns Hopkins University.

December 3: Miss Nutting chairs the first meeting of the Endowment Fund Committee, established with the approval of the board of trustees. The committee proposes to raise $1 million.

1916

May: Bessie Baker, 1902, appeals to nurses to join the Red Cross and the Johns Hopkins base hospital unit being organized "in the event of war."

May 26: At the annual meeting of the alumnae association an extended discussion takes place before the decision is made to let

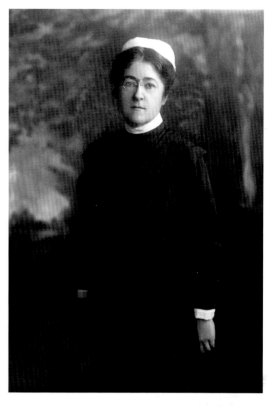

Elsie Mildred Lawler, 1899, was still a young woman when she became, in 1910, superintendent of nurses and principal of the School of Nursing, posts she held for thirty years.

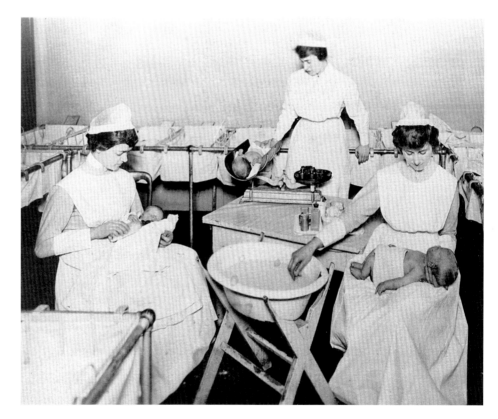

Students usually enjoyed clinical time caring for infants. They performed tasks such as feeding, weighing, and bathing newborn babies.

nurses decide for themselves whether they prefer to wear white or black shoes with the Johns Hopkins uniform. Although black shoes have always been required by the dress code, Ruth Brewster Sherman, 1901, mentions that, with the newly updated uniform, nurses could wear white shoes in the summer "because they are cool." Virginia McMaster Foard, 1896, adds, "When the Johns Hopkins Hospital uniform was made, white shoes were not in vogue. Now they are an absolutely common thing. South of Virginia everyone wears white shoes."

1917

June 9: With more than one hundred nursing alumnae already in Europe serving with the Red Cross, General Hospital No. 18, which includes many Johns Hopkins nurses and doctors, sets sail for Europe on the *Finland* after the United States declares war on Germany in April. They arrive in France on June 28 and set up a permanent base hospital at Bazoilles-sur-Meuse. Several other base hospitals open there, and together they treat 20,000 sick and wounded patients before the war ends.

Richard White (a great-nephew of Johns Hopkins), Dr. Hugh Young, George K. McGaw, and George Cator give a cottage on the Severn River on Nottingham Point in Sherwood Forest "for the pleasure of the student nurses." The cottage, which features a large living room with fireplace, three

bedrooms, a sleeping porch, and full kitchen, accommodates ten to twelve students. Each spring Christine Dick, 1899, the custodian of the keys, prepares the cottage for occupancy. Golf, tennis, horseback riding, swimming, rowing, and canoeing are always available, as well as occasional movies and club dances. Many use it as a quiet place to study for the state board examinations.

Enrollment increases to 232 students in response to a request from the Council of National Defense to increase numbers of trained nurses.

1918

March 11: Adelaide Nutting attends a meeting of the Johns Hopkins Hospital Historical Club to describe her visit with Florence Nightingale at her home in London shortly before Nightingale died in 1910. Nutting recalls that Miss Nightingale "held her hand and plied her with questions."

Captain Harvey B. Stone, chief of surgery at the Johns Hopkins Base Hospital in France, writes home: "The work is full of interest. The patients, most of them at least, are fine fellows, very grateful, and with lots of fun in them. They are usually delighted to get here, where the nurses give them excellent care, and where they get cleaned up, well fed and cheered into good mental tone. Their devotion to the nurses is really touching. Their letters home, which we have to censor, are full of praise and respectful devotion to these

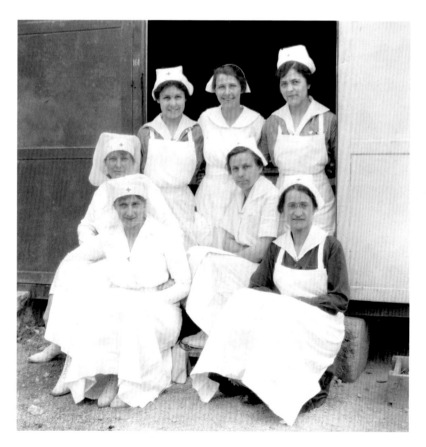

Alumnae, such as these Red Cross nurses at an evacuation hospital in France, cared for the sick and wounded even before the United States entered World War I in 1917.

fine women. I think that most of our patients would give their lives up gladly before they would let any harm come to a nurse. And the nurses deserve it every bit. They work very hard, are intensely interested in their cases, and help tremendously in keeping up the morale and civilization of a community otherwise entirely masculine and a bit inclined to be hard-bitten in its views of life and things and people."

Adelaide Nutting chairs a committee for the National League for Nursing Education when it publishes *The Standard Curriculum for Schools of Nursing.*

Miss Lawler's annual report notes that the school continues to grow. "The question of accommodation for the nurses continues to be a problem. In order to find rooms for the larger class admitted, a third house was rented, and we now have 410, 412 and 706 North Broadway all occupied by nurses."

March to December: The hospital and school persevere through hundreds of cases of influenza during a pandemic that kills millions worldwide. In November the alumnae magazine reports that "our nurses are not only overwhelmed by work but alarming numbers are ill with the disease." Four students and two alumnae die before the epidemic subsides. "The most tragic part of the situation is the number of deaths among the troops. Nine thousand five hundred and forty-nine Americans have been killed in battle in a year, in less than a month nearly seven thousand have died from influenza in camp hospitals, while the total deaths from diseases of all sorts in the Expeditionary Forces in France are only 2,149."

1919

February 3: The Johns Hopkins nursing unit sails from France. Two nurses die from illnesses during the voyage.

August: The alumnae magazine reports that Anna D. Wolf, 1915, Miss Lawler's assistant superintendent and an instructor at the school for the past three years, has left to take charge of the training school for nurses to be established with Peking Union Medical College in China. Wolf graduated from Goucher College in 1911 and, with the help of a scholarship from Johns Hopkins, earned a master's degree from Columbia University in 1915.

1920

The Rockefeller Foundation Committee on Nursing and Nursing Education includes Johns Hopkins Hospital president Dr. Winford Smith. Johns Hopkins is one of twenty-three schools of nursing studied for what becomes the Goldmark Report of 1923.

November: The alumnae magazine says Miss Nutting will "secure a woman trained in publicity work" to raise funds for the endowment, as per Smith College's successful campaign to raise $4 million. "Her principal duties should be to largely prepare the booklet, whatever pamphlets may be necessary, to write articles for the papers and magazines, prepare, or select for use, good stories regarding nurses' work, attend to all necessary printing, to cooperate and assist in every way, with the Publicity Committee." Miss Lawler says she would use the $1 million endowment to make essential improvements to the school. "The first thing would be a building and class-rooms for nurses. An assembly room large enough to house all the nurses would be nec-essary. A reading room, a library, and all the facilities for study and reading, etc. We would have a Florence Nightingale Memorial room in which to house all our treasures."

1921

February 26: Johns Hopkins University Presi-dent Frank Goodnow endorses the formal launching of the endowment fund and tells those attending a reception that "nursing education must of necessity be preeminently practical, and this would rank nursing schools with vocational schools—but on no account should the fact that the education of nurses is practical rather than academic debar it from taking its place in the great universities. There is a place for it here." Dr. Henry Hurd, who was present at the opening of the school in 1889, also endorses the concept of affiliating the nursing school with the university and expresses hope that nursing "would be regarded as other learned professions."

May 12: Dr. Howard Kelly presents the school with "the chair in which Florence Nightingale spent so much of her life" at commencement, which takes place in the Phipps Clinic, rather than its garden, because of rain.

May: The alumnae association opens the Gate House Shop to raise money for the endowment fund, which has accumulated $43,000. The shop, which is run by Helen Wilmer Athey, 1905, sells magazines, notepa-per, postcards, candy, and the organdy nurses' caps worn by Hopkins alumnae. Mary Lent, 1895, suggested using the small structure at the Broadway entrance to the hospital, origi-nally the porter's lodging and then the night watchman's. When the medical school opened in 1893, the gatehouse became the registrar's office, then a bookstore, and then sleeping quarters for hospital employees.

Alumnae continue to achieve distinction. This year Clara Noyes, 1896, is president of the American Nurses Association; Anna Jammé, 1897, president of the National League for Nursing Education; and Elizabeth Fox, 1914, president of the National Organization for Public Health Nursing.

Tuition doubles from $50 to $100.

1923

Loula Kennedy, who joined the faculty in 1921, recommends to students that they begin pub-lishing a yearbook. Publication of the *Routine* continues until 1932.

November: A new uniform for Johns Hopkins nurses is described in the alumnae magazine. Its skirt has five gores and measures two yards in width around the bottom; it must not be more than eight inches from the floor. The sleeves are shirtwaist length with a three-inch cuff with buttons. The uniform includes a bibbed apron. Nurses may choose black or white lace-up oxford shoes. The organdy cap,

which remains unchanged, is to be pinned on both sides with white beaded pearl pins, and the hair must be worn up and under the cap. Sweaters in inconspicuous colors are permit-ted. The only allowable jewelry is the alumnae pin or inconspicuous collar or cuff pins, and a wrist or chain watch, but no bracelets or rings except wedding rings.

1924

January 9: The Woman's Clinic is dedicated at the hospital, made possible by a generous gift from Mrs. Lucy Wortham James, of New York.

May 14: In a discussion about the complexity of trying to raise endowment monies while the university and the hospital are also solicit-ing funds from donors like the Rockefeller Foundation, the question of closer affiliation with the university arises again. Miss Nutting says she recently discussed the subject in "an informal conference" and "she could not discover any insuperable obstacle to estab-lishing a suitable relationship. The President of the University seemed entirely open-minded, and, in view of the fact that the University already offers courses leading to degrees for teachers, social workers, business-men and women, it seemed reasonable to expect that plans could, without great difficulty, be worked out which would offer somewhat similar opportunities to suitably qualified nurses, and then open up to them, as to other women engaged in no more important work, the resources and advan-tages of the University." Miss Nutting resigns as chairman of the endowment committee with regret because of illness; she becomes honorary chair.

Miss Lawler reports that students are now being admitted in three groups and that the Nurses' Home is crowded to its utmost capacity.

The endowment continues to grow, slowly, to $87,000.

1925

February: Blanche Pfefferkorn, 1911, writes an article entitled "On Nursing Education" for the alumnae magazine. She notes that training schools are a "mediaeval and ancient form of vocational preparation, the so-called apprenticeship system" and points out that medicine and law have moved on from this tradition to more professional education. Pfefferkorn emphasizes that there is a difference between training and education. Education "aims to develop those mental powers which have to do with independent, intelligent thinking, whereas [training] is largely a product of repeated and oftentimes unrelated acts with too little concern for the 'whys and wherefores.'" She presciently con-cludes that "the hospital apprenticeship sooner or later is doomed."

The May issue of the magazine gives a report about the new dormitory for nurses—Hampton House—to be built on the west side of Broadway between McElderry and Monument Streets. It will be eight stories high and accommodate 241 students.

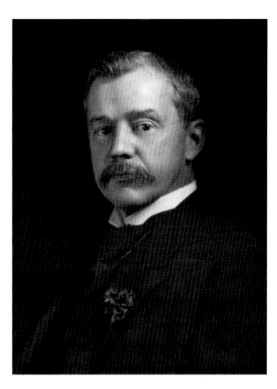

In 1921 Dr. Howard Kelly gave the nursing school a chair once owned by Florence Nightingale. Three years before, he had sur-prised the school with a bound volume of original Nightingale letters, which the alumnae magazine called "a wonderful gift, so generously conceived and so perfectly carried out."

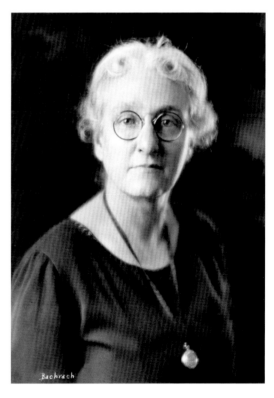

During World War I, Clara Noyes, 1896, oversaw the activities of American nurses serving in Red Cross facilities, as well as nurses serving in the U.S. Army and Navy. She became presi-dent of the American Nurses Association in 1921.

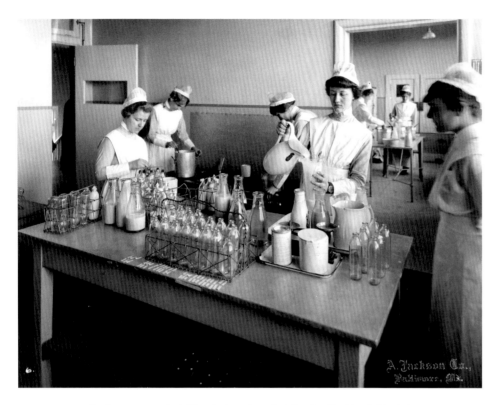

Student nurses worked diligently throughout the Johns Hopkins Hospital, including two rooms in the basement of the Harriet Lane Home used exclusively for preparing a protein milk formula.

Summer: The Gate House Shop receives electricity but still no running water. The alumnae managing the shop boast, "We have a good water supply when it rains and the lake at our doorway upon these occasions is full of charm and we are considering keeping gold fish. These with our window boxes would make us appear pleasantly rural and make our customers who must stay in town in summer think of the 'great open spaces.'"

1926

June 24: Students move into Hampton House, except those who will finish in November and probationers, who are still in the original Nurses' Home.

October 21: Students, faculty, alumnae, and friends of the School of Nursing gather to celebrate the dedication of Hampton House. Adelaide Nutting tells the editors of the *Routine* that Isabel Hampton Robb would be pleased to have the new building named in her honor. "Many, many times I heard her denounce in vigorous English the arrangement in the old home by which every resident there was compelled to go through the hospital in order to get out into the street. That seemed to her an unpardonable waste of time and strength, and a curious relic of military tradition in a modern institution."

1927

Harold Knight, of London, in Baltimore to paint portraits for the medical school and university, presents his portrait of Elsie Lawler, principal and superintendent of nurses since 1910. For ten years Miss Lawler

was president of the Maryland State Association of Graduate Nurses, a post she recently resigned. The new portrait is to hang with Isabel Hampton Robb's in Hampton House.

The Carnegie Building, which houses the dispensary, opens.

1928

January 27: A special committee of the Johns Hopkins nurses' alumnae meets with the hospital trustees to present a report on the committee's work since its formation in May 1926. Subjects include plans for significant changes in the curriculum, in both theory and practice; reports on nursing education elsewhere; public health; graduate and postgraduate study; and the possibility of affiliating with the university. "There are in this country to-day about forty-two schools having at least a working university relationship, while two schools are parts of the university, each organized as separate and distinct units, with all the rights and privileges of the schools of medicine, law, or education," the report explains, adding that "to see our school a part of the Johns Hopkins University has been the ambition and hope of its alumnae." The report goes on to say that the current school's staff is underpaid, underprepared, and has too heavy a teaching load. The School of Nursing "is used almost exclusively as the nursing service of the hospital and is unduly subservient to its demands." The committee points out that developments in the school have not kept pace with those in the hospital and recommends that a new committee be formed, with representatives of both hospital and university trustees, the alumnae, and the School of

Nursing, to try to establish an affiliation with the university "on the closest terms the policies of its organization will permit."

May 14: As a result of the January 27 meeting, the trustees appoint a committee consisting of two trustees, two members of the medical board, two alumnae, the superintendent of nurses, the director of the hospital, and Dr. William Welch representing the School of Hygiene. At its first meeting the new committee appoints subcommittees to study what the preparation of a nurse should be and to determine the ideal makeup of the nursing service of the hospital. Another committee will determine immediate needs of the hospital and school.

A writer for the *Routine* gloats, "A visible sign of growth and progress in our school has been realized this year in the acquisition of a group of classrooms on the fourth and top floor of the Surgical Building. Away from the din and bustle and confusion of the busy life in the hospital, we feel on top of the world with all the air and sunlight and hope which that implies. And we have a right to be proud of our quarters, snatched as they were from the envious medical school by our advocate Dr. Smith and made over so attractively to meet our needs."

1929

May 7: The fortieth anniversary of the Johns Hopkins Hospital is celebrated. The hospital that opened with 250 beds now has 743. In the hospital's first year, 1,825 patients were treated; in 1928, the number was 11,697. In forty years, the hospital has administered to 947,000 patients in wards and 3,250,000 in the dispensaries.

After fifteen years the endowment fund committee announces that it has surpassed $100,000. Part of the difficulty in meeting the $1-million goal was attributable to the restrictions placed by hospital trustees on who may be approached for support, since the trustees compete for contributions from the same sources. The trustees dictate that the endowment must come from alumnae and friends. Almost $25,000 was raised through the Gate House Shop.

The alumnae association votes to rename the endowment fund "The M. Adelaide Nutting Endowment Fund for the Johns Hopkins Nurses' Alumnae Association."

October 15. The William H. Wilmer Ophthalmological Institute, the first such institute in the United States associated with a university, is formally dedicated. It is under the direction of Dr. William Holland Wilmer, of Washington, D.C.

Maude Magill Bagwell, 1929, discovers that life in Hampton House is "very restricted for students." Years later she recalled, "There was a 10:00 P.M. curfew and all lights in the nursing quarters had to be out by 10:30 P.M. Some of my classmates used to talk of studying in their closets or under bedcovers, using flashlights to avoid breaking the curfew, which was a punishable offense. If we came in late from a date, even a few minutes after curfew, we had to enter by the hospital's main desk and be escorted by a nursing supervisor through the tunnel to the nurses' home and to our rooms, such an event always bringing an official reprimand. The entrance door to the nursing home was locked promptly at 10 P.M. each night and not opened until the next morning."

October 17: The Welch Library opens to serve all three schools on the medical campus.

1930

September 2: Judge Henry D. Harlan, chairman of the hospital trustees, writes a letter announcing the creation of an "Advisory Board for the Supervision of the Training School of Nurses" whose particular purpose is to consider the curriculum, a development Johns Hopkins University President Joseph Sweetman Ames recommends. The advisory board will meet monthly during the academic year. Its eleven members will comprise two doctors from the medical advisory board, one faculty member from the Advisory Board of the School of Hygiene and Public Health, the directors of the hospital and the School of Nursing, the president of the university, a member of the nursing school staff, two members at large, and two alumnae elected by the association. The new board meets for the first time on December 18.

1931

The new advisory board holds a two-day meeting to review opinions gleaned from a survey of deans of medical schools, nurses, physicians, social workers, and laypersons. The survey includes comments about the school, which they believe is "prepared to conduct post-graduate work on a high educational level." A long message from Miss Nutting is read, then resolutions are passed that disregard the conclusions of the survey. Dr. Ames requests Dr. Smith to submit figures at the next meeting giving the approximate cost of the nursing school separate from the cost of the nursing service at the hospital.

The first turtle derby is run in a large circle on the tennis court with turtles that are descendants of those kept in the early days of the hospital by Benjamin Frisby, doorman at the hospital from 1889 to 1933. Contestants are released from a large wire sterilizing cage positioned in the middle, and the first turtle to cross the line wins. Each department sponsors a contestant and contributes to the purse. The winner is "Sir Walter," pride of the brain surgeons, who takes this year's cash prize. Races in following years attract several thousand spectators and more than fifty brightly painted, cleverly (and sometimes raunchily) named entries, some of them from Hopkins men in other states or countries. In the 1933 race, a large grey rabbit wanders slowly toward the circle's edge while "Panic II," the entry of the Phipps Clinic, trudges steadily outward and wins, thereby reinforcing the lesson of the tortoise and the hare. Future races are broadcast over national radio and featured in newsreels. Proceeds are contributed to charitable causes.

1932

The alumnae magazine reports that the hospital now offers courses covering practice and theory for nurses in operating-room technique, psychiatry, pediatrics, obstetrics, and ophthalmology. The editor remarks "that no remuneration is given and students live outside the Hospital at their own expense, receive definite instruction through carefully arranged class and lecture schedules, is a clear sign that such courses are now regarded primarily as educational, rather than utilitarian, as was usually the case in the past. Practice necessarily forms an essential part of the instruction, yet a sharp contrast is offered by these courses to those given in many institutions in the past where the student worked long hours, was given a regular salary, board and lodging, and little or no classroom instruction." Referring to the nationwide Depression, she continues, "During this period of economic stress, when many nurses have leisure forced upon them, they could not be better occupied than to take advantage of such educational opportunities, thereby adding to their equipment for better days, which we are sufficiently optimistic to believe will surely arrive."

Students publish the final edition of the *Routine*.

September: The Depression motivates a larger number of well-qualified women to apply to the school. Of the seventy-five new students, thirty-three have college degrees and just thirteen have only high school diplomas. The others have from one to three years of college experience or have taken business or secretarial courses.

September: An agreement between the Johns Hopkins University School of Hygiene and Public Health and the Baltimore City Health Department establishes the Eastern Health District in a one-square-mile area of the city near Johns Hopkins Hospital. The district becomes a base for broad public-health and research programs conducted with financial support from the Rockefeller Foundation and the U.S. Public Health Service. Public-health nurses are trained and graduate students in the School of Hygiene and Public Health gather data for thesis research. Residents of the Eastern Health District are contacted individually and information is gathered on living conditions, general health, and diseases, especially tuberculosis and diphtheria. Child-health studies and epidemiological studies on infectious and chronic diseases are an important component of the research. In 1936 Dr. Thomas B. Turner and his staff conduct a study of syphilis that results in papers of national import.

1933

Hester K. Frederick, 1912, publishes "The Relation of the School of Nursing to the Hospital Administrative Unit as It Affects the Student Nurse." She reports that Miss Lawler supervises 116 graduate nurses, who act as assistants, instructors, supervisors, and head nurses, and 92 general-duty graduate nurses. There are 225 student nurses in the Hopkins school, as well as 48 affiliating student nurses from other schools and 15 postgraduate students taking supplementary courses in the hospital. Frederick explains that each service is maintained in its own building and has a separate staff, with a supervising nurse in charge and with assistants and head nurses within the unit, and that all nursing staffs are coordinated through the nursing school office.

The Nutting Endowment Fund finances the salary for two years of the first public-health instructor in the school, "thus making it

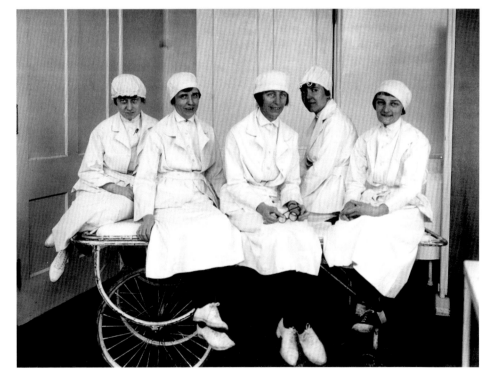

Nurse anesthetist Margaret G. Boise (center) posed with members of the nurse anesthetist class of 1922, who joined an elite group in the Department of Surgery.

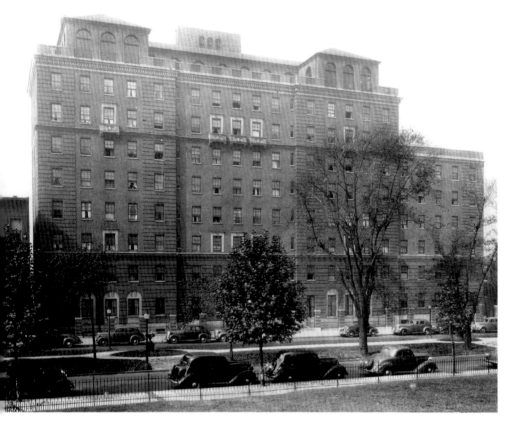

Students occupied the new Hampton House dormitory in 1926; by the next decade additional rooms were needed, and the first addition opened in 1938.

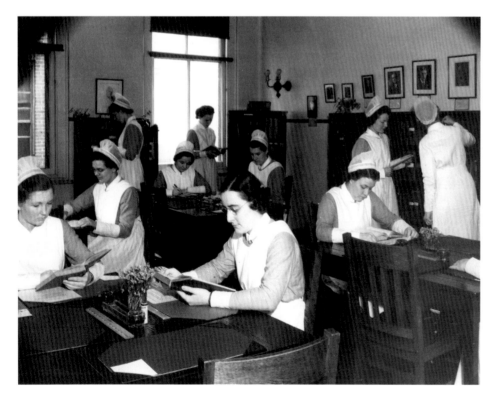

In the late 1930s nursing students and alumnae took advantage of a reference library on the fourth floor of the old surgical building.

possible for us to begin this work at a time of financial stress when it is obvious that it could not have been undertaken otherwise." The following year the school forms an affiliation with Baltimore's Eastern Health District, and students work in the field for a two-month period. As a result, more graduates choose to specialize in public-health nursing.

May 26: Members of the Alumnae Association of the Johns Hopkins Hospital Training School for Nurses of Baltimore City vote to change the organization's name to the Johns Hopkins Nurses Alumnae Association, Incorporated.

An infirmary opens in the Thayer Building where nursing students go for complete physicals when they arrive and where chest x-rays are done annually on all students. There is no dental or vision coverage. The infirmary's services are free and available to all nurses on the staff of the hospital, as well as to nursing students, dieticians, anesthetists, postgraduates, and affiliating students. If warranted, cases are transferred to the regular hospital service.

1934

K. Virginia Betzold, 1932, joins the nursing school faculty.

The Women's Auxiliary Board of the hospital funds two full-time nursing instructors for ward teaching, in the Halsted surgical ward and in the Osler medical clinic. This system permits the head nurse to concentrate on her administrative and housekeeping duties, records, and doctors' rounds while remaining available to the ward instructor as needed.

1935

The Johns Hopkins University bestows an honorary master of arts degree on Elsie Lawler in recognition of twenty-five years of "outstanding work as a nurse, teacher and administrator."

1936

A survey of the alumnae reveals a preference to keep control of the Nutting Fund rather than turn it over to the trustees of the hospital.

Ernestine Wiedenbach, 1925, writes about the new trend toward an eight-hour workday for private duty nurses but notes that the Johns Hopkins Hospital still "tenaciously cling[s]" to the twelve-hour schedule. At Hopkins, almost half the private duty nurses who respond to a ballot on the subject prefer the status quo. The concern is that the change would result in less work and a smaller annual income for private duty nurses. Nine other hospitals in Baltimore have made "this most sensible" change to the eight-hour schedule.

1937

January 30: In a reversal of their preference of the previous year, the alumnae association transfers $130,000 in bonds from the Nutting Fund to the trustees of the hospital. According to the magazine, "the principal reason the Alumnae voted to give their fund to the Trustees, as we understand it, is to demonstrate the value of an endowment, even a small one, and thus open the way for an approach to an adequate endowment." Years later, Helen Wilmer Athey remembered, "I shall never forget Mr. Leeke, the hospital treasurer, opening each of our bonds, taken from the safe deposit box, to be sure that no coupons had been unduly cut off."

April: Hospital trustees approve funding to permit nurses to work an eight-hour day, six days a week, with additional pay so that their income will not suffer from working fewer hours. General-duty nurses have one full day off; head nurses have only one afternoon a week off, but they will have every other Sunday off instead of one Sunday a month. To accomplish this, eight general-duty nurses and twenty ward helpers, ward clerks, and maids are hired. All general-duty nurses with six months of employment receive a $5-a-month raise. By May 1 one department has already instituted a forty-eight-hour week for all graduates.

May 27: Miss Lawler explains that the Nutting Fund was transferred to the custody of the hospital trustees "as a nucleus of an Endowment Fund for the School of Nursing. By the terms of acceptance the interest will be used to provide funds for additional educational expansion and the expenditures will be directed by the Advisory Committee of the School of Nursing."

The Johns Hopkins University awards thirty points of credit toward a bachelor of science degree to graduates of the training school who enroll in the Teachers College at Homewood. It is possible to earn this degree in one year, and tuition for nursing staff at the Johns Hopkins Hospital is half the usual rate. Anna D. Wolf, 1915, an alumna representative on the advisory board, reports that "accreditation of the nursing curriculum by the university has led to the matriculation of several students for the continuation of their university work. This plan should be a real benefit to the students as time goes on and should bring the school into closer relationship with the university."

June: Isabelle C. Diehl, 1934, becomes the first nursing graduate to earn her BS degree from the Johns Hopkins University.

The alumnae association begins sponsoring research and oral histories conducted by Edith Ware on the life of Isabel Hampton Robb.

1938

February 23: Nurses move into the new wing of Hampton House, which has 124 rooms and connects on each floor with the original building. The nurses' residences on Wolfe St. are no longer needed. Hampton House now accommodates 359 women.

1939

To mark the fiftieth anniversary of the school, alumnae are offered copies of a commemorative book called *Within the Gates*. The book includes sixty-eight photographs and costs $1 plus 10¢ postage.

The Advanced Standing Committee of the Johns Hopkins University conducts a survey of the nursing school and concludes that "the administration of the school is efficient, the instruction competent, the facilities adequate, the students in the main, earnest and attentive, and the personnel of the student body of high quality. The teaching methods also compare favorably with those in ordinary college instruction." This strengthens the argument for awarding credit toward a BS degree.

October 3: The first patient is admitted to a new infirmary exclusively for nurses, created in the former bridge between the Halsted and Thayer Buildings. There are eleven private cubicles, and each has a window with southern exposure.

December 5: The board of trustees regretfully accepts Elsie Lawler's resignation.

1940

February 28: Anna D. Wolf accepts the board's offer for her to succeed Miss Lawler as superintendent of the school.

The Johns Hopkins Hospital begins forming another General Hospital No. 18. Initial plans call for 45 medical officers, 120 nurses, and 400 enlisted men.

Helen Wilmer Athey, 1905, who manages the Gate House Shop where nurses purchase their caps, warns buyers that the caps currently on sale are of inferior quality because "imported organdy is held up by war conditions. If, in about a month, you find caps made of domestic material are not holding their shape, it is useless to tell us at the shop of your troubles. Please communicate directly with either Hitler or Chamberlain."

August 31: Miss Chisolm, "our faithful registrar for so many years," is the last resident to leave the Nurses Club at 219½ E. North Ave. The house is in ill repair and members decide not to invest money in the old building. Over the years, it became a permanent residence for many alumnae.

The registry office moves to 315 E. North Ave. and the alumnae office moves to 330 N. Charles St., an office building downtown, where mail is delivered four times daily.

Helen Waid, 1934, reports on the ongoing debate about eight-hour versus twelve-hour shifts for nurses. Patients prefer a twelve-hour workday because they form a closer bond with their nurses. Waid notes that with shorter schedules more nurses are required, which increases record keeping.

November 3: Miss Lawler gives a tea honoring Anna Wolf in Hampton House.

First patients are treated in the Halsted and Osler Buildings.

1941

Nurses enlisting in the new military hospital unit being organized by Johns Hopkins must be Red Cross nurses. To date, 16,000 are enrolled in the American Red Cross. Reserve members must be less than forty years old, unmarried, and graduates of an approved three-year nursing school connected with a hospital. Until the United States enters the war on December 8, response among Hopkins nurses is slow.

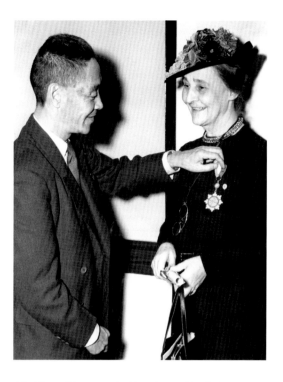

Alice Fitzgerald, 1906, received broad recognition for her accomplishments during a long international career in nursing. On October 24, 1940, Dr. F. C. Yen presented Fitzgerald with a medal for work with the American Bureau for Medical Aid to China.

Senior nursing student Marie Lowe, 1941, reports that a constitution has been drafted to create a student government. "We are anticipating a plan by which the faculty and students may be drawn closer together to work for the advancement of all school relations."

The last class to receive organdy caps at commencement graduates.

September: Beginning with the incoming class of 1944, students have a new uniform—a blue dress without an apron, with elbow-length sleeves and cuffs, and an attached white collar. Students wear brown shoes, tan hose, and a special washable student cap. A long-sleeved uniform with a white turned-back cuff is worn at formal occasions like teas, convocations, and commencement. Preclinical students (formerly known as probationers) wear tan lab coats over civilian clothes while uniforms are being custom-made for them. Students will pay about a hundred dollars for their uniforms over three years.

October 14: Faculty organizes and adopts bylaws. Nurses with the rank of head nurse and above are voting members of the new faculty organization. Monthly meetings, each to discuss a separate theme, are planned.

November 7: Miss Wolf tells alumnae a month before the United States enters the war that because of defense contract work, Baltimore has become a boom city with a population of more than a million people. This increases the number of patients in the hospital. There is also a high turnover in nursing personnel because other employers offer better pay. She announces that the federal government now provides funds in order to increase the number of student

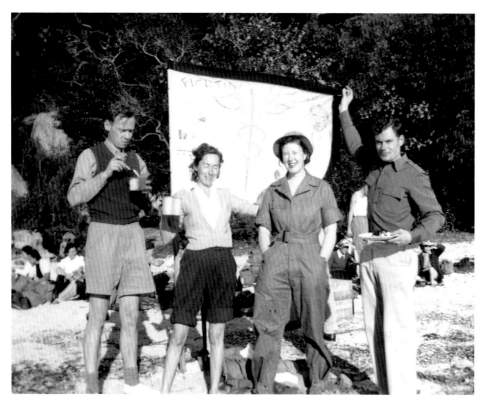

Hopkins nurses and doctors served with two hospital units in World War II. Members of the "fighting 118th" found time in 1944 to relax on the beach on Leyte Island in the Philippines.

nurses. "The Red Cross has stated that they will need eleven thousand more nurses this year, and we cannot too strongly urge our Hopkins nurses to join the Red Cross nursing service."

Students initiate a new tradition, the candlelight service, to mark the end of their preclinical period. The occasion is the first time they wear their new uniforms.

1942

The hospital makes preparations for possible blackouts. Emergency operating rooms with every modern feature are set up in the basement of the dispensary building under the accident ward for use in the event of an air raid. Most windows are fitted with removable fiberboard to create blackout panels.

February 18: The largest spring class in the history of the school expands student enrollment to 265.

February 19: One hundred two of the 120 nurses required to fill the ranks of General Hospital No. 18 are now in place. The alumnae magazine reports that twenty-eight come from the hospital staff, so "the depletion of our educational and service groups will be serious, however, we are relying upon our alumnae to help us and are confident we may secure a sufficient number to tide us over this critical period." Other nurses in the military unit come from Church Home and Hospital, Sinai, St. Joseph's, Union Memorial, and other hospitals outside Baltimore and Maryland.

April 10: The surgeon general sends word that Johns Hopkins will lead two hospital units instead of one, and he needs the names of the head physicians and nurses the next day. He disqualifies Mildred Struve, 1926, the chief nurse since the unit's reactivation, because of impaired vision in one eye. Mary Sanders, 1934, assistant to Miss Struve, replaces her. The next day, Jane Pierson, 1932, agrees to leave Kentucky for Baltimore the following week. Sanders heads General Hospital No. 118 and Pierson leads No. 18.

April 20: More than three hundred people come to the train station on a cold and rainy night to bid farewell to the first contingents of nurses and doctors to leave Baltimore. General Hospital No. 18 goes to Camp Jackson, Columbia, South Carolina; No. 118 goes to Camp Edwards, Falmouth, Massachusetts.

June 4: No. 18 reaches Melbourne, Australia, then quickly moves on to Sydney. By August 3, the unit forms an alliance with the Royal Prince Alfred Hospital and is ready to receive patients.

June 12: No. 118 arrives in Auckland, New Zealand.

August: General Hospital No. 18 moves to the Fiji Islands. By late October they are treating patients in a converted school. Personnel live in grass huts with thatched roofs, four, six, or eight persons to a hut, depending on its size. Although skeptical at first, they soon realize that the structures are cool and comfortable. They discover that on Fiji, it rains seven months out of the year, sometimes for three weeks at a time.

Jessie B. Black, 1930, chair of the library committee, reports that through the years the nursing school has accumulated many "rare and priceless" books and pamphlets on nursing history that are kept in the school's library. Black says that plans are under way to publish a pamphlet with a cataloged list of the collection.

1943

May: General Hospital No. 118 moves to a new facility near Sydney, which gradually expands to accommodate a thousand patients. The majority of patients suffer from medical conditions like malaria rather than battle wounds (a situation also faced much of the time by No. 18).

Summer: Johns Hopkins participates with the nursing schools at the University of Maryland, Union Memorial, Church Home and Hospital, and the Hospital for the Women of Maryland in a joint preclinical program at Goucher College. Jessie Black takes a leave of absence from her position as associate director at the Johns Hopkins Hospital School of Nursing to become dean of the program, which expects to admit 100 students. At summer's end, 47 students enroll at Johns Hopkins. The Goucher program is based on a similar curriculum at Bryn Mawr College, which Hopkins participated in during 1941 and 1942.

Because of the nursing shortage brought on by the war, more than $100,000 from the federal government is earmarked for housing an increased number of student nurses. At Johns Hopkins the funds make possible the addition of two floors to the west wing of Hampton House.

Charlotte Fischer, 1928, writes to the alumnae magazine from General Hospital No. 18: "Really we could not have picked a more beautiful spot. . . . We are celebrating our year on this island by having a large party in the new Recreation Hall. . . . The nurses have nice quarters . . . in grass houses built by the natives."

Mildred Struve, 1926, and Miriam Ames, 1914, both members of the faculty, receive Rockefeller Travel Grants to visit other nursing schools for ideas on improving the curriculum at Johns Hopkins. They return with numerous suggestions, including studying the records created by nurses in the Eastern Health District.

October: The newest group of students swells enrollment to the largest in the school's history: 418. They hail from forty-four states, Washington, D.C., and five foreign countries—Chile, Colombia, Mexico, Panama, and Hawaii.

December 2: Several nurses in the 118th are promoted to first lieutenancies and Mary Sanders is elevated from lieutenant to captain.

1944

February 3: Elizabeth McLaughlin writes from the Fiji Islands to describe conditions there. Each nurse gets one week's leave every four months. There are several options where to spend their free time—a beach cottage, a house in the mountains, or a trip to a different island.

February 16: Anna Wolf notes that the young women graduating this day are a mixture of the twenty members of the class who registered on February 12, 1941, one of the smallest classes in the school's history, and members of the first wartime class, who participated in an accelerated program. The new graduates join the recently created U.S. Cadet Nurse Corps, and every member of the class is a member of the American Red Cross Nursing Service; some join the army and navy immediately.

February 17: Dr. H. Alvan Jones tells the alumnae about conditions in General Hospital No. 18, which he recently left. He reveals that the unit is now back in Auckland, New Zealand, and injured troops are shuttled to the hospital from the Fiji Islands. Men associated with the 18th are quartered in a military camp but the nurses are billeted in private homes. The nurses receive a daily stipend since they are not provided with military housing, but their host families refuse payment for their room and board. As a group, the nurses decide to contribute the money to a crippled children's hospital.

April 4: The board of trustees determines that only graduates of nationally or regionally accredited colleges and universities will be admitted to the School of Nursing beginning in October. They cite the difficulty of providing a curriculum appropriate for students with varying amounts of education as the primary reason for the change. An analysis of recent classes reveals that those with more preparation are likelier to complete the program and earn higher salaries. The faculty hopes this move might secure divisional status with the Johns Hopkins University since the emphasis there has always been on graduate study. The hospital trustees also recommend to the trustees of the university that the school become a division of the university immediately, "to the end that graduates of the School of Nursing shall be entitled to receive an appropriate Master's Degree."

September: As military engagements move northward in the Pacific, General Hospital No. 18 moves to the India-Burma theater of operations. No. 118 shifts its location to Leyte Island in the Philippines.

Students who recently completed the summer Preclinical Nursing Program at Goucher sign a newly adopted honor code during orientation. Student Ann Strickland, 1945, reports that "the group received it most enthusiastically." Students will be asked to re-sign the pledge in six months and recommit themselves.

October 11: The new class of fifty-six nursing students, selected from ninety-seven applicants, is the first composed exclusively of college graduates.

Students on rotation in the Harriet Lane Home participate in the new Child Life Program, which encourages pediatric patients to participate in organized activities.

1945

January 29: Christine Dick dies. The cottage at Sherwood Forest, which she managed along with the other nurses' residences for more than twenty-five years, is named in her honor.

February 13: First Lady Eleanor Roosevelt addresses nurses at Johns Hopkins on the care of the wounded overseas. She combines humorous anecdotes with gruesome details about the lives some nurses are leading in military service.

After serving thirty-five months in the Pacific and the Far East with General Hospital No. 18, the last Johns Hopkins personnel in the unit return to the United States having lost no members. (A hospital unit No. 18 still exists, but no one from Johns Hopkins is in it.)

Summer: The hospital lacks two hundred graduate nurses. As a result the two-months' program of public-health nursing becomes an elective because students are needed in the hospital for service. Miss Wolf reports that senior students are substituting for graduate head nurses, assistant head nurses, and "even for assistants in supervision and instruction."

September 14: Thirty-nine new students, all of whom participated in three months of preclinical training at Bryn Mawr College, are admitted, continuing the trend toward much smaller postwar classes.

The alumnae association discontinues its library and gives more than five hundred professional books, bound periodicals, reports, pamphlets, and announcements of historical interest to the school.

December: German prisoners of war thoroughly clean rooms in the Main Nurses' Home. Newly sanded floors, fresh paint in some rooms, new wiring, and new furniture improve appearances.

1946

May: The hospital trustees approve a forty-eight-hour workweek for nursing students. The new curriculum requires two and a half years to complete and includes twenty-four weeks of preclinical training, twelve weeks of psychiatric nursing, and sixteen weeks of pediatrics. Beginning with the June 1947 class, students will resume eight weeks of public-health training. Changes will be implemented gradually as graduate nurses become more available for patient care.

April 1: Dr. Edwin L. Crosby replaces Dr. Winford Smith when Smith retires after thirty-five years as director of the hospital.

April: Mildred Struve, 1926, and Miriam Ames, 1914, publish an editorial in the alumnae magazine that emphatically elucidates the necessity for a university school of nursing. They explain that the reputation of the Johns Hopkins Hospital, while excellent, is not enough to compete with the credentials being offered by other schools. "The time has come when we can no longer hope to secure the well qualified student with a good cultural background unless in return we can offer her the full advantage conferred by collegiate schools, namely, full academic credit and an academic degree." They stress that an adequate endowment is essential and that the hospital trustees should grant authority to seek support from educational foundations and individuals interested in nursing.

The alumnae association votes to discontinue the Johns Hopkins Nurses' Registry,

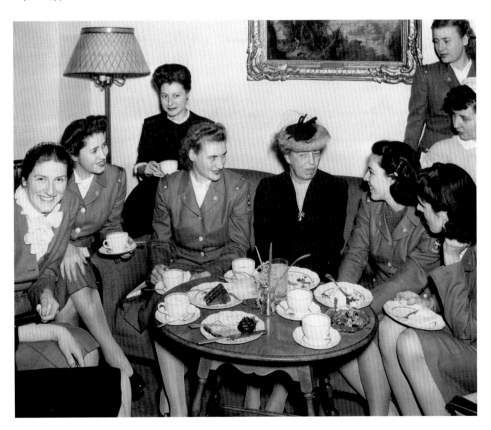

Mary Earnest, 1945, reported that on February 13, 1945, Eleanor Roosevelt encouraged nurses to "see once more how they could contribute to the solution of present and postwar problems."

in existence since 1896. Hopkins nurses are encouraged to join with a central directory "to promote the interests of all nurses and the public."

June 1: The beginning salary for general staff nurses at the hospital is $180 per month. After two or more years, the salary reaches a maximum of $200. Head nurses and assistants in instruction are paid $200 as a beginning salary and $210 during the second year of service. Assistant directors receive $280. Ten dollars per month is added for those on evening or night service for one month or more. Graduate nurses can rent a single room in the Main Nurses' Home for $25 per month; a single room with a private bath is $40. Charges for rooms, personal laundry, and meal tickets may be charged against the current month's salary.

June 27: A new alumnae committee meets for the first time to discuss the possibility of publishing a history of the school. Previously there had been discussions about a biography of Isabel Hampton Robb, but the committee makes a history of the school its priority.

October: An article in the alumnae magazine spells out policies for the use of the Christine M. Dick Cottage in Sherwood Forest. Student nurses have preference over all others for use of the retreat. "No men may be invited to the cottage. This means fathers, husbands, brothers, other relatives and friends." Dresses are required for dinner in the clubhouse; otherwise, informal attire is recommended. A new refrigerator requires defrosting twice a month. Students are warned not to hitchhike but to go to the cottage by train and bus. The round-trip fare is $1.65 and the trip takes more than two hours each way.

As the result of nursing shortages, three senior students are named assistant instructors and given supervisory assignments. Ten

students are assigned as head nurses and 159 more become assistant head nurses or general staff nurses.

October 14: In her convocation address, Anna Wolf vents her ongoing frustration with the long work hours demanded of student nurses and the heavy workload, which has not lessened since the end of the war. "Such a system perpetuates an apprentice system of education in nursing, long deplored not only by nursing leaders but by educators in other fields of general and professional education." The practice, she feels, is stifling hopes for an affiliation with the university and discourages degree holders from applying to the school. Nonetheless, her nursing students "have shown an unusually fine attitude and maintained high morale." Wolf notes the many special challenges that members of the class of 1946 face since they deal with so many war-related shortages. She worries that they have received less than adequate instruction. "We are not particularly proud of what we have given them or of our guidance. We have done the best we could in the face of the present social and economic conditions of our country and the continued approbation of a school as a service agent." Wolf sees no hope for improvement until nursing education and nursing service are separated.

November: A new nursing-aide program begins in the Wilmer Clinic and soon spreads throughout the hospital. High school graduates able to pass a short course in elementary nursing arts are employed to work in teams with fully qualified nurses. The alumnae magazine reports that many of the new aides are African-American women, who are well received by patients "both colored and white, and rarely has there been difficulty due to racial differences." The program eases difficulties caused by the shortage of professionally trained nurses.

1947

March: Trustees authorize a forty-four-hour schedule for nursing students, including both classes and clinical time, for the class of 1949. They also raise tuition to $400 for the thirty-two-month program.

The Gate House Shop Committee gives a station wagon to the students as a tribute to Christine Dick. The car is to be used for trips to the Sherwood Forest cottage.

Summer: By mid-year 199 people have already sent in subscriptions at $10 each for the "first edition" of the history of the school. The alumnae magazine endorses the project. "We think our history is going to be a must on everyone's reading list whether her interest be in medical, historical, biographical, philosophical or sociological literature. In fact our history will have not only a fulsome share of all these within its pages, but will also be rich with the deeply gratifying 'human interest' aspects that are so great a part of our heritage and tradition."

1948

January 11: The great demand for professional nurses makes it impossible to maintain the school's short-lived admissions standard requiring a college degree. After the hospital board of trustees reduces the qualifications for admission to a high school diploma, Johns Hopkins University President Isaiah Bowman and Dr. Edwin L. Crosby, director of the hospital, announce that the university will confer the degree of bachelor of science in nursing on graduates of the Johns Hopkins Hospital School of Nursing through McCoy College. Candidates for the degree are required to have completed at least two years of work at an approved college or university before entering the nursing school.

Dean Francis H. Horn of McCoy College declares that the new relationship between his university division and the diploma school "is believed to be unique in higher education in America." The arrangement is extraordinary because half the course work is to be accomplished at other institutions, and "the Hospital and the University are separate corporations, therefore, the University will be conferring its degree upon individuals who may never have taken a single hour of work within its halls." He notes that this arrangement acknowledges that Hopkins' "sound program of nursing education is the equivalent of upper division college work." One reason for the unusual arrangement is that the Johns Hopkins University is all male at the undergraduate level, except in McCoy College.

Summer: The admissions office reports a marked increase in the number of applications to the school since the announcement of the affiliation with McCoy College and the university.

June 14: Anna Wolf announces the recent appointment of Ethel Johns, former editor and business manager of the Canadian Nurse, as editor of the forthcoming history of the school of nursing. Jessie Black McVicar, former associate director of the school and nursing service, is to be associate editor.

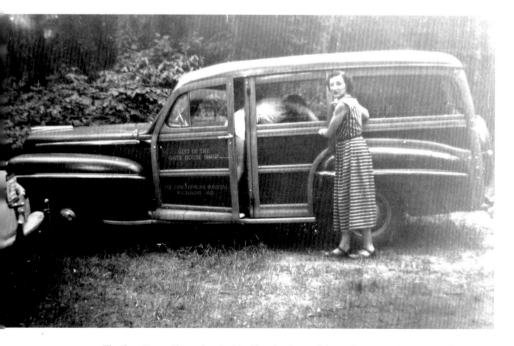

The Gate House Shop advertised itself on the doors of the station wagon it gave to students in 1947 to transport them to and from their cottage in Sherwood Forest.

The class of 1928 establishes the Elsie M. Lawler Scholarship Fund on the occasion of its twentieth reunion.

September 22: Two-thirds of students who register say they intend to matriculate for the BS degree from the Johns Hopkins University. Twenty-three new students already have a bachelor's degree.

October 3: Mary Adelaide Nutting dies in New York. She entered the first class of the Johns Hopkins Hospital Training School for Nurses on October 31, 1889, at the age of thirty. She became the school's second director in 1894 and left in 1907 to join the faculty of Teachers College at Columbia University, where she later became the first nurse appointed to a full professorship at an American university.

The 1948–49 circular for McCoy College clarifies that the basis for awarding the BS degree is not retroactive. Graduates of the school of nursing prior to 1948 who have completed the necessary college work are eligible for the degree after finishing thirty credits at McCoy College. Previous work from an accredited school will be evaluated to determine whether it can be counted toward the degree.

1949

May 30: The library of the School of Nursing is dedicated in honor of Loula E. Kennedy, 1903, a member of the faculty from 1921 to 1946.

June 7: Lucile Petry, 1927, is appointed assistant surgeon general of the U.S. Public Health Service with the rank of brigadier general. She is the first woman named to the position. During World War II she held the rank of navy captain and was head of the U.S. Cadet Nurse Corps.

October: The presidents of the university and hospital boards of trustees announce a reorganization of the governance of the hospital, the School of Medicine, the School of Hygiene and Public Health, and the Welch Library. Dr. Lowell J. Reed, vice president of the university in charge of medical affairs for the past three years, is named to a newly created position, vice president of the Johns Hopkins University and Hospital. This is the first time that the hospital and the university's medical divisions have been placed under unified administration.

November: Julia Harris, 1950, explains the significance of the candlelight ceremony in Hurd Hall, the first time new students wear their full uniforms. It is not a capping ceremony because, unlike training schools in which students enter for a probationary period, all students who enroll at Johns Hopkins have already been accepted as students. They begin in lab coats only because their uniforms have not yet been made for them. The candles carried by the students are a symbol of the light that Florence Nightingale carried in her work among the sick and wounded. Harris tells the new students that Miss Wolf and members of the student body, "symbolically passing to you the inspiration of the lady with the lamp," will light their candles. The next year Mabel Gerhart, 1953, writes in her scrapbook about how she and

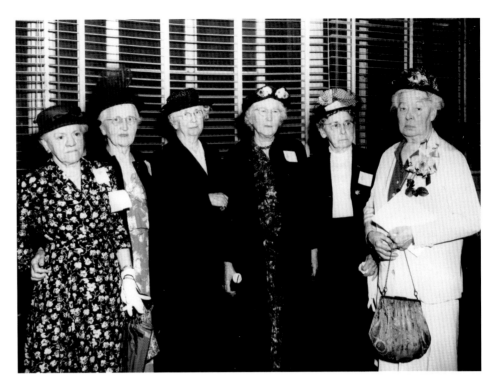

On May 29, 1951, members of the class of 1901 returned, not just for their fiftieth reunion but also for the dedication of an educational unit in the old Nurses' Home.

her classmates looked before the ceremony, when they were still wearing the rented lab coats. "With our brown uniform shoes and hose, the group of us probably looked like one big dark cloud in the hospital halls."

Annabelle Gleason Brack, 1929, chairman of the Writing of the History Committee announces that Blanche Pfefferkorn, 1911, has expressed an interest in writing the history of the school covering the years 1907 to 1950. Ethel Johns is already working on the years 1867—the year Johns Hopkins wrote his will—to 1907. The committee hopes to receive Johns's manuscript by September 1951. Johns is working in Vancouver, British Columbia.

1950

Mildred E. Barnard, 1950, cares for a patient on Osler 2, who has advanced tuberculosis. The day before he dies, Barnard sits down and listens to the "rambling, incoherent stories of his life." Later, she realized that this patient named Walter had taught her "more than any instructor or textbook. Beneath his repulsive appearance and manner, Walter showed me we shared a common humanity. We were both human beings struggling to make sense of our lives. And he was literally dying to be heard. Nursing often seems to be a matter of tearing around to get things done, but our efficiency may take us away from people who need us most. For our sake as well as theirs, let's slow down and take the time to listen. In recognizing patients as human beings, we affirm our own humanity as well."

September 20: New facilities honoring the memory of M. Adelaide Nutting open on the ground floor of the old Nurses' Home. Fourteen renovated rooms for class and lab

work, ten offices for faculty, and a new educational auditorium constructed from the World War II–era east dining room make up the new educational unit. There are twenty-three patient units and a utility room for lab practice. On May 29, 1951, various rooms are dedicated to students of Nutting who went on to influence the development of the school, including Elsie Lawler, 1899, the superintendent of the school for thirty years; Amy Miller, 1900, the first full-time instructor; and Helen Wilmer Athey, 1905, who gave the money for the east wing of the Nurses' Home.

1951

The advisory board shifts the emphasis in recruitment away from the need for a college degree as a requisite for entering the school. They also seek legal counsel regarding the admission of men because Johns Hopkins' will expressly states that the training school associated with the hospital be for "female nurses." The board decides to accept affiliating male nurses "in the near future."

Margaret E. Courtney, 1940, becomes the new assistant director of the School of Nursing. A graduate of American University before coming to Johns Hopkins as a nursing student, she received a master's degree in nursing education from Columbia in 1948.

Student Mary Gurthrie, 1951, describes the curriculum in the alumnae magazine. For the six-month preclinical period, the workweek consumes five and a half days with a maximum of six hours per week in hospital wards. Courses include nursing arts, anatomy, physiology, microbiology, chemistry, physics, dietetics, dosages and solutions, and social psychology. By the time the course of study is

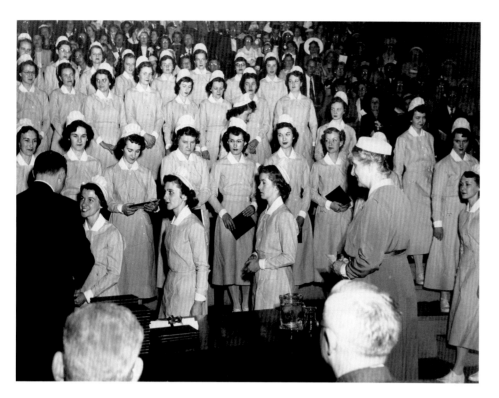

Anna D. Wolf proudly watched as hospital director Edwin Crosby presented diplomas to members of the class of 1951, some of whom possessed a bachelor's degree.

complete, the nursing student has had five months each of medical and surgical nursing (including two months in the operating room), four months in pediatrics, and three months each in obstetrics and psychiatry. Students devote one month each to ophthalmology, gynecology, and urology. "Much stress is laid today in the conception of adequate health care and preventative medicine," according to Guthrie. "Nurses today are taught the importance of teaching preventative measures in disease in their two months' public-health nursing experience."

The alumnae association's History Committee makes a plea to members for suggestions about alumnae whose achievements are exceptional. "It is appalling how little biographical data are available about graduates of our school. Several attempts have been made in the past to secure this, but your overweening modesty and selfless concern with today's and tomorrow's nursing needs must have prevented you from giving proper thought to history's need for autobiographical information."

1952

May 26: The alumnae association votes unanimously to accept sweeping changes to the code of ethics originally adopted in 1896. The new guidelines—instead of a regimented code—entitled "Some Ethical Concepts for Nurses," eliminate the subservient attitudes espoused by the initial code and embrace a new approach: "The nursing ethics of each nurse are a part of her individual character as a person, manifest in her nursing service and in every situation in which she is identified

as a nurse. Her ethics are deeply personal." The report emphasizes that ethical decisions are affected by many conditions. In the new version, the nurse's relation with a physician is considered in a section called "The Nurse's responsibility to her co-workers." Physicians and nurses are presented as colleagues who are both "responsible, legally and professionally" for treatment of the patient, though their obligations are different. The nurse is urged to "exercise independent judgment, in appropriate circumstances, with regard to therapy prescribed by a physician" and to take actions that may question treatment recommended by a physician—an enormous change from the 1896 code.

September 15: The Dispensary Visiting Nurse Service closes. Established in September 1934 to provide a place for students to practice public-health nursing in the field, the service is no longer needed because of a new agreement with the Baltimore City Health Department for a formal affiliation between the School of Nursing and the Eastern Health District. The Dispensary Visiting Nurse Service provided experience in morbidity nursing and maternity and child health but was limited to observations in clinics and school health services.

The National League for Nursing is established, combining the functions and services of the National League for Nursing Education, the National Organization for Public Health Nursing, and the Association of Collegiate Schools of Nursing.

1953

The board of trustees determines that, as of graduation 1954, scholarships will no longer

be awarded to seniors. Instead, those who have "demonstrated outstanding ability in class work and nursing practice" will graduate with honors and be given up to $2,400 a year to continue their professional education. While it is not a requirement for the award, it was hoped that the recipients would return to Johns Hopkins Hospital for employment after studies are complete.

Anna D. Wolf becomes the first president of the Maryland League for Nursing. The new organization will work closely with the Maryland Nurses Association.

The manuscript by Ethel Johns and Blanche Pfefferkorn on the nursing school's history is accepted by the Johns Hopkins Press, which plans to print 1,200 copies at $4.50 each.

1954

The alumnae magazine clarifies that the Johns Hopkins Hospital pin is to be worn not by all graduates but only by members of the alumnae association. "A nurse who has been a member of the Association and who allows her membership to lapse has forfeited her right to wear the pin of the Alumnae Association."

May 24: Miss Wolf announces that because many applicants are coming directly from high school, the preclinical term has been increased from twenty-five to thirty-six weeks. Those with two years of college still have a twenty-five-week term. There is no longer any minimum or maximum age for admission.

An advertisement for the Gate House Shop lists some of its prices. Organdy caps are 60¢; hosiery is $1; collars, which must be ordered directly from Marvin Neitzel Corporation in Troy, New York, with a minimum order of three collars, are 34¢ each. On November 22, the Gate House Shop Committee votes to increase the price of the Hopkins cap, their most popular item, to 75¢.

The Johns Hopkins Hospital School of Nursing, 1889–1949, by Ethel Johns and Blanche Pfefferkorn, is selling briskly, and the Johns Hopkins Press reports that it is one of their best sellers.

December: The alumnae association's board accepts the recommendation of its Publication Committee and votes to discontinue the alumni directory. Rising costs and frequent changes of address make the directory, which was published every five years, no longer practical.

1955

Anna D. Wolf announces that her retirement will take effect on July 1.

Hochschild Kohn and Co. offers a Johns Hopkins nurses' cape, made of navy blue broadcloth and lined with lighter blue flannel, for $25. Capes may be ordered through the nursing school office. There is also a dark blue coat and cap of water-repellent wool to be worn by public-health nurses. The cap and coat have a JHH insignia embroidered on them. Coats may be rented for $2 and caps for 50¢ for an eight-week assignment. The wool coats can be purchased for $33 and caps for $3.

May 21: A new chemistry laboratory is dedicated to the memory of Lavinia L. Dock, the first instructor appointed by Isabel Hampton to the School of Nursing.

Mary Sanders Price, 1934, becomes the director of the School of Nursing and the hospital nursing service. Mary Farr, 1941, who served under Price in General Hospital No. 118 in World War II, remembers that "there was no chief nurse in the army who enjoyed more affection and respect, not only among her own nurses, but among the many who were on detached service with the 118th." Farr notes that Price is "remembered for her kindness and fairness." Price's husband, Dr. Harry Price, DD, was an army chaplain during the war. With his wife's appointment, Dr. Price is named director of clergy services at the Johns Hopkins Hospital. They live in Hampton House.

November: Mrs. Price succeeds in reducing the number of hours nursing students are required to work in the hospital.

1956

The alumnae association revises its bylaws and changes its name to the Alumnae Association of the Johns Hopkins Hospital School of Nursing, Inc.

1958

Director Mary S. Price announces the demise of the thirty-two-month program because there are so few applicants with two years of college.

May: Members of the alumnae association vote to transfer $50,000 from the Sick Benefit Fund to an education fund to enable members with financial need to pursue full- or part-time study in nursing.

1959

April 28: The advisory board agrees to pay one half of the salary of Assistant Director Margaret Courtney in order for her to be given a part-time appointment on the McCoy College faculty. The money will come from the Nutting Endowment Fund and be used in the hope that the Johns Hopkins University will develop a program in general nursing leading to a baccalaureate degree.

Gertrude Jones of New York State becomes the first African American to graduate from the Johns Hopkins School of Nursing.

July 1: Following a number of administrative changes, hospital director Dr. Russell Nelson announces a new administrative subdivision called Materials Management. On September 1, 1957, a new facility opened that centralized the acquisition and dispensing of supplies. Nurse Janet Beach supervised the construction and equipping of central supply, which does not fall under nursing services. Graduate nurse John Meloche succeeded Miss Beach in 1958. This new development relieves the professional nursing staff of the responsibility of preparing and maintaining an inventory of sterile and other supplies, related budgetary activities, and fetching and delivering supplies. The changes increase efficiency and economy

for the hospital and allow nurses to concentrate their efforts on patient care.

1960

Spring: Caps are no longer available from the Gate House Shop and must be ordered from the White Crown Company in New York. Mrs. Bowersox, who had been making the caps, became ill and had to stop making them. This development is a blow to the finances of the Gate House Shop, as is the shift of bus routes from Broadway to Monument St., which greatly lessens foot traffic into the Broadway entrance to the hospital, as people no longer stop in the shop to buy candy bars and cigarettes. On July 1, after thirty-nine years of providing many services to the hospital community and supporting the alumnae association, the Gate House Shop closes. The building is demolished in 1964.

Several members of the Turtle Derby Committee approach the hospital administration about building an outdoor swimming pool for the professional staff and medical, nursing, and public-health students. A three-month campaign raises $43,000, which is matched three-to-one by the university, the School of Medicine, and the School of Hygiene and Public Health. The pool is built behind Hampton House and north of the medical residence hall.

December: The Thayer and Finney floors for semiprivate patients open on the newly constructed top floors of the Osler and Halsted Buildings. Each service accommodates thirty-three patients. Porches on the lower floors have been enclosed to create room for another thirty-three beds. These additions bring the total number of beds in the hospital to 1,030.

1961

The new 125-member class, which includes future dean Martha Norton Hill, is one of the largest in history. Elizabeth Moser, 1926, gives the convocation address and quotes Adelaide Nutting: "We need to realize and to affirm anew that nursing is one of the most difficult of arts; compassion may provide the motive, but knowledge is our working power. Perhaps, too, we need to remember that growth in our work must be preceded by ideas and that any conditions which may suppress thought must retard growth. Surely, we will not be satisfied in perpetuating methods and traditions. Surely, we shall wish to be more and more occupied with creating them."

1962

The alumnae magazine reports that "this year Hopkins exhibited a fast-moving well-spirited [basketball] team representing all three classes." The season includes nine games, each played against nursing students from different hospital schools in the Baltimore area.

February 20: Elsie M. Lawler dies at age 88 after living in the Marburg Building for many years. Agnes J. Doetsch, 1931, cared for Miss Lawler during her long illness.

May 1: Dorothea Robertson becomes executive secretary of the alumnae association.

September 23: Graduation exercises for the School of Nursing take place in Shriver Hall on the Homewood campus of the Johns Hopkins University—a first. Jessie Black McVicar, 1939, tries to visualize the future. "One cannot resist the temptation to dream. And to hope that very soon the School of Nursing will become an integral part of the University."

1963

May 25–26: University President Milton Eisenhower convenes a meeting at Higgins Mill Pond to explore the possibility of developing a bachelor's program in nursing at the university.

June 5: The alumnae association gathers in the Welch Library's main reading room, a faculty club at the time, for cocktails, dinner, and a fashion show of nursing student uniforms from 1905, 1920, 1933, 1943, 1944, and 1963, which were donated by alumnae for the collection being assembled for the school's historical library.

1964

February 1: Helen Wilmer Athey, 1905, one of the founders and a moving force behind the success of the Gate House Shop, dies and leaves an insurance policy worth $3,535 to the alumnae association, which votes to apply the money to the Sick Benefit Fund.

April 2: Milton Eisenhower meets with the Advisory Board of the School of Nursing and tells the members that the Ford Foundation turned down the university's grant request for money to finance a university nursing program.

September 18: On the seventy-fifth anniversary of the hospital, Lucile Petry Leone, 1927, the chief nurse officer of the U.S. Public Health Service, affirms her appreciation of the opportunities afforded by a Johns Hopkins education. "I believe I speak for every Hopkins nurse here when I say that we are grateful for what we learned in this school about the care of patients and about the ethics of our profession. We are proud of the role of our school and of its nursing and medical leaders in the early history of nursing education in the United States. We learned the meanings of service and respect for science as we saw it applied to human need by great physicians. And when we think long thoughts of science and people now we are likely to recall a wonderful teacher we had at the Hopkins. For all this and for the efforts to bring nursing education to its full potential here—efforts always persistent, sometimes ingenious, though not always successful— for all this we speak our gratitude tonight."

1965

McCoy College is renamed the Evening College of the Johns Hopkins University.

The Dick Cottage in Sherwood Forest is sold.

Dr. Margaret Courtney, 1940, becomes associate director of the School of Nursing when K. Virginia Betzold, 1933, retires from the position after twenty-two years.

The American Nurses Association produces a position paper on nursing education, which calls for professional nursing education to take place in institutions of higher learning rather than hospital diploma schools.

The administration bans the wearing of pierced earrings while in uniform.

1966

The class of 1966 introduces the first school ring. When other alumnae express interest, the seniors vote to make the ring available to all alumnae. The ten-carat gold ring sells for $22.25.

September: First-year students are bused to the Homewood campus to take classes in the liberal arts at the Evening College, for which they receive college credit. Margaret Andrews, a first-year student, comments that the classes at Homewood mean "grass and trees and boys. What more could a girl ask for?" Emphasis in courses taught at the hospital shifts to reflect changing approaches to patient care and evolving dynamics among personnel in the health care professions.

1967

Alumnae representatives to the advisory board report that university President Milton Eisenhower has appointed Dr. Russell Morgan, chairman of the Department of Radiology, to chair a special committee to consider how nursing education might become a function of the university. Dr. Morgan comments that the university is considering options "not only in the preparation of nurses, but of workers for other allied medical sciences as well. Consideration will be given to the education of several groups together, which would save on costs, duplication of courses, and in other ways. The baccalaureate level for preparation of these workers would be the first consideration."

November 4: The alumnae association gives Dr. Nelson a standing ovation when he asserts his strong support for a program of baccalaureate nursing education in the Johns Hopkins University. "You have not only my personal support," he declares, but he confirms that trustees of the hospital support the idea, "and we will do more than shout about it. We [will] do all we can with the financial resources that the Hospital has that it can commit to nursing." Dr. Nelson, while acknowledging alumnae concern that nursing education "would get lost" in the new college as it has been proposed, says he is sure that will not happen because "nursing here is much too strong." He assures the alumnae that non-nursing professionals will not become involved in the nursing curriculum.

Dr. Sarah E. Allison, 1953, makes a proposal to Director of Nursing Mary S. Price, Director of the Hospital Dr. Russell Nelson, and hospital administrator David Everhart for the development of an institute for nursing at Johns Hopkins Hospital; the proposal is accepted.

1968

February 28–March 2: Johns Hopkins University President Lincoln Gordon convenes a conference of the senior medical faculty to discuss plans for comprehensive medical programs for East Baltimore and the new city of Columbia, Maryland, as well as the proposed school of allied health services, which eventually becomes the School of Health Services.

March: Consultants, including Dorothea Orem, Joan E. Backscheider, Mary B. Collins, Ann Poorman Donovan, and M. Lucille Kinlein, join Dr. Sarah Allision for the first planning sessions for the hospital's proposed institute of nursing, later named the Center for Experimentation and Development in Nursing. According to Allison, the focus will be on analyzing workflow to pinpoint when and where nurses are performing non-nursing activities and redirect their energies into clinical areas. Clerical concerns are redirected to unit clerk staff so that nursing personnel can concentrate on assessing, assisting, teaching, guiding, and supporting patients.

June: Dr. Russell Morgan further explains plans for a new division of the university to prepare "allied medical professions." The new school will have a status equivalent to that of the Schools of Medicine and Hygiene and Public Health, and nursing will be a department within the school. Partial funding will come from the federal government through the Allied Health Professions Personnel Training Act. Mary Sanders Price is on the planning committee.

Because of an inquiry implying that the Sick Benefit Fund might be construed as an insurance fund, the alumnae association, at a special twenty-minute meeting, passes a resolution to amend the charter of the corporation to meet Internal Revenue Service requirements, thus assuring the tax-exempt status of the organization.

April 6: Just thirty minutes after the first disruptions begin in Baltimore after the assassination of the Rev. Martin Luther King Jr., the Johns Hopkins Hospital declares operation yellow to be in effect. Because the number of emergency patients is so high, nursing students assume new roles, including delivering meals for the dietary department. Sandra Stine Angell, 1969, later remembered: "We could see small fires being set in a lot of the businesses along Monument St. west of Hampton House. Then it became apparent what was happening. We had National Guardsmen on the roof of Hampton House and we were told not to walk past open windows. We were supposed to travel over to the hospital through the tunnels."

Herb Zinder and Jim Levya become the first male students to attend the Johns Hopkins Hospital School of Nursing. The new freshman class also includes five former Upward Bound participants. Although two additional men register for classes the following year, only Zinder and Levya complete the program, graduating in 1971.

October 12: At the seventy-sixth annual meeting of the alumnae association, Martha Norton Hill, 1964, suggests that an effort be made to involve various heads of nursing departments in the hospital in planning for the new "College of Allied Health Sciences."

1969

Development of the nursing component of a Diabetic Management Clinic begins under the direction of Mrs. Emma Ventura. The Center for Experimentation and Development in Nursing staff and the nursing staff in the outpatient department assist Ventura in her planning.

Dr. Dennis Carlson, a surgeon with international health care program experience, becomes the director of Health Services Research and Development Center at Johns Hopkins. He is asked to develop educational programs for the School of Health Services.

June 21: For the first time, nursing school graduation takes place in the new Turner Auditorium, and it occurs in June rather than September.

Louise Fitzpatrick, 1963, writes a challenging essay in the alumnae magazine in which she asserts, "We may be called upon to admit once and for all that diploma education, even our own, has outlived its usefulness and is no longer a benefit to nursing. It will not be easy to state openly that The Johns Hopkins School of Nursing no longer serves the purposes of technical or professional nursing education. Perhaps the greatest contribution we as alumnae can make to further the cause of the nursing profession, the goals of the potential nursing student and the health of the community is to request that our doors be closed."

October 11: University President Lincoln Gordon addresses the alumnae association and acknowledges that "the current school is obsolescent and the question is not whether we should change and create something new—the question is: what—how—when?"

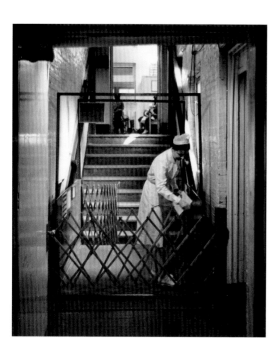

When the Department of Pediatrics moved to the Children's Medical and Surgical Center in 1964, the hospital continued to use the Harriet Lane Home for various purposes. Shortly before the building was demolished in 1974, an alumna nurse closed the gate of the Inclinator elevator for the last time.

1970

June 2: Johns Hopkins Hospital announces that it will close the School of Nursing in 1973. Mary Sanders Price retires as director, effective June 30. The position of director of the School of Nursing and the hospital nursing service, which has always been combined, is divided. Dr. Margaret Courtney, 1940, becomes director of the school and Doris M. Armstrong takes over as director of the Department of Nursing Services at the Johns Hopkins Hospital.

June 4: The school's advisory board recommends an alternative plan, suggesting that the original school be closed and a baccalaureate program for nurses be created in the Evening College of the Johns Hopkins University. This idea is commended to Lincoln Gordon "to convey to appropriate bodies in the University for further exploration." The first two years of liberal arts preparation could take place at any accredited junior or four-year college. The hospital would continue to provide facilities and supportive services, and clinical nursing courses would take place in East Baltimore, while other upper-division nursing courses would be given at the Homewood campus. This plan never became a reality.

As president of the alumnae association, Betty Scher, 1950, writes, "The meaning is clear. The Johns Hopkins *Hospital* School of Nursing, established in 1889, in three years will probably be no more. It has been inevitable; and certainly the reasons are sound. No longer can our school, offering diploma nursing education, attract and conscientiously accept sufficient numbers of superior applicants to merit continuing our quality programs. Should our school lower its requirements, graduate less-than-the-best nurses? Or should she close her doors and retire with dignity? All of us should completely reject lowering our standards! It is a sad thing that is happening, but it is right."

On learning of the impending closure of the school, Dr. I. Ridgeway Trimble, associate professor of surgery at the Johns Hopkins School of Medicine, writes to Dr. Russell A. Nelson, "As one associated with the Johns Hopkins Hospital over forty years, I have through the years become more and more convinced that our School of Nursing has, through the high quality of its students and graduates and their example of professional skill, devoted duty and their tireless work, contributed every bit as much as have physicians to the dignity, the accomplishments, and the renown of the Hospital and the Medical School."

The alumnae magazine reports that Dr. Nelson has reassured the association about the future of the Nutting Fund and that "he and the Board consider this a sacred trust and it will be used as it was originally intended when the transfer was made from the control of the Alumnae Association to the Board of Trustees."

November 30: The last candlelight service takes place in Hurd Hall. Barbara Bernhard, 1971, tells those assembled that although they are "privileged and last" they should not feel discouraged or sad. "Since . . . this service replaced the capping event resulting after the probation period, Candlelight has represented

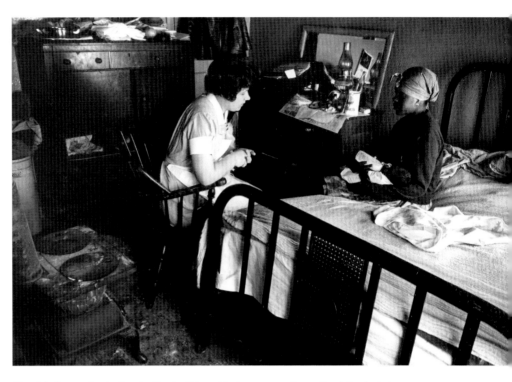

Shortly before graduating in 1964, Carolyn Griggs visited a young mother and her infant in their East Baltimore home as part of her training in public-health nursing.

the time when each student nurse first dons her blue uniform and white cap to proudly assume her position in learning at The Johns Hopkins School of Nursing." She encourages them to lift their spirits. "As you light your candles tonight, may they keep burning as a personal inspiration to each of you in your search for responsibility, knowledge, and honor within the horizons of nursing."

The class of 1972 is no longer required to wear the highly starched uniform worn by their predecessors. The new uniform is made of Perma-Press blue/gray fabric and is shorter than previous uniforms.

December 18: The university and hospital jointly announce the formation of the Center for Allied Health Careers, to be headed by Dr. Dennis G. Carlson. The formal announcement states that "priority consideration will be given to the field of nursing."

1971

When James Levya and Herb Zinder graduate, the alumnae association changes its bylaws to reflect the new reality and votes to rename itself the Alumni Association of the Johns Hopkins Hospital School of Nursing, Inc.

September 13: The executive committee of the university board of trustees approves a series of recommendations to create a new division that will include nursing as a program. The *Johns Hopkins Gazette* reports "that the creation of a school for training in nursing and other allied health services" is approved in principle, "it being understood that the entire cost of developing and maintaining such a school is contingent on obtaining funds for that purpose."

October 7: School of Nursing advisory board members express concern about the limited representation of nurses on the proposed advisory board for the new school.

December: A nursing subcommittee to help plan the new school includes Doris Armstrong; Dr. Margaret Courtney; Dr. Kay Partridge and Dr. Anna Scholl, both assistant professors in the School of Hygiene and Public Health; Nell Kirby, an instructor in surgery; Mafalda Lochow, assistant director of nursing for outpatient services at the hospital; and LoisAnn Furgess, 1959, president of the alumni association. They submit a proposal to the advisory board of the proposed school that includes two options. One recommends a program in which the master's degree would be the first professional degree, while the other calls for the development of an upper-division baccalaureate program.

Sarah Allison reports on the status of the Nutting Fund, which continues to grow with new contributions and interest earned. On June 30, its book value is $404,797.75 and its market value is $662,898. The alumni association asks for a legal analysis "to determine the purpose, acceptance, and restrictions made" on its use. Hospital President Dr. Russell Nelson concludes that control of the fund remains with the advisory board of the School of Nursing. However, when the school ceases to exist, he agrees to create a mechanism between the hospital and the alumni association to assure that alumni will have a voice in determining how the funds are used. Allison urges her readers, "Let us maintain our vigilance and the power of the purse!"

The Center for Experimentation and Development in Nursing initiates a nurse-managed

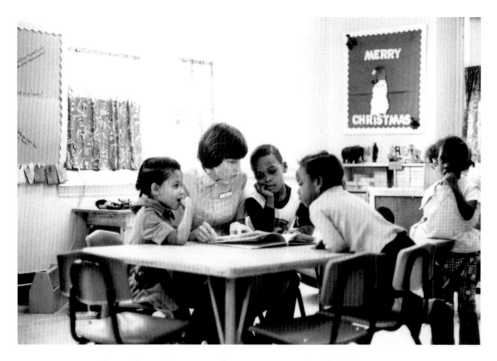

While a student in the Nursing Education Program in the School of Health Services, Karen Shank Santmeyer, 1978, wore her student uniform as she read a holiday story to neighborhood children.

clinic at the hospital for patients suffering from congestive heart failure. A similar project is instituted in the Woman's Clinic.

1972

Three members of the Center for Experimentation and Development in Nursing staff are involved in a tragic automobile accident while traveling back to Baltimore from Washington after an editorial meeting. Joan Backscheider and Mary Collins are killed and Sarah Allison is seriously injured. Dr. Allison's long convalescence and the loss of her staff, along with rapid changes in the hospital's administration, lead to the closure of the center in 1974.

In keeping with the new name of the association, the title of its seventy-one-year-old publication changes to *Johns Hopkins Nurses Alumni Magazine*. Only two issues appear in 1972. A new newsletter, published for the first time in April, contains the first reference to the newly named School of Health Services.

Dr. Nelson retires as president of the hospital. University President Steven Muller, who is also the titular head of the hospital, names Dr. Robert Heyssel executive vice president and administrator of the hospital.

March 9: President Steven Muller names Dr. Malcolm Peterson dean of the new School of Health Services, effective immediately. Prior to this time, Peterson was director of the Johns Hopkins Health Services and Research Development Center in the Office of Health Care Programs at the hospital.

1973

The Robert Wood Johnson Foundation grants $3 million to be given over three years to the School of Health Services.

The alumni association compiles a 600-recipe cookbook, *On Duty in the Kitchen*.

June 15: President Steven Muller presides over a ceremony in Turner Auditorium marking the closing of the Johns Hopkins Hospital School of Nursing. Lucile Petry Leone, 1927, retired assistant surgeon general with the U.S. Public Health Service, addresses the assembled guests and expresses her gratitude to Johns Hopkins, "for giving me a bias favoring clinical education, for confirming my belief that nursing is a humanitarian force and for feeding my knowledge and respect for science, all of which have guided my actions in a rich career."

June 16: An overflow crowd witnesses commencement for the class of 1973 in Turner Auditorium. Steven Muller presents diplomas to forty-one graduates, all wearing uniforms identical to those worn by the first graduates, in 1891. Each carries a bouquet of long-stemmed red roses given by hospital physicians, similar to those given to the first class by Dr. Osler. Cathy Novak, president of the student council, receives the Anna D. Wolf Award and is presented with Anna Wolf's personal alumni pin. Sue Appling receives the Elsie Lawler Award.

June 16: After graduation members of the alumni association meet for a spirited discussion about the organization's future. They consider several possibilities, including the association's dissolution. The suggestion that garners the most support involves merging with the alumni association of the Johns Hopkins University, but a decision is postponed until such time as a special meeting permitting the use of absentee ballots can be called.

November 15: President Steven Muller appoints Dr. Henry Seidel chairman of the committee to search for an educator to head

the Nursing Education Program in the School of Health Services. Muller also asks the committee to draft a preliminary statement on the nature of the program. Doris Armstrong, Dr. Turner Bledsoe, Dr. Arthur Bushel, Dean Marion Murphy from the University of Maryland, Dr. Kay Partridge, Dr. Malcolm Peterson, Dr. Mary Betty Stevens, Dr. Jean Straub, and alumni association representative Genevieve Wessel, 1963, are committee members.

Plans are announced to raze the old Nurses' Home (also known as the Main Residence) in early 1974, and the historical collection is sent to the Welch Library for storage.

1974

May 11: The alumni association votes to reaffirm the intent of the Nutting Fund: to advance education in nursing at Johns Hopkins. Their highest priority is to establish a full professorship in nursing in the new school, to be called the M. Adelaide Nutting Chair of Nursing.

August 1: The Maryland Historical Society opens an exhibition of uniforms and other memorabilia relating to Hopkins nursing. These items were transferred to the society "on semi-permanent loan" earlier in the year, when the Main Residence was demolished. Betty Cuthbert, 1943, later reported that "the exhibit attracted interest from many visitors other than nurses."

September 23: Dr. Kay Partridge, a faculty member in the School of Hygiene and Public Health and Doris Armstrong's assistant director in the Department of Nursing Services in the hospital, becomes director of the Nursing Education Program at the School of Health Services. She tells the alumni magazine that "it is rare to have the opportunity to have occasion to bring together resources and talent with a great historical foundation to build on. Hopkins was very creative the first go around and we'd like to do that again. Maybe we'll have a different type of graduate, but hopefully she'll be just as distinguished." Partridge was a member of the search committee.

1975

April 18: Provost Harry Woolf presents Anna D. Wolf, 1915, with the Johns Hopkins University Alumni Association's Heritage Award. In May President Steven Muller honors K. Virginia Betzold, 1933, with the same award, making them the first women to receive the honor.

June 25: President Muller presides over the final meeting of the Advisory Board of the School of Nursing. The purpose of the meeting is to determine the disposition of the Nutting Fund and to dissolve the board. Upon approval of the recommendation, Dr. Muller declares that "interest from the Fund could be transferred immediately as of July 1, 1975, to the university." However, he "could not say how or when the principal of the Nutting Fund would be transferred from the hospital to the university."

The bylaws committee reports that "the disbanding of the Advisory Board of the School of Nursing was the last official function of the School of Nursing"; therefore, the alumni association's corresponding bylaw must be reworded to "The object of the Association shall be to promote the advancing of nursing education" and mention of the hospital school be removed.

September: The first class of nursing majors is admitted to the School of Health Services. Four men are among the thirty-two students, who range in age from nineteen to forty.

1976

Joan M. Sutton, 1963, describes her experiences as a representative of the nurses' alumni association on the executive committee of the university's alumni association. "Recently I overheard one member of the Executive Committee say to another, 'You know, those Hopkins nurses are not only attractive; they're very intelligent, too.'" Sutton assures her fellow nursing alumni that "we truly have been welcomed, warmly received, and made to feel that we are a very important and respected group within the University Alumni Association."

September 18: Members of the alumni association vote to change the organization's name to the Johns Hopkins Nurses' Alumni Association, Inc., so that graduates of the School of Health Services will feel included. Other modifications are made to the seal and the qualifications for membership.

Doris Armstrong resigns as director of nursing services at the Johns Hopkins Hospital to become the vice president for nursing at Hartford Hospital in Connecticut. Pauline Musco becomes acting director.

1977

Hospital Executive Vice President Dr. Robert Heyssel appoints Martha Sacci vice president for nursing and patient services at the Johns Hopkins Hospital. Sacci had been at the New England Medical Center Hospital.

April 29: Dr. Kay Partridge meets with the Visiting Committee for the Nursing Education Program to evaluate the program's progress and discuss issues relating to the upcoming meetings with the National League for Nursing's accreditation team. Doris E. Roberts, who chairs this meeting, later explained the purpose of the committee in a letter to Malcolm Peterson. "We have functioned largely as a consulting group to Kay, challenging her to promote clarity in programming while supporting and encouraging progressiveness in the curriculum." Roberts also noted, "I have enjoyed working with Kay and support her efforts to build a creative program." The Visiting Committee recommends that the NLN accreditation visit be postponed.

May 16: Betty Cuthbert, 1943, Connie Waxter, 1944, and Joan Sutton, 1963, meet with Dean Malcolm Peterson to discuss concerns regarding possible misuse of the Adelaide Nutting Endowment Fund.

May 27: The first students to complete the Nursing Education Program in the School of

Health Services join their fellow Johns Hopkins University graduates for commencement on the Keyser Quadrangle on the Homewood campus. The thirty degree candidates from the School of Health Services must finish a six-week summer course after the ceremony before receiving their diplomas. Alumni President Connie Waxter presents each candidate with a nursing cap and expresses "the delight of the Alumni Association, recognizing that this event marks the fulfillment of a goal long worked and hoped for."

June 1: Dean Malcolm Peterson writes to Dr. Kay Partridge requesting her resignation. Later that day, a special meeting of a majority of the faculty of the Nursing Education Program concludes with a vote unanimously supporting Partridge's leadership. They write to Provost Richard Longaker, "We believe that her removal at this time will jeopardize the future of nursing education at The Johns Hopkins University and has implications for the survival of the School of Health Services."

June 8: Kay Partridge resigns as director of the Nursing Education Program. Much later, she reflected on this surprising development. "I loved Hopkins and so it was an honor to be able to step in and try to make a contribution to keep nursing alive. I certainly didn't see it as a long-term thing that I would do ten or twenty years. I certainly didn't expect to be fired either, and so abruptly, but I was happy to do it for that reason. I knew it was going to be a tough, tough sell."

June 9: Faculty of both the Nursing Education Program and the Health Associate Program (the other section of the School of Health Services) give Dean Malcolm Peterson a vote of no confidence and demand his resignation. Peterson offers a letter of resignation to University President Steven Muller, who declines to accept it.

June 22: Dr. Margaret Courtney, 1940, takes over as director of the Nursing Education Program in the School of Health Services in addition to continuing her duties directing nursing classes offered by the Evening College.

November 22: Edith D. Nikel, president of the Maryland State Board of Examiners of Nurses, writes to Margaret Courtney to inform her that the Nursing Education Program "has been granted final approval and will continue to be on the list of Maryland Schools and Programs of Nursing Approved by the Maryland State Board of Examiners of Nurses."

The School of Health Services reports a $700,000 deficit in fiscal year 1977; a similar loss is anticipated for fiscal year 1978.

1978

January: After the administration of the university determines that "there is no alternative but to recommend to the University's Board of Trustees that the newest division of the University, the School of Health Services, be closed as it is presently constituted, effective June 30, 1978," the board follows this recommendation.

In the midst of this discouraging news, the alumni magazine offers a hopeful thought from M. Adelaide Nutting: "The system,

method and institutions we cherish today may fade and pass, but the developed mind and imagination of future nurses will be able to create new ways—they will not be afraid of their own ideas."

February 26: Margaret Courtney, acting director of the Nursing Education Program, and Ross Jones, vice president for institutional affairs of the university, meet with nursing alumni to explain that the university plans to continue nursing education at Hopkins "with a freestanding administrative entity, having an autonomous nurse leader reporting directly to the Provost of the University." Courtney hopes that the new school will open in 1980, just a year after commencement for the last graduates of the School of Health Services in 1979. Jones explains that, in the Hopkins tradition of decentralization, the new nursing program will have to "generate its own funds to be economically viable."

1979

May 7: Provost Richard Longaker writes to Margaret Courtney and the few remaining members of the faculty as the operations of the Nursing Education Program come to an end. "On behalf of the Johns Hopkins University I wish to express my appreciation for your perseverance in meeting commitments to the students of the Faculty of Health Services. We are very aware that this final year has been unusually difficult for all concerned so that your loyalty has been highly valued and is duly noted." And in a handwritten, personal note to Dr. Courtney: "You will not be surprised to know how deeply in your debt the University is—not even to mention my personal gratitude. Many, many thanks."

May: The third and final class graduates from the Nursing Education Program of the School of Health Services.

1980

January: Dean Roman J. Verhaalen of the Evening College explains the benefits of the new, revised program the college offers to "adult learners" in nursing. "Not only is the University responding to an identified community and professional education need, but, by placing the program in the Evening College, the needs and special characteristics of the adult learner are being recognized."

1981

May: Betty Cuthbert reports in the alumni magazine on meetings with President Muller concerning the future of the Nutting Fund and of nursing education at Johns Hopkins. The agreement with the university stipulating that the funds be used to establish a chair in nursing had a five-year time limit for negotiations, which was up in July 1980. Cuthbert makes an impassioned plea to alumni to stay the course and not give up; she also encourages alumni to make provisions for the fund in their estate planning.

July 10: Dr. Carol J. Gray, associate dean of the School of Nursing at the University of Texas Health Science Center, is named director of the Evening College's Division of Nursing, effective January 1.

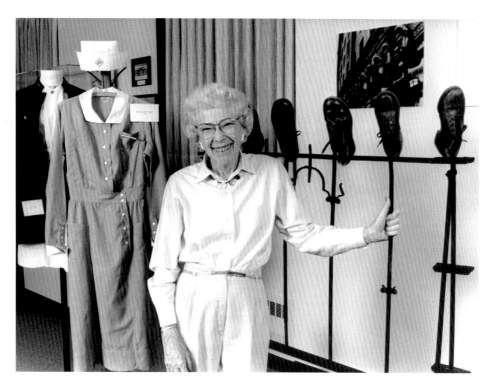

Betty Cuthbert, 1943, who preserved hundreds of artifacts relating to Hopkins nursing, smiled with pleasure at a 1989 exhibit, which included "duty booties" impaled on fence posts like those at Hampton House.

1982

Dr. Gray conducts a feasibility study, which leads to the charter for the Consortium for Nursing Education, Inc., funded by the Johns Hopkins, Church, and Sinai Hospitals.

September 19: Betty Cuthbert announces in the association's annual report that "for the first time, the need for a school of nursing at Hopkins is recognized and supported by groups other than nurses."

October 29: Dr. Carol Gray reports to the alumni association's annual meeting about ongoing plans to establish the School of Nursing. She says she has been asked to accept the position of dean. However, since the school will not open until 1984, she recommends a further search for the right leader. Later, the Consortium for Nursing Education, Inc., and the Johns Hopkins University announce the appointment of Carol Gray as dean of the new Johns Hopkins University School of Nursing.

1983

July 26: The Maryland State Board of Examiners of Nurses unanimously approves plans for the establishment of the Johns Hopkins University School of Nursing. The University of Maryland expresses concern about the advisability of establishing another university nursing school in Baltimore, but Dean Gray emphasizes that the Hopkins school will "draw from a national pool of student applicants and faculty" and not compete with the state university, nor does she anticipate problems finding clinical opportunities for students in area hospitals.

December: The Johns Hopkins University submits a proposal for its new School of Nursing to the Maryland State Board of Higher Education.

1984

January: Sue Appling, 1973, describes plans for the new School of Nursing in the magazine. "With Dr. Gray's guidance, the school will have an innovative structure. A consortium has been formed to include Hopkins University, and Hopkins, Sinai, and Church Hospitals, all providing financial and administrative support and a broad range of clinical practice sites. The nursing education offices will be located on the East Baltimore campus in the Phipps Building, although a multi-campus concept, using the facilities of all four consortium affiliates, will be employed. As a degree granting division of the University, the school will open its doors in September 1984 to a class of about fifty students. The future will see an expansion to one hundred upper division participants and the eventual formation of a graduate program."

Marjorie Clowry Dobratz, 1960, responds to photographs depicting new nursing "fashions," which appeared in the previous issue of the magazine. "The nursing cap, akin to the veil worn by the religious and signifying obedience, has been shelved. The caps lie on the shelves, a relic to the struggle within the profession to free ourselves from the image of the passive, dependent person who no longer wishes to be viewed as a subservient individual. The nursing pin, likewise, has become optional and is seen less frequently, especially in the acute care settings where complex and highly skilled procedures are performed. In

these settings, one is evaluated only for competence, rather that the school once graduated from."

September 6: Thirty-three students, ranging in age from 21 to 41, begin classes at the Johns Hopkins University School of Nursing. Two hold master's degrees in education and more than half are pursuing a second baccalaureate degree. Explaining the multifaceted approach of the curriculum, Dr. Stella Shiber, coordinator of clinical services for the school, explains, "We believe experience with patients and technology is a vital part of academic programs for students preparing for a nursing career."

September 23: As the Johns Hopkins University dedicates its new School of Nursing, President Steven Muller tells the assembled guests, "The combination of imagination and disciplined purpose led to the decision to establish the School of Nursing." He then offers "a special word to the members of the Johns Hopkins Nursing Alumni Association, here and wherever they may be. More than ten years ago we pledged to you that Johns Hopkins would return to a full program of nursing education—explicitly, completely, and with distinction. Today we formally redeem that pledge, and we thank you for your support and understanding."

1985

January: Alumni association president Sandra S. Angell, 1969, announces that issues concerning the M. Adelaide Nutting Fund are settled and the search is under way to fill the M. Adelaide Nutting Chair, the first professorship in the new School of Nursing. The person selected for the position will specialize in nursing education. Angell thanks Betty Cuthbert and Joan Sutton, who championed the alumni's cause through years of negotiations with the university. She also reveals the reactivation of the History Committee, whose chief goal is to update the history of the school written by Johns and Pfefferkorn and published in 1949.

May: Dean Carol Gray announces that Dr. Elaine Larson will be the first to hold the M. Adelaide Nutting Chair in Nursing Education. "This appointment fulfills a dream of the individual in whose name the Chair was established and makes clear the commitment of the Johns Hopkins Hospital Nurses Alumni whose generous contributions over seventy years made the Chair a reality," Dean Gray writes to Dr. Steven McClain, the associate provost who served on the search committee for the Nutting Chair.

July 5: Anna Dryden Wolf, 1915, director of the school from 1940 to 1955, dies at age 95 in St. Petersburg, Florida.

September 30: Dean of the School of Medicine Richard S. Ross writes to Dean Carol Gray to "strongly support a Master's Program for nursing in the School of Nursing."

October 8: Dr. Stella Shiber informs Dr. Arlowayne Swort, associate in administration, that the school is receiving one to three requests a day for information about graduate programs and that most callers, many from out of state, assume there is already a graduate program in place.

Autumn: The first issue of the School of Nursing's newsletter, *Nursing News*, appears.

Computer courses are among the requirements of the new curriculum, making the school one of the first to provide the skills nurses would need to meet the new demands of information technology systems.

December 20: Mary Sanders Price, 1934, director of the school from 1955 to 1970, dies at age 80 in Selingsgrove, Pennsylvania.

1986

May 30: Twenty-eight members of the first class of the Johns Hopkins University School of Nursing graduate on the Homewood campus. Dean Carol Gray announces that most of the graduates have accepted positions at hospitals participating in the consortium: two will go to Church, three to Sinai, and twelve to Hopkins.

The Johns Hopkins Nurses' Alumni Association changes its bylaws to open membership to graduates of the Johns Hopkins University School of Nursing.

Dr. Arlowayne Swort designs a graduate degree curriculum emphasizing acute care and long-term care rather than traditional medical specialties. "We will train nurses not only as expert clinicians but also as professional nurses who can manage patient care," Swort explains. "Nurses have to know about personnel management, fiscal management, budgets, cost evaluation, and resource allocation. They need to know more about health policy and about how health institutions and the government function so that they can participate in the decision-making process." A challenge grant from the James S. McDonnell Foundation helps to launch the initiative.

December 10: The I. Ridgeway Trimble MD Lecture Hall is dedicated in the Phipps Building in the memory of the surgeon who was a longtime champion of nursing education at Johns Hopkins.

In her first year as the first occupant of the M. Adelaide Nutting Chair in Clinical Nursing, Dr. Elaine Larson initiates or consults on twenty research and program studies at Hopkins, Sinai, and Church Home and Hospital. She secures two grants, teaches students, and plans several studies. For several years, Larson has studied handwashing habits among hospital employees. "Though we have known for over a century that the hands of health care personnel are the most important mechanism by which hospital-acquired infections are spread, studies have shown that physicians and nurses do not always wash their hands between patient contacts," Larson says.

1987

March 18: K. Virginia Betzold, 1933, who joined the faculty in 1934 and was associate director of the school from 1943 until she retired in 1965, dies. A memorial service is held in Trimble Auditorium.

September: The first students enter the master's degree program, which is explained in the alumni magazine. "The program is designed to educate nursing leaders who will develop not only a strong clinical focus, but also will be able to manage the implementation of health care. Indeed, the program is ideal for nurses wishing to achieve a dual major as a clinician and manager. Students will also gain a broad perspective of the health care system by participating in courses such as Ethics of Health Care Policy and Economics of Health Care. In addition, graduates will have a firm grounding in research courses and three credits in biostatistics. All students will be able to then synthesize and apply research knowledge by developing and implementing an original research project culminating in a written thesis." The program takes four semesters and one summer to complete.

Dr. Arlene Butz and Dr. Denise Korniewicz become the first postdoctoral fellows. Their fellowships are sponsored by Johnson & Johnson/SURGIKOS, and their efforts, under the direction of Dr. Elaine Larson, will concentrate on ways to improve infection control.

Martha Sacci retires as vice president for nursing and patient services at the Johns Hopkins Hospital and is succeeded by Linda Arenth.

1988

Caroline Pennington, 1918, gives $1 million to endow a chair to honor the memory of Elsie Lawler, who was superintendent of nurses at the hospital and led the School of Nursing from 1910 to 1940. "The establishment of the Elsie Lawler Chair conjures up a very human image of the past and a personal challenge for the future," according to Dean Carol Gray. "The gift will serve as a constant reminder that we must educate nurses who are as compassionate as they are intelligent, and as sensitive to others as they are skilled."

1989

Dr. Dorothy Gordon, on the faculty since 1985, is named the first Elsie M. Lawler Professor.

Fund-raising begins for the Anna D. Wolf Chair to mark the occasion of the centennial of the beginning of nursing education at Johns Hopkins.

Elizabeth Brizendine, 1945, chairman of the History Committee, reports with regret that the updated history of the school will not be ready in time for the centennial celebration of nursing education at Hopkins. "At present, the manuscript is being revised and the process is taking longer than anyone can imagine," she tells the alumni. "The committee will continue to work for an early publication of a worthy history and you will be advised of future happenings."

June 1: Seventeen students, all with bachelor's degrees, enter the first accelerated class, a program designed to be completed in fifteen months. The students range in age from 22 to 46. The class includes one former Peace Corps volunteer in Niger, an attorney, and a former field artillery officer in the army.

September 21: The school celebrates the establishment of its first laboratory enabling students and faculty to accomplish "basic scientific research that can be directly applied to clinical practice," according to Dr. Elaine Larson. Equipment in the lab, including two microscopes and a centrifuge, is the gift of Margaret Hanson VandeGrift, 1943, whose husband was a longtime Hopkins pathologist.

1990

Enrollment in the second class of accelerated students jumps to sixty. Ten of the new students are men, eight have master's degrees, three are former Peace Corps volunteers.

August 8: Melinda Rose begins working with the association as its alumni coordinator. She later becomes associate director of alumni relations.

October: New bylaws are adopted by the membership to streamline the association and bring it in line with the original charter of 1892.

1991

April 12: A chartering ceremony is held for the Johns Hopkins School of Nursing chapter of Sigma Theta Tau, the international nursing honor society.

May 21: The Hon. Paul D. Coverdell, director of the Peace Corps, Interim Provost M. Gordon "Reds" Wolman, and Dean Carol Gray sign an agreement creating a program for returning Peace Corps volunteers to study nursing at Johns Hopkins either before or after their service overseas. It is the first such program in nursing in the United States.

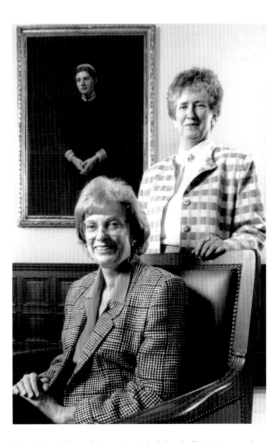

Dean Carol Gray of the university's School of Nursing posed in 1989 behind Linda Arenth, the hospital's vice president for nursing and patient services. A portrait of Isabel Hampton Robb, their predecessor a century before, hung behind them.

Fall: The alumni association publishes the first issue of the *Vigilando*, the new title for the alumni magazine. Plans are announced for the formation of an Archives Committee, which will work with the staff of the Alan Mason Chesney Medical Archives. The committee will address "the issues of preserving our history and promoting the distinguished contributions that Hopkins nurses have made to nursing, medicine, and health care."

The Joan D. Sutton Award is established in memory of a member of the class of 1963 who served on the faculty of all three nursing schools at Hopkins. The recipient will be a student who is dedicated to professional nursing, clinical excellence, and interdisciplinary practice. Sutton died earlier this year at the age of 51. "Students learned not only about illness when they studied under Joan Sutton, they learned about the care of patients. She had a great concern for the patients. Joan was always over-extended for time, but that never stopped her from caring," remembers her friend and colleague Betty Cuthbert, 1943.

1992

The Johns Hopkins Nurses' Alumni Association celebrates its first one hundred years.

April 7: Hospital President Dr. Robert Heyssel informs Johns Hopkins University President William Richardson that "the Johns Hopkins Hospital Board of Trustees has voted the land on [North] Wolfe Street bordered by McElderry, Jefferson, and Washington Streets be used for a permanent site for a School of Nursing."

A scholarship fund is created to honor Dr. Robert M. Heyssel on his retirement after twenty years as head of the Johns Hopkins Hospital. Dr. Heyssel has been a steady

advocate of nursing and nursing education at Hopkins.

November: University President William C. Richardson and James A. Block, the new president of the Johns Hopkins Hospital, meet with Dean Carol Gray and the faculty of the School of Nursing to discuss plans for the future. Richardson talks enthusiastically about the need for a new building for the school since its current home, the Phipps Building, is slated to be razed to make way for a new cancer center. Until the new building can be built, the school will have temporary quarters on the third and fourth floors of the 1830 Building, on Monument St.

December 1: Alumni, faculty, staff, and friends gather to celebrate the gift of two adjoining row houses on Washington St. from former longtime faculty members Mary Farr Heeg, 1941, and Betty Liggett Cuthbert, 1943. Their former residences become the new home of the Center for Nursing Research faculty, directed by Dr. Martha Norton Hill, 1964.

Linda Arenth, vice president for nursing and patient services at the Johns Hopkins Hospital, dies. Karen Haller is named acting vice president.

The Endowed Bed Fund and the Sick Benefit Fund are liquidated owing to changes in federal tax laws. Four hundred thousand dollars from the Endowed Bed Fund is given as a gift to the Johns Hopkins University School of Nursing toward its building fund.

1993

Dean Carol Gray announces her retirement at the end of the 1993–94 academic year. The magazine declares the gratitude of the alumni. "Few leaders of any school of nursing have achieved as much in as short a time. The enrollment in the programs has increased

from an initial 28 students to a current student body of over 300. Besides the regular baccalaureate program, the school has added a 'fast track' baccalaureate program, a master's program, a postdoctoral program, and a doctoral program to begin in the fall of 1993. In addition, she has forged an alliance with the Peace Corps, has assembled a superb faculty, and has built an endowment that exceeds most of the schools of nursing in the country."

The first five students enter the newly established doctoral program. In each successive year, a new cohort of five additional students will join the program.

Maryann Fralic becomes vice president for nursing and patient services at the Johns Hopkins Hospital.

As she prepares to leave the deanship, Carol Gray tells the alumni magazine, "I have always been committed to ensure nursing's place in private universities. Were it not represented there would suggest that nursing is different from other professions. It is not. To have the opportunity to establish a university program in nursing at Hopkins, with its legacy and rich history, was an opportunity I could not refuse."

Dr. Jackie Campbell, an expert in the area of domestic violence, is named as the first professor to hold the Anna D. Wolf Chair. The professorship is not fully funded until 2003.

1994

February 24: The first annual Nightingala takes place in the Glass Pavilion on the Homewood campus. The event raises awareness of nursing among the Baltimore corporate community. Proceeds are used to support continuing education, advanced preparation for nurses, and the building fund for the School of Nursing.

September 1: Dr. Sue K. Donaldson becomes the second dean of the Johns Hopkins School of Nursing. Donaldson comes from the University of Minnesota Schools of Nursing and Medicine, where she had been a professor since 1983.

A $3-million gift from the Jacob and Annita France and the Robert G. and Anne M. Merrick Foundations enables plans for the new School of Nursing building to move forward. "The school has grown in countless ways, especially in the area of enrollment, academic programs, and research opportunities," Dean Donaldson says. "It would be tragic if our progress were hindered by space limitations. The new building will allow us to spread our wings and move boldly into the future."

The Lillian D. Wald Community Nursing Center, named to honor the founder of American community nursing, opens at the Rutland Center in East Baltimore. Founded and directed by Assistant Professor Marion Isaacs D'Lugoff, the clinic offers complete physical examinations and routine preventive pediatric services, immunizations, and lead screening to uninsured children. Adult services at the Rutland Center and a second site at St. Bernardine's Catholic elementary school in West Baltimore are added in 1997. Later Wald clinics, at the G.A.T.E. (Gaining Access to

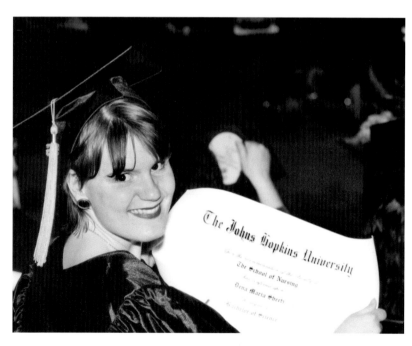

At her commencement, Dena Sheetz, 1996, proudly unfurled her bachelor of science degree from the Johns Hopkins University School of Nursing.

Employment) program and the House of Ruth, a shelter for women and children recovering from domestic violence, increase services offered to Baltimore residents and clinical opportunities for students and faculty of the School of Nursing. In 2000–2001, some 3,320 patients visit the various Wald clinics, all at no cost to the patient.

November: Dean Sue Donaldson reports that, after a four-day visit, representatives from the National League for Nursing recommend that the School of Nursing's doctoral programs be fully accredited. "This is a rare accomplishment for any program and especially noteworthy, given that the school is only eleven years old." Donaldson explains that the endorsement "is a stamp of approval demonstrating that we have met specific national criteria for excellence. Most federal and other operating agencies require NLN accreditation."

December: The first three participants in a new eighteen-month master's degree program offered in conjunction with the School of Hygiene and Public Health complete the requirements for their degrees. "The MSN/MPH is a powerful set of degrees to have," explains the chairwoman of the joint program's steering committee, Dr. Jacqueline Agnew, "particularly now, when there is so much emphasis on health care delivery that is not in an acute care setting."

1995

March: *U.S. News and World Report* ranks Johns Hopkins' graduate programs in nursing 14th among more than 225 comparable programs in the United States.

The school joins with the Department of Nursing at the hospital to create the Institute for Johns Hopkins Nursing. The new entity promotes and supports nursing practice through joint professional educational opportunities and innovations in nursing research.

May: Seniors in the traditional baccalaureate class establish a new tradition. At a formal ceremony someone special to each student fastens his or her school pin on the proud graduate. Statistics professor Ronald Berk shares anecdotes written by grateful graduates about special moments they experienced at the school, as well as their appreciation for the emotional and practical support they received. On July 7 Assistant Dean Sandra Angell, 1969, presides over a similar ceremony for the accelerated class where they receive their pins as well as their diplomas.

May 25: Lucile Petry Leone, 1927, becomes the first nurse to receive an honorary doctoral degree from the Johns Hopkins University. Leone was the first director of the U.S. Cadet Nurse Corps, which was created in 1943 to address the nursing shortage caused by World War II. In 1948 she became the chief nurse officer and assistant surgeon general in the U.S. Public Health Service. She remained in that office until her retirement in 1966. Dean Donaldson declares that Lucile Petry Leone "is one of this century's true role models for the nursing profession. We take great pride in the fact that she started her remarkable career at Hopkins."

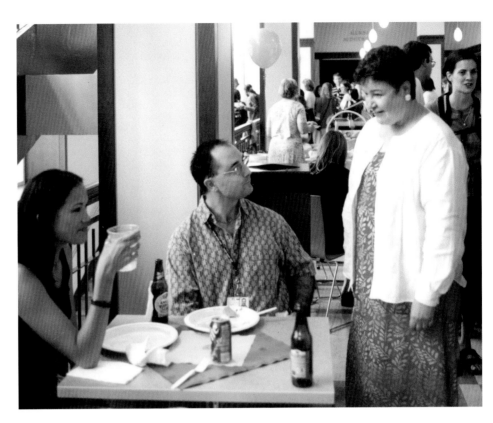

Dean Sue K. Donaldson welcomed returning students at a 2002 picnic in the café of the Anne M. Pinkard Building, for which she raised most of the funds.

June 10: Membership in the alumni association is redefined in the bylaws to welcome nursing graduates of McCoy College and the Evening College.

July: The Harry and Jeanette Weinberg Foundation pledges $20 million to the hospital to support construction of a new cancer treatment center. The new facility opens in 2000 and is named in the Weinberg's honor.

Autumn: The Nutting Fund is valued at more than $2.5 million. It is the largest endowment fund in the school and supports the only nursing chair in the United States created by an alumni association. The school has seventy additional endowment accounts, totaling $19.3 million—the second largest total in the country for a nursing school.

A new joint master's degree combining nursing and business is offered in cooperation with the School of Continuing Studies, formerly the Evening College. "As the job market for nurses with unique skills continues to expand, it is critical that we prepare the leaders to fill these positions," Dean Donaldson declares. Faculty member Jacqueline Dienemann explains that the new degree "aims to prepare nurses to manage nursing services and integrated health services successfully."

Tuition increases from $14,000 to $15,000 per year.

Dean Donaldson announces that the School of Nursing will receive $1 million toward the new building from Michael Bloomberg, as part of his record-breaking $55-million gift to the university.

1996

June 6: More than five hundred guests watch as ground is broken for the new School of Nursing building. To date, major gifts have been received from numerous sources, including the France/Merrick Foundations, the E. Rhodes and Leona Bowman Carpenter Foundation, Michael Bloomberg, and several anonymous donors. Speaker of the House Casper Taylor, representing the Maryland General Assembly, which contributed $2.5 million toward the building, says "there is no question that what we're doing here today is absolutely essential and it is a great contribution to the existing education and health care structure in the state of Maryland."

Mary Frances Keen, 1970, becomes the first nursing alumna and the first woman elected president of the Johns Hopkins University Alumni Association. Keen was president of the Johns Hopkins Nurses' Alumni Association in 1980 and 1981.

1997

Dr. Martha Norton Hill, a specialist in hypertension and the director of the Center for Nursing Research, becomes the first nurse and nonphysician elected president of the American Heart Association.

December 20: Occupancy of the new School of Nursing building begins as furniture, books, and equipment are delivered from the six different sites where the school had been conducting business. The new building is named the Anne M. Pinkard

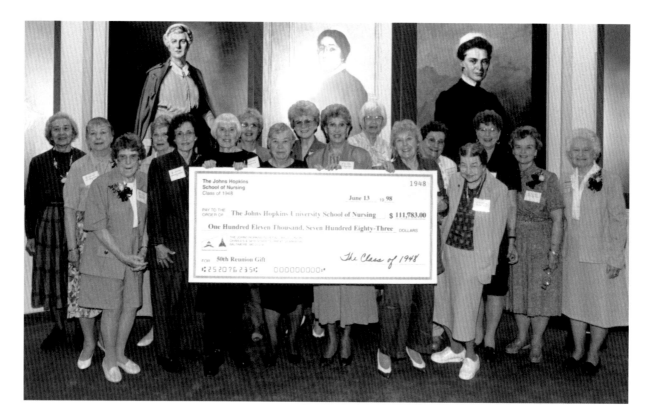

Reunion classes have been extraordinarily generous to the School of Nursing. In 1998 members of the class of 1948 presented a check for $111,983 as they stood before portraits of Anna D. Wolf, Elsie Lawler, and M. Adelaide Nutting.

Building to honor longtime Baltimore philanthropist and former Hopkins hospital and university trustee Anne Merrick Pinkard. Mrs. Pinkard served as the first chair of the Consortium for Nursing Education in 1983 and worked closely with Dean Carol Gray as plans for the university-based school were developed. University President William Brody calls the naming highly appropriate: "It is a place that will foster education, compassion, and a love for learning—all of the things I know Nan Pinkard holds dear."

1998

May 21: As she receives her master's degree, Dara Lawrence Geiser, 1991, reminds her classmates that "the Hopkins nursing education exposed us to many challenges. We have developed the courage to be leaders, the flexibility to adjust and grow from change, and the courage to pursue our dreams." Geiser points out their place in the continuum. "Hopkins nursing graduates are executives, running their own clinics, conducting and publishing their own research, and using today's technology strategically. The School of Nursing has expanded our courage, taught us not to give up when obstacles are stacked high, and we, as Hopkins alumni, will pass this courage on."

June 11: The Anne M. Pinkard Building is dedicated.

October: Dr. Fannie Gaston-Johansson, an expert in pain management, becomes the first African-American woman with both tenure and a full professorship at the Johns Hopkins University. Dr. Gaston-Johansson, who joined

the faculty in 1993, is the director of International and Extramural Affairs at the school and holds the Elsie M. Lawler Chair.

Maryann Fralic resigns as vice president for nursing and patient services at Johns Hopkins Hospital, and Karen Haller assumes the position.

1999

Returned Peace Corps volunteer Marni Sommer remembers her experiences as a member of the accelerated class of 1999. Sommer acknowledges the influences on her education. "The faculty and administration inspire and push us to think about the system, to become leaders in the field, and not to shrink from changing the status quo." Her classmates, Sommer says, "feel passionate about helping others," and she is proud to join the "dedicated nurses of America who have been taught, inspired, and molded by the traditions of the Johns Hopkins School of Nursing."

June 18: Margaret Courtney, 1940, the last director of both the diploma school and the Nursing Education Program in the School of Health Services, dies in Wilmington, Delaware.

Karin Coyne and Susan Immelt, 1977, become the first students to complete the doctoral program. Immelt believes the program affects everything she does professionally. "The difference between having a PhD and not having a PhD [becomes evident] in terms of how I approach teaching problems, clinical problems, any kinds of issues. You have a

broader perspective about how you deal with things because you're always thinking about how do I really know this procedure? How do I really know that this is the best way to teach these students? Why should I change this way of doing things? Is there really a reason to do that? That's how you think about things in every part of your life. Now, I'm always asking myself 'How do I know that?' and 'How would I show that it ought to be done differently?'"

2000

April 3: The Johns Hopkins University School of Nursing ties for the number five position in the rankings of graduate schools in *U.S. News & World Report*. Reflecting back on this achievement, Dean Donaldson "considered that another miracle, quite frankly, because the school was young and the other schools in the top ten had existed for decades with thousands of graduates and we had just a few hundred. This school and this faculty and the institute and everything played into that visibility and that quality and that excellence. So I would say, Hopkins is held in very high regard by the other nurse leaders."

The school begins offering a doctoral degree in nursing science with classes held exclusively during the summer. Candidates focus on clinical and financial outcomes measurement, health care economics, clinical nursing informatics, and applied research. This is the only DNSc program in Maryland.

The alumni association and the Alan Mason Chesney Medical Archives join forces to arrange and preserve all historical records relating to nursing education at Johns Hopkins. Phoebe Evans Letocha begins assessing a wealth of material that has been squirreled away in the attics and basements of those concerned about protecting for posterity official and unofficial records, scrapbooks, photographs, and artifacts. Dean Sue Donaldson encourages the archives project: "The history of an institution is really the avenue to its future, and it is critical that we leave a well-documented history to inspire all of the future Hopkins nurses."

2001

January and February: The Discovery Health Channel airs a five-part series entitled *Nurses*. The television programs, shot exclusively at Johns Hopkins, emphasize the teamwork characteristic of Johns Hopkins Medicine and show many instances where nurses are crucial in decision-making and execution of health care activities.

April: Dr. Sue K. Donaldson announces that she is stepping down as dean to return to research and teaching. Dr. Martha Norton Hill becomes interim dean in July.

The World Health Organization and the Pan American Health Organization designate the Institute for Johns Hopkins Nursing as a Collaborating Center for Information Systems in Nursing Care to concentrate on clinical nursing informatics needs and trends.

As a result of the terrorist attacks on the United States on September 11, the faculty begins discussions about expanding courses related to disaster nursing. Stephen Gonsalves, a 1997 graduate of the Family Nurse Practitioner Program, spends two weeks on assignment with the U.S. Public Health Service at Ground Zero in New York City, the site of the attacks on the World Trade Center. "I was prepared to mend the physical damages. But I soon came to understand that the traumatized, weary rescue workers needed help on a more emotional level. They needed a listening ear, a therapeutic touch, and the presence of someone who cared. And that is what nursing is all about."

2002

May 5: After a national search, President William Brody announces that Martha Norton Hill, 1964, is the new dean of the School of Nursing, making Hill the first alumna to be dean of the university school.

Johns Hopkins ranks in the top ten among nursing schools nationwide for research funding from the National Institutes of Health. One $2-million grant to faculty member Dr. Linda Pugh funds research to determine the cost effectiveness of promoting breastfeeding. Other areas of research being pursued at the school include domestic violence, health issues among Korean Americans, asthma management, hypertension care and control, symptom management, and patient strategies for coping with pain.

October 2–4: The School of Nursing successfully hosts the National League for Nursing's accreditation committee.

A gift of $2 million from the Leonard and Helen R. Stulman Charitable Foundation establishes an endowed professorship in mental health and psychiatric nursing.

The School of Nursing establishes the Center for Health Disparities Research in partnership with the North Carolina Agricultural and Technical State University School of Nursing and wins a $2.3-million grant from the National Institute for Nursing Research. This is one of eight grants that join the resources of research-intensive universities like Hopkins with minority universities.

2003

In cooperation with the alumni association, the School of Nursing launches the new *Johns Hopkins Nursing Magazine*, edited by Kate Pipkin. The new publication, which will "track Johns Hopkins nurses and tell the story of their endeavors in the areas of education, practice, and scholarship, including research and national leadership," according to its mission statement, goes to alumni and friends of the school as well as 275 media outlets.

With a pass rate of more than 97 percent of graduates who take the National Council Licensure Examination for Registered Nurses, Johns Hopkins produces more new nurses than any other nursing school in Maryland.

In the 2003–4 academic year the student body increases by 10 percent. The incoming baccalaureate class includes members from thirty states, the District of Columbia, India, and Ghana. Enrollment of twenty-nine doctoral candidates is an all-time high. There are now nine full professors and thirteen associate professors on the faculty, with a total faculty comprising eighty-one full-time and ninety-five part-time members.

September 17–19: Tropical storm Isabel causes cancellation of some events and creates considerable drama during homecoming. The annual meeting takes place as planned on Saturday morning, September 20.

2004

February 26: To mark the 20th anniversary of the university school and the 115th year of nursing education at Johns Hopkins, the Milestones Celebration begins with a symposium on health care issues affecting the aging population.

August: Johns Hopkins Nursing and Peking Union Medical College form a partnership to create the first doctoral nursing education program in China. The goal is to create nursing leaders in China for clinical programs, nursing research, and health care administration. This global link renews the longtime bond between Hopkins and the PUMC, where Anna D. Wolf helped to establish a collegiate nursing program from 1919 to 1925.

2005

January: To help combat the nationwide nursing shortage, the school inaugurates a new seventeen-month accelerated program, which begins with forty-eight students.

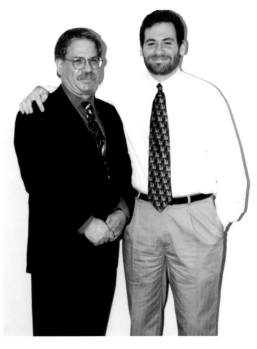

Herb Zinder and his son Matt were the first father and son alumni in nursing at Johns Hopkins. In 1971 Herb Zinder became one of the first two men to graduate from the hospital school; Matt Zinder received his degree from the university school in 1999.

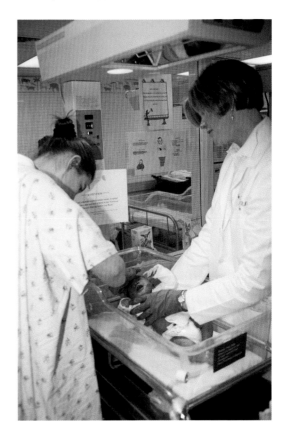

Betty Jordan supervised Emily Bahne, 2001, as she examined a newborn infant in the birthing center of Johns Hopkins Hospital on February 25, 2000.

Acknowledgments

MAME WARREN
Director
Hopkins History Enterprises
The Sheridan Libraries of the Johns Hopkins University

Many people contributed to bringing this book into print. As far back as 1978, members of the class of 1945 established a "history fund" to preserve records and memorabilia of the Johns Hopkins Hospital School of Nursing. In 1985 the Johns Hopkins Nurses' Alumni Association named Betty Bietsch Brizendine, Gertrude Wooddy Mitchell, and Mary Louise Frock Miller, all members of the class of 1945, and Miriam Buchaca Stockbridge, 1948, to serve on a committee with the goal of publishing a companion volume to Ethel Johns and Blanche Pfefferkorn's classic *The Johns Hopkins School of Nursing, 1889–1949.*

No doubt the committee's work was facilitated by the tenacity of Betty Liggett Cuthbert, 1943, whose accomplishments enrich almost every page of this book. "When they tore down the nurses' library, Betty Cuthbert took boxes of some of the important books and archives and stored those things at her house," remembered former associate dean Stella Shiber. "The library really had some very important, historically significant things." Indeed, the endnotes and the bibliographical note at the back of this book illustrate the breadth of the historical records Cuthbert helped preserve. "If it hadn't been for Betty, a lot of those things would have been lost," Shiber explained. "Betty was hoping for the day when somebody would value and take care of these things. She truly was, in a literal sense, the 'keeper of the flame.' Hopkins was her life." Complementing Cuthbert's efforts, in 1993–94 Professor Ada Davis inventoried other materials relating to Hopkins nursing, which had long been stored in the Nightingale Room of the Welch Library.

In 1998 a new book committee formed, this time with Sue Appling, 1973, who continued Cuthbert's archival endeavors, at the helm. The new committee, which included Betty Scher, 1950, Sue Wright, 1962, Pat Sullivan, 1977, and Phyllis Naumann, MSN 1994, engaged Linda Emerson Sabin, 1967, to compose chapters about the history of the hospital school from its beginning through the 1960s, when its end was clearly in sight. Sarah Allison provided indispensable guidance for these chapters. Later, Fran Keen, 1970, agreed to take on the turbulent 1970s, which included the closing of the diploma school and the short life of the Nursing Education Program in the School of Health Services, in which Keen was an instructor.

As Drs. Sabin and Keen were wrapping up their work, the committee turned to Nancy McCall, archivist, and Phoebe Evans Letocha, coordinator of processing and research, at the Alan M. Chesney Medical Archives for advice about publishing the manuscript. Nancy and Phoebe were aware of the wealth of visual material in the nursing collections and knew this book could become something very special. They showed *Johns Hopkins: Knowledge for the World*, the book I had produced for the 125th anniversary of the university, to committee members. Liking what they saw, the committee commissioned me to edit the existing manuscript, thoroughly review all possible sources for illustrations for the book, and bring the story up to the present by conducting oral history interviews with people who could speak about various aspects of the history of nursing education at Johns Hopkins.

I quickly plunged into the project by reviewing copies of the *Johns Hopkins Nurses Alumnae Magazine*, which began publication in 1901. Over the years, the editors highlighted the latest developments in nursing and the Hopkins medical institutions and featured articles about the earlier history of the school. The magazine led me to other sources and fairly soon I was awed by the accomplishments of both the school and its graduates. The chronology at the back of this book includes many of the details and anecdotes I gleaned from my reading, and from timelines previously assembled by Linda Sabin and Phoebe Letocha.

Throughout my endeavors, members of the book committee and the alumni board have been extraordinarily supportive and responsive. Having committee members scrutinize each chapter as it was edited gave me confidence that we were getting the full story, and doing it well. Their feedback revealed them to be careful readers, each with a broad understanding of Hopkins nursing and alumni history.

In the Office of Development and Alumni Relations, Melinda Rose and Jackie Gray were there for me time and again, providing essential information and answering esoteric questions, making sure that I had all the backing needed for various necessary tasks. Their colleague Shirley Brooks became my photo agent, inquiring about potential illustrations when she talked with alumni, and I am grateful to Shirley for bringing several photographic gems to these pages. In the Office of Communications, Lynn Schultz-Writsel and Ming Tai shared dozens of photographs depicting life in the university school, many of which were taken under the direction of Lynn's predecessor, Kate Pipkin.

The Chesney Medical Archives became my second home through much of this project. Gerard Shorb and Marjorie Kehoe often worked patiently with me as I conducted research. Phoebe Letocha and Anthony Dellureficio, who are the persons most familiar with the riches of the Johns Hopkins Nursing Historical Collection, delved into its unprocessed depths to share hidden treasures, ensuring that they will now be part of the public record. I am also deeply indebted to Phoebe and her colleague Andrew Harrison, who spent countless hours pulling photographs from many collections and researching their provenance so that they could be released for publication here. They were assisted by Michael Miers, Alexia Robinson, and Elisabeth Sultzbaugh. Ellen H. Winslow of Johns Hopkins PathPhoto

proficiently produced digital images of photographs from the Chesney Archives.

James Stimpert, university archivist and my colleague at the Sheridan Libraries, made available the records of the Office of the Provost. Examination of these files revealed considerable detail about the somewhat murky history of the short-lived School of Health Services, which I shared with author Fran Keen. There was also fascinating background material on the evolution of the Johns Hopkins University School of Nursing.

Alumni responded generously to my call for photographs and memorabilia. Mary Farr Heeg, 1941, Ethel Rainey Ward, 1947, Joan Tunnicliffe Hurlock and Mabel Gerhart Hollowell, both of the class of 1953, Mary Warfield MacSherry, 1954, and Herb Zinder, 1971, provided snapshots, adding a personal touch. Particular thanks go to Betty Scher, 1950, who kept a photo album of her time at the School of Nursing, which included an abundance of pictures of her instructors and classmates in lectures, in clinics, and at leisure. Jeanie Aydelotte, Patrice Sturm Gerster, Deborah Holmes, Bonnie LeHew Samter, and Kathy White, all members of the class of 1973, rallied to a plea for photographs from the final days of the hospital school. Richard Masek sent a portrait of his sister, Joan Masek Sutton. Professor Ron Berk, who has been shooting routine and special events at the university school almost since its inception, gave me access to his hoard of prints and color slides. At the Enoch Pratt Free Library, Jeff Korman welcomed me and gave access to the visual resources of the expansive photographic collection in the Maryland Department, where I found a few important images available nowhere else.

In addition to the chapters written by Linda Sabin and Fran Keen, text came from various sources. Gert Brieger graciously composed an astute and scholarly introduction. A memoir written by Frances Schlosser Scherer, 1944, and a scrapbook with diary

entries kept by Mabel Gerhart Hollowell, 1953, were special discoveries that give a vivid sense of what it was like to be a student then. The voices that appear on these pages reflect many hours of interviews with particularly thoughtful alumni and friends of the various schools of nursing. Sandra Stine Angell, Sue Appling, Ada Davis, Donna Dittberner, Sue Donaldson, Paula Einaudi, Maravene Deveney Hamburger, Mary Farr Heeg, Robert Heyssel, Martha Norton Hill, Trudy Jones Hodges, Lois Grayshan Hoffer, Susan Carroll Immelt, Bernard Keenan, Kate Knott, Elaine Larson, Maureen Maguire, Medea Marella, Stephen McClain, Betsy Mumaw McGeady, Steven Muller, Cathy Novak, Kay Partridge, William C. Richardson, Betty Borenstein Scher, Frances Schlosser Scherer, Stella Shiber, Benita Walton-Moss, Ethel Rainey Ward, Connie Waxter, and Herb Zinder sat down with me to record their insights into the past, present, and future of nursing education at Johns Hopkins.

All those hours of tape were meticulously transcribed by Barbara Muller, who later donned a different hat to become an incomparable proofreader. Barbara Lamb made elegant suggestions and contributions as copyeditor. Both did their best to tidy up unruly punctuation. I am grateful for every comma and semicolon, and if any errors persist, no doubt they are the result of my stubborn resistance to correction. Robert Wiser is the newest member of this team. As the book's designer, he was responsible for weaving many disparate visual and textual elements into a coherent whole. Cathy Sabol accurately assembled the index of names and subjects. At Johns Hopkins University Press, Bob Brugger expertly shepherded the book through the evaluation process, and Ken Sabol managed this complex printing job to great effect.

It has been a privilege to work with so many talented people to bring *Our Shared Legacy* to you.

Notes

Abbreviations

AMCMA
Alan Mason Chesney Medical Archives, The Johns Hopkins Medical Institutions, Baltimore, MD

FHJA
Ferdinand Hamburger Jr. Archives, Milton S. Eisenhower Library, The Johns Hopkins University, Baltimore, MD

JHNHC
Johns Hopkins Nursing Historical Collection, which is housed in the Alan Mason Chesney Medical Archives, The Johns Hopkins Medical Institutions, Baltimore, MD

JHNAM
Johns Hopkins Nurses' Alumnae Magazine

J&P
Ethel Johns and Blanche Pfefferkorn, *The Johns Hopkins Hospital School of Nursing, 1889–1949* (Baltimore: Johns Hopkins Press, 1954).

Introduction
GERT BRIEGER

1. Florence Nightingale, *Notes on Nursing: What It Is and What It Is Not* (London: Harrison, 1859), 6.

2. Martineau quoted by Katherine Williams, "From Sarah Gamp to Florence Nightingale: A Critical Study of Hospital Nursing from 1840 to 1897," in *Rewriting Nursing History*, ed. Celia Davies (London: Croom Helm, 1980), 55.

3. Philip A. Kalisch and Beatrice J. Kalisch, *American Nursing: A History*, 4th ed. (Philadelphia: Lippincott Williams & Wilkins, 2004).

4. Nightingale, *Notes on Nursing*, 6.

5. Susan M. Reverby, *Ordered to Care: The Dilemma of American Nursing, 1850–1945* (London: Cambridge University Press, 1987), 43.

6. Letter to trustees, March 10, 1873, in Alan M. Chesney, *The Johns Hopkins Hospital and the Johns Hopkins School of Medicine*, vol. 1, *The Early Years, 1867–1893* (Baltimore: Johns Hopkins Press, 1943), 15.

7. A. M. Harvey, G. H. Brieger, S. L. Abrams, and V. A. McKusick, *A Model of Its Kind: A Centennial History of Medicine at Johns Hopkins* (Baltimore: Johns Hopkins University Press, 1989), 1: 26–27.

8. William Osler, "Doctor and Nurse," in *Aequanimitas and Other Papers* (New York: Norton, 1963), 34. This paper originally appeared in the *Bulletin of the Johns Hopkins Hospital* in 1891.

9. Janet Wilson James, "Writing and Rewriting Nursing History: A Review Essay," *Bulletin of the History of Medicine* 58 (1984): 568, 571.

10. See especially Barbara Melosh, *The Physician's Hand: Work, Culture, and Conflict in American Nursing* (Philadelphia: Temple University Press, 1982); Reverby, *Ordered to Care*; Karen Buhler-Wilkerson, *No Place Like Home: A History of Nursing and Home Care in the United States* (Baltimore: Johns Hopkins University Press, 2001); Davies, ed., *Rewriting Nursing History*; Ellen C. Lagemann, ed., *Nursing History: New Perspectives, New Possibili-*

ties (New York: Teachers College Press, 1983); Barbara Mortimer and Susan McGann, eds., *New Directions in the History of Nursing: International Perspectives* (London: Routledge, 2005).

11. *Nursing and Nursing Education in the United States* (New York: Macmillan, 1923) and the discussion in Kalisch and Kalisch, *American Nursing*, 1st ed., 332–37.

12. Gert H. Brieger, "Why the University-Based Medical School Should Survive: A Historical Perspective," *Academic Medicine* 72 (1997): 362–69.

13. October 17, 2005, 3.

14. Vern L. Bullough and Bonnie Bullough, *The Emergence of Modern Nursing*, 2nd ed. (New York: Macmillan, 1969), v.

15. Ethel Johns and Blanche Pfefferkorn, *The Johns Hopkins Hospital School of Nursing, 1889–1949* (Baltimore: Johns Hopkins Press, 1954).

Chapter One: An Auspicious Beginning
LINDA SABIN

1. Dr. Winford Smith, *JHNAM* 14 (July 1915): 194.

2. Ada Davis, interview by Mame Warren, March 9, 2004.

3. Paula Einaudi, interview by Mame Warren, July 28, 2003.

4. Davis, interview.

5. Ibid.

6. Charles J. M. Gwinn to the Trustees of the Johns Hopkins Hospital, per instructions of Johns Hopkins, March 10, 1873. Ethel Johns and Blanche Pfefferkorn, *The Johns Hopkins Hospital School of Nursing, 1889–1949* (Baltimore: Johns Hopkins Press, 1954), 8.

7. John S. Billings to the trustees, in 1874, quoted in J&P, 12.

8. J&P, 54.

9. Henry Hurd, "The Relation of the Training School for Nurses to the Johns Hopkins Hospital," *The Johns Hopkins Hospital Bulletin* 1 (Dec. 1, 1889), quoted in Victor Robinson, *White Caps* (Philadelphia: J. B. Lippincott, 1946), 263.

10. Alan Mason Chesney, *The Johns Hopkins Hospital and the Johns Hopkins University School of Medicine: A Chronicle*, vol. 1, *Early Years, 1867–1893* (Baltimore: Johns Hopkins Press, 1943), 40–41.

11. Isabel Hampton Robb, "Aims of the Johns Hopkins Hospital School for Nurses," in *Educational Standards for Nurses, with Other Addresses on Nursing Subjects* (Cleveland: Koeckert, 1907), 36–37.

12. Ibid., 39; Isabel Hampton, "The Johns Hopkins Hospital Training School for Nurses," *Trained Nurse* 7 (July 1891): 37–40.

13. Philip A. Kalisch and Beatrice J. Kalisch, *The Advance of American Nursing*, 3rd ed. (Philadelphia: J. B. Lippincott, 1995), 71–72.

14. Josephine (Teeny) Waldhauser, interview by Ethel Johns, October 25, 1948. Waldhauser was head waitress in the Nurses' Home dining room for twenty-seven years. According to

Johns, Waldhauser was "possessed of a photographic memory"; she was undoubtedly an important informant for the coauthor of the original history of the school. JHNHC.

15. J&P, 232–33.

16. Ibid., 120–21.

17. Kalisch and Kalisch, *The Advance of American Nursing*, 216.

18. Agnes Ysobel Irvine to Adelaide Nutting, August 16, 1899, Mary Adelaide Nutting Papers, JHNHC.

19. Colonel Dallas Bache, "The Female Nurse in the Army," *Journal of the Military Service Institution of the United States* (1899): 15–18.

20. William Welch to Adelaide Nutting, March 21, 1903, Mary Adelaide Nutting Papers, JHNHC.

21. J&P, 177–79.

22. Elsie Lawler to M. Adelaide Nutting, undated, in the Mary Adelaide Nutting Historical Nursing Collection, fiche 2109–19.

23. Maravene Hamburger, interview by Mame Warren, August 27, 1999. For many years, outpatients at Johns Hopkins were treated in the dispensary. Dr. Russell Nelson later became president of the Johns Hopkins Hospital and a champion of Hopkins nursing.

24. Ibid.

25. Report of the Director of the School of Nursing, January 16, 1941, Minutes of the Advisory Board of the School of Nursing, 175, AMCMA.

26. Dr. Winford Smith, interview by Ethel Johns, 1948.

27. "In Appreciation of Miss Lawler," *JHNAM* 39 (July 1940): 116.

28. Betty Scher, interview by Mame Warren, June 26, 2004.

29. Hamburger, interview.

30. Minutes of the Board of Trustees of the Johns Hopkins Hospital, October 8, 1940, 5: 316–17, AMCMA.

31. "Twenty-fifth Anniversary of the Johns Hopkins Hospital, 1889–1914," *Bulletin of the Johns Hopkins Hospital* 25 (Dec. 1914): 360–61.

32. Anna D. Wolf, interview by Sarah E. Allison, February 25, 1976, Sunny Shores Villas, St. Petersburg, Florida. "Anna D. Wolf" biographical file, AMCMA; *JHNAM* 48 (July 1949): 120.

33. Loula Kennedy, "Hester King Frederick," *JHNAM* 40 (July 1941): 116–18.

34. Robb, "Aims of the Johns Hopkins Hospital School for Nurses," 39.

35. There is another story about the origin of the cap. According to a student who participated in the planning, three people actually worked on the cap, which was made of fine organdy and stitched by Susan Read.

36. J&P, 67–68.

37. Elsie M. Lawler, interview by Ethel Johns, March 30, 1948, "Elsie Lawler" biographical file, AMCMA.

38. Ibid.

39. Helen Athey, "Almost Fifty Years Ago," *Vigilando* 94 (Winter 1996): 12–13.

40. Effie Jane Taylor, "Address to the Alumnae Association," *JHNAM* 41 (Oct. 1942): 167.

41. Wolf, interview.

42. "A Day on Ward E: Johns Hopkins Hospital, 1928–1929," *Vigilando: The Alumni Magazine* 91 (Winter 1991): 10–11.

43. Lucile Petry Leone, "Our Heritage and Challenge of the Future," *JHNAM* 64 (Mar. 1965): 9–10.

44. Ibid.

45. "A Day on Ward E: Johns Hopkins Hospital, 1928–1929."

46. K. Virginia Betzold, interview by Betty Brizendine, March 4, 1985.

47. Elsie Lawler, "Reminiscences," *JHNAM* 44 (Jan. 1945): 22.

48. Thomas Turner, *Heritage of Excellence: The Johns Hopkins Medical Institutions, 1914–1917* (Baltimore: Johns Hopkins University Press, 1974), 262.

49. Yssabella G. Waters to [Lillian] Wald, undated, "Spanish-American War" file, JHNHC.

50. C. G. Link, "Heroines of the Recent Spanish-American War," *Atlanta Journal*, September 26, 1898. JHNHC, 90–159.

51. Ibid.

52. Contract for Charity Babcock for Services as a Nurse, JHNHC, box 10.

53. Lavinia Dock, Sarah Elizabeth Pickett, Clara D. Noyes, Fannie F. Clement, Elizabeth G. Fox, and Anna R. VanMeter, *History of American Red Cross Nursing* (New York: Macmillan Co., 1922), 139–50.

54. Ibid., 151.

55. "Gertrude Muldrew," *JHNAM* 17 (May 1918): 58.

56. Linda Sabin, "Clara Dutton Noyes, 1869–1936," in *American Nursing, A Biographical Dictionary* (New York: Garland Press, 1988), 242–43.

57. Dock et al., *History of American Red Cross Nursing*, 486.

58. John Finney, *A Surgeon's Life* (New York: G. P. Putnam's Sons, 1940), 175.

59. Ibid., 489.

60. Ibid., 492.

61. Ibid., 489–90.

62. Grace Baxter, "Letters from Our Correspondent in Italy," *American Journal of Nursing* 1 (Feb. 1901): 407.

63. Ibid., 3 (June 1903): 737–38.

64. Edith Cavell was an English nurse who brought the Nightingale approach to nursing education to Belgium before the war. A German firing squad shot her in October 1915 for providing relief to allied soldiers.

65. "The Story of an American Red Cross Nurse," *JHNAM* 67 (June 1968): 43.

66. Alta Elizabeth Dines, "Katherine Olmstead, 1912–1964," *JHNAM* 63 (Sept. 1964): 93–94; Signe Cooper, "Katherine Olmstead," *American Nursing, A Biographical Dictionary*, 247–48.

67. Vern L. Bullough, "Ellen LaMotte," *American Nursing, A Biographical Dictionary*, 204.

68. Ellen LaMotte, *The Backwash of War* (New York: G. P. Putnam's Sons, 1916), 3–4.

69. Ibid., 134.

70. The Registry Committee files, JHNHC, 90–159, 1896–1913; Editorials, "Our Registry," *JHNAM* 26 (May 1927): 48–49.

71. Lilli Sentz, "Mary E. Lent," *American Nursing, A Biographical Dictionary*, 211–12; "Pioneers in Public Health: Mary Elizabeth Lent," *Trained Nurse and Hospital Review* 80 (May 1928): 3.

72. Ethel M. Damon, "Pioneer in Public Health: Mabel Wilcox," *Paradise of the Pacific*, 1952 Annual, JHNHC.

73. The Maltese cross was originally worn by members of religious orders in the Middle Ages. These early nursing orders used the Maltese cross to symbolize the eight beatitudes of the members of the order: "1. Spiritual joy. 2. To live without malice. 3. To weep over thy sins. 4. To humble thyself to those who injure thee. 5. To love justice. 6. To be merciful. 7. To be sincere and pure of heart. 8. To suffer persecution." Ruth Brewster Sherman, "The Sign of the Cross and the Nursing Insignia," *JHNAM* 71 (Jan. 1972). Note: This article first appeared in the July 1937 issue of the *JHNAM*, 5; J&P, 363.

74. J&P, 333.

75. History of the Endowment Fund, JHNHC.

Chapter Two: Rapid Change
LINDA SABIN

1. "Editorials: Hopkins Nurses, Your Own Nurses Need You," *JHNAM* 40 (Apr. 1941): 60.

2. Sarah E. Allison, "Anna Wolf" (Paper presented at the International Nursing History Conference, St. Johns, New Brunswick, Canada, 1992). Much of the information about Miss Wolf included in this chapter and in chapter three is based on the work of Dr. Allison.

3. Anna D. Wolf, interview by Sarah E. Allison, February 25, 1976.

4. Sarah E. Allison, "Anna Wolf's Dream: Establishment of a Collegiate Nursing Education Program," *Image* 25 (Summer 1993): 127–31; biographical research and notes on Anna Wolf by Sarah E. Allison, JHNHC.

5. Sarah E. Allison, "Higher Education for Nurses: The Vision of Anna D. Wolf," unpublished paper, 8–9. Sarah Allison Research Papers, box 1, JHNHC.

6. Minutes of the Board of Trustees of the Johns Hopkins Hospital, March 5, 1940, 287–88.

7. Sarah E. Allison, editorial note added to the transcription of interview with Anna D. Wolf.

8. J&P, 146–47.

9. Betty Cuthbert, "Progress or Decline?" *JHNAM* 66 (Sept. 1967): 56–62.

10. Ibid; Monica Thompson and Constance Waxter, interview by Janie Brown, July 14, 1987.

11. "Memorandum Concerning a University School of Nursing, March 21, 1941," Administrative Files and Minutes of the Advisory Board of the School of Nursing, March 27, 1941, AMCMA.

12. Mary Kuntz, "Fiftieth Anniversary Memory Book, Class of 1943, the Johns Hopkins Hospital School of Nursing," JHNHC.

13. Anna D. Wolf, "Our Opportunities," *JHNAM* 40 (July 1941): 128–29.

14. Wolf, interview.

15. J&P, 247.

16. Minutes of the Advisory Board of the School of Nursing, March 25, 1943, AMCMA.

17. K. Virginia Betzold to Sarah E. Allison, July 11, 1982, JHNHC.

18. Joan Verlee DeYoung, "Fiftieth Anniversary Memory Book, Class of 1945, the Johns Hopkins Hospital School of Nursing," JHNHC.

19. Robert H. Dombro, "Helen Schnetzer Child Life Program," *JHNAM* 63 (Mar. 1964), 7–13; Augusta Tucker, *It Happened at Hopkins* (Baltimore: Women's Board of the Johns Hopkins Hospital), 98.

20. Wolf, interview.

21. Philip A. Kalisch and Beatrice J. Kalisch, *The Advance of American Nursing*, 3rd. ed (Philadelphia: J. B. Lippincott, 1995), 546, 552.

22. J&P, 251–52.

23. Mildred Struve, interview by Sarah E. Allison, May 23, 1991.

24. Francis Horn, "Unorthodox Academic Wedlock," *JHNAM* 47 (Apr. 1948): 37–39.

25. Anna D. Wolf, "A Message from the Director of the School of Nursing and Nursing Services," *JHNAM* 47 (Apr. 1948): 35–37.

26. Esther Lucille Brown, *Nursing for the Future* (New York: Russell Sage Foundation, 1948): 100, 116, 132, 168–70.

27. Anna Wolf, "Editorial: Nursing for the Future," *JHNAM* 48 (Jan. 1949): 6–7.

28. Wolf, interview.

29. Doris Diller, telephone interview by author, August 20, 1998.

30. Mary Goldthwaite, "Our Plan for a Memorial to Miss Christine Dick," *JHNAM* 44 (Jan. 1945): 88–89.

31. Betty Cuthbert, interview by Janie Brown, July 10, 1987.

32. "Turtle Derby," *JHNAM* 40 (July 1941): 137; "Turtle Derby Day," *JHNAM* 46 (Oct. 1947): 137.

33. Lee McCardell, "Johns Hopkins Takes Air-Raid Precautions," *JHNAM* 41 (Apr. 1942): 68–71.

34. Mary Agnes Gautier to Mr. James D. Gautier, Kreole, Mississippi, December 13, 1941. Mary Agnes Gautier Collection, Special Collections of the Louisiana State University Libraries, Baton Rouge.

35. "The Army Nurse Corps of General Hospitals Nos. 18 and 118," JHNAM 41 (July 1942): 104.

36. "Hail and Farewell," ibid., 105–6.

37. "Miss Lawler Visits General Hospitals Nos. 18 and 118," ibid., 111–12.

38. Elizabeth McLaughlin to the alumnae magazine, undated, JHNAM 42 (Oct. 1943): 169.

39. H. Alvan Jones's address to the alumnae association, February 17, 1944, JHNAM 43 (Jan. 1944): 39–40.

40. Captain Helen Weber to the alumnae magazine, November 21, 1944, JHNAM 44 (Jan. 1945): 12.

41. Edith A. Nunn to the alumnae magazine, JHNAM 45 (Jan. 1946): 3–4.

42. Mary Claire Cox to the alumnae magazine, undated, JHNAM 42 (Oct. 1943): 170.

43. "Mississippi Nurses Association Hall of Fame Induction, 1998" (Jackson: Mississippi Nurses Association, 1998). Mississippi Department of Archives and History, Jackson.

44. "School Activities," JHNAM 43 (Oct. 1944): 141.

45. "Elizabeth Smellie—1909," JHNAM 67 (June 1968): 54.

Chapter Three: Nursing at the Crossroads
LINDA SABIN

1. Philip A. Kalisch and Beatrice J. Kalisch, The Advance of American Nursing, 3rd. ed. (Philadelphia: J. B. Lippincott, 1995), 523–28.

2. Ibid.

3. Minutes of the Advisory Board of the Johns Hopkins Hospital School of Nursing, January 2 and 16, 1951, 73–82, AMCMA.

4. Ibid., January 2, 1951, 76, AMCMA.

5. Ibid., October 18, 1951, 99; ibid., October 20, 1953, 166, AMCMA.

6. Ibid., January 2, 1951, 80–82, AMCMA.

7. Kalisch and Kalisch, The Advance of American Nursing, 609–12, 621–28, 178–80.

8. "The New Educational Unit," JHNAM 50 (Jan.1951): 22–24.

9. Anna D. Wolf, interview by Sarah E. Allison, February 25, 1976. In an interview with the author on August 20, 1998, Doris Diller confirmed that, although Miss Wolf kept to herself when upset and did not let her feelings show, she did feel things very strongly.

10. Richard W. TeLinde, "Opportunities and Responsibilities in Nursing," JHNAM 52 (Jan. 1953): 7–11. Presented at convocation September 22, 1952. Convocation in this period was held on the occasion of the graduation of seniors and the arrival of incoming freshmen.

11. Wolf, interview.

12. Minutes of the Advisory Board of the Johns Hopkins Hospital School of Nursing, December 18, 1951, 102, AMCMA.

13. Margaret Bridgeman, Collegiate Education for Nursing (New York: Russell Sage Foundation, 1953).

14. Minutes of the Advisory Board of the Johns Hopkins Hospital School of Nursing, October 18, 1953, 158–66, AMCMA.

15. Wolf, interview.

16. Minutes of the Advisory Board of the Johns Hopkins Hospital School of Nursing, October 18, 1953, 158–66, AMCMA; Wolf, interview.

17. Mary Jane Donough, interview by author, August 5, 1998.

18. Minutes of the Advisory Board of the Johns Hopkins Hospital School of Nursing, December 15, 1953, AMCMA.

19. Ibid., September 15, 1952, 125–26, AMCMA.

20. Kalisch and Kalisch, The Advance of American Nursing, 594–95, 602–3.

21. Wolf, interview.

22. Minutes of the Advisory Board of the Johns Hopkins Hospital School of Nursing, April 28, 1953, AMCMA. During the years following this decision, many nurses who made significant contributions to the school received help in their advanced education, including Margaret Courtney and Sarah Allison.

23. Minutes of the Advisory Board of the Johns Hopkins Hospital School of Nursing, April 20, 1954, 188, AMCMA.

24. Anna D. Wolf, verbatim transcription of record handwritten in pencil and sent to Sarah Allison, April 16, 1976. In the author's possession.

25. Sarah E. Allison, "Higher Education for Nurses: The Vision of Anna D. Wolf," unpublished paper, 39. Sarah Allison Research Papers, box 1, JHNHC.

26. Annual reports on the activities in the school, published in JHNAM, 1951–55.

27. Minutes of the Advisory Board of the Johns Hopkins Hospital School of Nursing, October 26, 1954, 196, AMCMA.

28. Wolf, interview.

29. Russell Nelson, interview by Janie Brown, June 3, 1987.

30. Esther Jacoby, interview by Janie Brown, July 13, 1987.

31. Margaret Courtney, interview by Janie Brown, July 7, 1987.

32. Esther Lucille Brown, Nursing for the Future (New York: Russell Sage Foundation, 1948). The Brown Report, written by social scientist Esther Lucille Brown, PhD, examined the social significance of nursing and charged that society was neglecting nursing education. She noted that nurses, unlike teachers, received little public support for education because most nurses trained in hospitals, which dimmed the professional prospects of diploma graduates who did not receive a degree. Brown pointed to severe shortages of practicing nurses and nursing students in the United States after World War II and warned that the system as it existed would fail to attract enough students to replenish the profession.

33. Minutes of the Advisory Board of the Johns Hopkins Hospital School of Nursing, May 1, 1956, 245–50, 270–72, AMCMA.

34. Ibid., April 26, 1954, 220, AMCMA.

35. Ibid., October 26, 1954, 198, AMCMA.

36. After her retirement in 1940, Miss Lawler lived in California for a time. When she became ill, she returned to Johns Hopkins and became a permanent resident in the Marburg Pavilion until her death in 1962.

37. Mary S. Price [address to the graduating class, May 21, 1956], JHNAM 55 (July 1956): 84–6.

38. Minutes of the Advisory Board of the Johns Hopkins Hospital School of Nursing, October 30, 1956, 270–72, AMCMA.

39. Ibid., December 30, 1955, 231, AMCMA.

40. Ibid., March 28, 1958, 315–17, AMCMA; Mary S. Price, "A Special Report from the Director of the School of Nursing, May 17, 1958," JHNAM 57 (Oct. 1958): 64.

41. Minutes of the Advisory Board of the Johns Hopkins Hospital School of Nursing, October 21, 1958, 319–25, AMCMA.

42. Ibid., October 20, 1959, 365.

43. Anna D. Wolf, "Notes from Office of Director of the School of Nursing and the Nursing Service," JHNAM (Apr. 1952): 61–64.

44. Betty Scher, class of 1950 memory books, JHNHC.

45. Student survey and memory books from the 1950s, and the student handbook, 1958, 48.

46. Graduate surveys returned, 1998–2000, to the alumni association; reunion memory books from the classes of 1950, 1951, 1953, 1954, and 1955.

47. Mary A. Goldthwaite, "Our Plan for a Memorial to Miss Christine Dick," JHNAM 44 (Apr. 1945): 86–89.

48. "The Christina [sic] M. Dick Cottage—Sherwood Forest," The Dome: The Student Handbook of the Johns Hopkins Hospital School of Nursing, 1958, 31–36.

49. Doris Higgins Thompson, "Memory Book of the Fortieth Reunion of the Class of 1951," 9.

50. Adele Sparks Birx, ibid., 2.

51. Trudy [Jones] Hodges, "Reflections," Vigilando 92 (Winter 1993): 6–7.

52. "Dedication—Chemistry Laboratory," JHNAM 54 (July 1955): 103–5.

53. Grace K. Stone, "Effie J. Taylor: Humanitarian and World Citizen," JHNAM 58 (Oct. 1959): 69–73.

54. "Miss Dunbar Retires," JHNAM 58 (Apr. 1959): 23.

55. Frances Reiter, "Preparation for Professional Nursing Practice," JHNAM 66 (Sept. 1967): 49–50. Dr. Richard Cabot of the Massachusetts General Hospital in Boston wrote extensively on medical issues; he visited JHH in 1903. Abraham Flexner conducted a landmark study of medical education in

North America in 1910 for the Carnegie Foundation for the Advancement of Teaching. Josephine Goldmark was secretary to the national Committee for the Study of Nursing Education, which published its report in 1923.

56. Barbara Donaho, keynote address, June 7, 1996, JHNAM 95 (Winter 1996): 8.

57. Anna Wolf portrait gift file, 1952, in alumni records 90–159, JHNHC.

58. Wolf, interview.

59. Betty Scher, "I Remember," Vigilando 92 (Summer 1993): 8.

60. "Proposed Revision—Code of Ethics," JHNAM 51 (Apr. 1952): 68–77.

61. The Johns Hopkins Hospital Nurses' Alumnae Association, Inc., "Some Ethical Concepts for Nurses" (1953), 25. The pamphlet included a reprint of the original code of ethics because it had "become so large a part of our heritage" and the committee felt it was "fitting that it be published with the revised version so that it will remain a living historical treasure"; ibid., 2.

62. Ibid., 3–4.

63. Ibid., 11–12.

64. Jessie Black McVicar, "History Is the Past, the Present, and the Future," JHNAM 53 (July 1954): 81.

65. "The Johns Hopkins Roll Call," JHNAM 53 (Apr. 1954): 57.

66. "Gate House Shop Committee Report," JHNAM 53 (July 1954): 99.

67. JHNAM 57 (Apr. 1958): entire issue.

Chapter Four: The Handwriting on the Wall
LINDA SABIN

1. JHNAM 59 (Oct. 1960): 86; JHNAM 63 (Mar. 1964): 15.

2. JHNAM 60 (Apr. 1961): 17.

3. "What's New at Hopkins," JHNAM 63 (Mar. 1964): 15.

4. Committee members were Dr. Richard Mumma, dean of McCoy College; Virginia Betzold and Margaret Courtney, representing the faculty of the School of Nursing; Dr. Paul Lemkau, of the School of Hygiene and Public Health; and Dr. Edward Stafford, a faculty member at the School of Medicine.

5. Minutes of the Advisory Board of the School of Nursing, December 20, 1960, 27, AMCMA.

6. Ibid.

7. Ibid., June 21, 1960, 2, AMCMA.

8. Ibid.

9. Ibid.

10. Ibid.

11. Ibid.

12. Higgins Mill Pond was a corporate retreat located near Cambridge, Maryland. It was given to the university during Milton Eisenhower's administration and sold after a few years because the cost to maintain it was prohibitive.

13. Informal memorandum of a meeting at Higgins Mill to discuss the possibility of establishing a collegiate school of nursing at the Johns Hopkins University, May 25–26, 1963, JHNHC.

14. Ibid.

15. Minutes of the Advisory Board of the School of Nursing, October 3, 1963, 126, AMCMA.

16. Ibid.

17. Ibid.

18. Agenda and Minutes of the Advisory Board of the Medical Faculty, October 21, 1965, AMCMA.

19. Minutes of the Advisory Board of the School of Nursing, June 10, 1965, AMCMA; K. Virginia Betzold, "A School of Nursing in the University—A Cherished Dream," JHNAM 66 (Sept. 1967): 72.

20. Betty Cuthbert, interview by Janie Brown, July 10, 1987.

21. The association's Committee on Education prepared the position paper, which was approved by the board of directors in September 1965. "American Nurses' Association's First Position on Education for Nursing," American Journal of Nursing 66 (Mar. 1966): 515–17.

22. "American Nurses' Association First Position Paper on Education for Nursing," JHNAM 66 (Sept. 1967): 43–48. Reprinted from the American Journal of Nursing, December 1965.

23. Frances Reiter, "Preparation for Professional Nursing Practice," JHNAM 66 (Sept. 1967): 49–50.

24. Report of the Committee on Allied Medical Professions, February 1967, JHNHC.

25. Sarah E. Allison, "Report to the Alumnae Association of the Johns Hopkins Hospital School of Nursing from Representatives to the Advisory Board of the School of Nursing for the Years 1966–1967," JHNAM 67 (Mar. 1968): 10.

26. In 1966 the School of Arts and Sciences was created by the merger of the School of Engineering Sciences and the Faculty of Philosophy.

27. Sarah E. Allison, "Annual Report to Alumnae Association, from the Representatives to the Advisory Board of the School of Nursing," JHNAM 68 (Dec. 1969): 92–93.

28. Ibid.

29. "The Seventy-seventh Annual Meeting," JHNAM 68 (Dec. 1969): 87–88.

30. Ibid.

31. Minutes of the Advisory Board of the School of Nursing, January 4, 1968, 125, AMCMA.

32. Donna Dittberner, interview by Mame Warren, May 18, 2002.

33. Ibid.

34. JHNAM 60 (Dec. 1961): 50.

35. Lena Van Horn, "NLN Convention: Interaction—Key to Progress," JHNAM 60 (July 1961): 35–37.

36. "Dr. Nelson Has a New Title," JHNAM 62 (June 1963): 40.

37. Mary Ellen Miller, "Finding Meaning When There's No Cure Possible," The Dome (Jan. 1993): 1.

38. Betzold, "A School of Nursing in the University—A Cherished Dream," 72–73.

39. Clyde Shallenberger, e-mail interview by author, April 15, 1999.

40. Martha Hill, interview by Janie Brown, July 28, 1987.

41. Sarah E. Allison, "A Center for Nursing: An Historical Record," Vigilando 99 (Spring 2000): 6.

42. Ibid.

43. Minutes of the Advisory Board of the School of Nursing, November 1, 1960, 19, AMCMA.

44. Ibid., June 21, 1960.

45. Ibid., May 1, 1962.

46. At no time during the history of the diploma program did the graduates fail to perform above national and state averages on licensing examinations.

47. Dittberner, interview.

48. Sandra Stine Angell, interview by Mame Warren, August 6, 2003.

49. Minutes of the Advisory Board of the School of Nursing, June 2, 1966, 31–32, AMCMA.

50. Martha Norton Hill, interview by Mame Warren, March 30, 2000.

51. Faculty member Joan Williams fractured her ankle.

52. JHNAM 62 (June 1963): 42.

53. Angell, interview.

54. Alice Kiger, "School of Nursing News," JHNAM 63 (Mar. 1964): 15–16. Ethel Ensor was the director of Hampton House in 1963.

55. Susan Barker, "School of Nursing News," JHNAM 60 (Dec. 1961): 51.

56. Ibid.

57. Minutes of the Advisory Board of the School of Nursing, October 7, 1965, 14, AMCMA.

58. Ibid.

69. Ida Graham Price, "Pediatric Nursing Supervision Practicum," JHNAM 62 (June 1963): 35.

60. Herb Zinder, interview by Mame Warren, March 10, 2004.

61. Ibid.

62. Ethel A. Brooks, "Let's Keep the Nurse in Nursing," JHNAM 62 (Mar. 1963): 11.

63. Dittberner, interview.

64. Zinder, interview.

65. Sybil MacLean, "President's Report," JHNAM 60 (December 1961): 56.

66. Jessie B. McVicar, "Editorial," JHNAM 61 (December 1962): 83.

67. Lucile Petry Leone, "The Spectrum of Education for Nurses," *JHNAM* 67 (September 1967): 51–55; Betty Cuthbert, "Progress or Decline?": 56–62.

68. Betzold, "A School of Nursing in the University—A Cherished Dream."

69. Rozella Schlotfeldt, "The Responsibility of the University for Preparation of Members of the Health Professions," panel response in The Alumnae Association of the Johns Hopkins Hospital School of Nursing, "Response to Change in Health Services: Papers from the Seventy-Fifth Anniversary Program, November 3, 1967, 39–40, JHNHC.

Chapter Five: Tension and Triumph
MARY FRANCES KEEN

1. Minutes of the Advisory Board of the School of Nursing, March 1970, 42–52, AMCMA.

2. Ibid.

3. When the first male nurses, James Levya and Herb Zinder, graduated from the Johns Hopkins Hospital School of Nursing in 1971, the alumni association honored this landmark event by changing its bylaws and name to the gender-neutral "Alumni Association of the Johns Hopkins Hospital School of Nursing, Inc."

4. Press release May 18, 1970, subject file, "JHH School of Nursing—closing 1973," AMCMA.

5. Minutes of the Advisory Board of the School of Nursing, June 4 and May 25, 1970, 64–71, AMCMA; Sarah E. Allison and Betty L. Cuthbert, "The Future of Nursing at Hopkins, an Alternative Proposal," *JHNAM* 69 (Sept. 1970): 58–60.

6. Sarah E. Allison and Betty L. Cuthbert, "Leave No Stone Unturned," in "Alumnae Association 1970" file, JHNHC.

7. "Center for Allied Health Careers," *JHNAM* 70 (Mar. 1971): 14–15.

8. Martha Hill, secretary, "Report of the Johns Hopkins Hospital School of Nursing Alumnae Sponsored Conference on Suggestions for the Future of Nursing Education for the Proposal for the Center for Allied Health Careers, held April 16, 1971," in "University School of Nursing Planning" file, box 14, accession 2000.131, JHNHC.

9. Dr. I. Ridgeway Trimble et al. to President Lincoln Gordon, December 19, 1970, subject file, "JHH School of Nursing—closing 1973," AMCMA.

10. "Report to the Alumnae Association of the Johns Hopkins School of Nursing from the Alumnae Representatives to the Advisory Board of the School of Nursing, 1970–1971," *JHNAM* 70 (Dec. 1971): 76; Minutes of the Advisory Board of the Johns Hopkins Hospital School of Nursing, October 7, 1971, 1–2.

11. On March 12, 1971, Lincoln Gordon abruptly resigned and the board persuaded former president Milton Eisenhower to serve as interim president until the inauguration of Provost Steven Muller as president on February 1, 1972.

12. "Report to the Alumnae Association of the Johns Hopkins School of Nursing from the Alumnae Representatives to the Advisory Board of the School of Nursing, 1970–1971," *JHNAM* 70 (Dec. 1971): 77.

13. Minutes of the Advisory Board of the Proposed School of Health Services, October 22, 1971. Office of the Provost, series 4, subseries 2, RG 03.001, box 23, "School of Health Services Minutes, 1971–78," FHJA.

14. "Dr. Peterson Appointed Dean," *JHNAM* 71 (July 1972): 9; Dr. Robert Heyssel, interview by Janie Brown, July 20, 1987, JHNHC.

15. "Report to the Alumnae Association of the Johns Hopkins School of Nursing from the Alumnae Representatives to the Advisory Board of the School of Nursing, January–September 1972," *JHNAM* 72 (Jan. 1973): 10.

16. "Name Approved for the School of Health Services," *Johns Hopkins Gazette*, April 27, 1972.

17. Russell Nelson, "Director," *JHNAM* 72 (July 1973): 42.

18. Steven Muller, "Closing Remarks," ibid., 43–44.

19. Memorandum to the Academic Council, School of Health Services, January 25, 1974. Office of the Provost, series 4, subseries 2, RG 03.001, box 23, "School of Health Services Minutes, 1971–78," FHJA.

20. Doris Armstrong, interview by author, June 2, 1999.

21. "Fahy to Direct New Nursing Program," *Johns Hopkins Gazette*, September 6, 1973, 2.

22. Kay Partridge, interview by Mame Warren, July 16, 2004.

23. Jon Franklin, "Hopkins Health School Hit by Internal Politics," *Baltimore Evening Sun*, June 22, 1977, subject file, "JHU School of Health Services—closing," AMCMA.

24. Malcolm Peterson to Kay Partridge, June 1, 1977. Office of the Provost, series 4, subseries 2, RG 03.001, box 24, "School of Health Services—Nursing School, January–June 1977," FHJA.

25. Partridge, interview.

26. Memorandum from the Executive Committee of the Faculty Assembly of the School of Health Services to Steven Muller, June 9, 1977. Office of the Provost, series 4, subseries 2, RG 03.001, box 24, "School of Health Services—Nursing School, January–June 1977," FHJA.

27. Glen Fallin, "JHU Names Interim Nursing Director," *Baltimore News American*, June 27, 1977.

28. The School of Health Services received monies primarily the Robert Wood Johnson Foundation.

29. Carolyne Davis, interview by author, June 4, 1999.

30. Unsigned personal memorandum, probably written by Richard Longaker, March 29, 1977. Office of the Provost, series 4, sub-series 2, RG 03.001, box 24, "School of Health Services—Nursing School, January–June 1977," FHJA.

31. Doris Roberts to Mary Nash, chair of the school's Curriculum Committee, September 6, 1977. Ibid., "School of Health Services—Nursing School, July 1977–1979." Dr. Roberts' statements are fully supported by the minutes of the April 29, 1977, meeting of the Visiting Committee.

32. Doris Roberts to Malcolm Peterson, June 17, 1977. Office of the Provost, series 4, subseries 2, RG 03.001, box 24, "School of Health Services—Nursing School, July 1977–1979," FHJA.

33. Malcolm Peterson to Steven Muller, June 15, 1977. Ibid., "School of Health Services—Nursing School, January–June 1977."

34. "Hopkins Appoints Margaret Courtney Acting Head of Nursing Program," press release, June 23, 1977. Ibid.

35. Minutes of the Academic Council, January 24, 1978. Ibid., "School of Health Services—Nursing School July 1977–1979."

36. JHU press release, February 21, 1978, subject file, "JHU School of Health Services—closing," AMCMA.

37. Catherine Novak, interview by Mame Warren, June 28, 2004.

38. Susan Appling, interview by Janie Brown, July 15, 1987, JHNHC

39. "Candlelight Ceremony," *JHNAM* 79 (Mar. 1971): 11.

40. Catherine Novak, "Student News," *JHNAM* 71 (July 1972): 11.

41. Novak, interview.

42. Vahle, Robin, "Graduation: Joy and Tears," *JHNAM* 72 (July 1973): 44.

43. Susan Immelt, interview by Mame Warren, June 22, 2004.

44. Reikenis, Gale and Linda Benson, "JHU NEP," Alumni Association of the Johns Hopkins Hospital School of Nursing Newsletter, April 1976.

45. Eileen Gallagher Leahy, interview by Linda Sabin, April 15, 1999.

46. Alumni Association Newsletter, October 1973.

47. Michael G. Ventura memo to Russell A. Nelson, MD, September 23, 1971, in the Minutes of the Advisory Board of the Johns Hopkins Hospital School of Nursing, 130–32.

48. Ibid., June 25, 1975.

49. "M. Adelaide Nutting Endowment History and Recommendations," in "Reports, Minutes" file, June 1971–June 1975, JHH School of Nursing Advisory Board—Minutes (Oct. 1963–June 1975), RG 1 series a & c, box 1, AMCMA.

50. Betty L. Cuthbert, "Budget—July 1, 1978–June 30, 1979," *JHNAM* 78 (Jan. 1979): 3.

Sandra Stine Angell, 1969, received a BSN degree in 1977 from the Evening College of the Johns Hopkins University. A former president of the Johns Hopkins Nurses' Alumni Association, she is now associate dean for student affairs at the Johns Hopkins University School of Nursing. She was interviewed on August 6, 2003.

Sue Appling, 1973, received the final Elsie Lawler Award at the historic last graduation of the Johns Hopkins Hospital School of Nursing. In 1984 she became one of the first faculty members hired by the Johns Hopkins University School of Nursing, leaving in 2004 to be a nurse practitioner in the Prevention and Research Center at Mercy Hospital. She was interviewed on November 24 and December 1, 2002.

Maude Magill Bagwell, 1929, wrote "Don't Fence Me In: Memoirs of Maude Magill Bagwell, RN," which was privately published by William F. Bagwell in 1992.

Deborah Baker, 1992, MSN 1997, is an adult nurse practitioner and administrator in the Department of Surgery at the Johns Hopkins Hospital and a clinical instructor in the master's degree program of the School of Nursing. She is the current president of the Johns Hopkins Nurses' Alumni Association.

Gertrude H. Bowling, 1915, wrote *Side-lights on Life with a Shock Team* about her experiences during World War I in France.

Gert Brieger, MD, PhD, was the William H. Welch Professor and director of the Institute of Medicine in the Johns Hopkins University School of Medicine from 1984 to 2002.

Ada Davis joined the faculty in 1987 with an expertise in nursing history. She was interviewed on March 9, 2004.

Donna Dittberner, 1966, was a faculty member of the hospital school and a former president of the alumni association. She was interviewed in Woodstock, Illinois, on May 18, 2002. She died on September 7, 2003.

Sue Donaldson became the second dean of the Johns Hopkins University School of Nursing in 1994. She joined the research faculty in 2001 and holds a joint appointment as a professor of physiology in the School of Medicine. A fellow of both the National Academy of Nursing and the Institute of Medicine, National Academy of Sciences, she was interviewed on January 16, 2002.

Paula Einaudi was director and associate dean for development at the Johns Hopkins University School of Nursing from 1995 to 2000, following seven years as associate director. Now the vice president for development at Marymount University in Arlington, Virginia, she was interviewed on July 28, 2003, in Columbia, Maryland.

Dara Lawrence Geiser, 1991, MSN 1998, gave a graduation address on May 21, 1998. She is the assistant director of care management at the Kennedy Krieger Institute.

Carol Gray was the first dean of the Johns Hopkins University School of Nursing. Prior to that appointment in 1983, she had been on the nursing faculty or administration of five universities. She came to Johns Hopkins from the University of Washington, where she was on the faculty. She was interviewed for *Vigilando* as she prepared to leave the deanship in 1993.

Maravene Deveney Hamburger, 1937, worked in the Johns Hopkins Hospital after World War II, particularly with the "blue baby" patients of Dr. Alfred Blalock and Dr. Helen Taussig. She was interviewed on August 27, 1999.

Mary Farr Heeg, 1941, worked in the Johns Hopkins Hospital after graduation and served with General Hospital 118 in World War II. In 1951, after receiving a master's degree from the University of Chicago, she joined the faculty of the Johns Hopkins Hospital School of Nursing, where she taught in the Osler Clinic until her marriage in 1969. She was interviewed on July 21, 2003, in Vassalboro, Maine.

Robert Heyssel was the chief executive of the Johns Hopkins Hospital for twenty years, until he retired as president in 1992. He was interviewed in Seaford, Delaware, on November 28, 2000. He died on June 13, 2001.

Martha Norton Hill, 1964, earned her BSN degree from the Evening College in 1966. She served as a faculty member in the diploma school, the School of Health Services' Nursing Education Program, and the university school. She received a PhD degree from the Johns Hopkins School of Public Health and gained national recognition when she became the first nurse and the first nonphysician to serve as president of the American Heart Association. Hill directed the Center for Nursing Research until she became the third dean of the Johns Hopkins University School of Nursing in 2002. She was interviewed on March 30, 2000, and March 23, 2005.

Trudy Jones Hodges, 1959, received her baccalaureate degree from Johns Hopkins University upon graduation from the diploma school because she had previously completed two years at New York University. She worked at the Johns Hopkins Hospital until she left to pursue a master's degree at Teachers College, Columbia University. The first African-American president of the Maryland Board of Nursing, she retired as chairman of the nursing program at the Community College of Baltimore. She was interviewed on March 12, 2004.

Who We Are

Only nursing degrees earned at the Johns Hopkins Hospital School of Nursing or the Johns Hopkins University have been cited with the narrators' names. Unless noted otherwise, interviews were conducted by Mame Warren in Baltimore, Maryland.

Lois Grayshan Hoffer, 1962, worked at Johns Hopkins Hospital and in Harford County after becoming a registered nurse. She has remained active in the Johns Hopkins Nurses' Alumni Association and served on numerous committees as well as the board. She was interviewed on August 9, 2004.

Susan Carroll Immelt, 1977, was in the first class of the Nursing Education Program in the Johns Hopkins University School of Health Services, and in 2000, she became one of the earliest recipients of a PhD degree from the Johns Hopkins University School of Nursing. A faculty member at the school, she was interviewed on June 22, 2004, in Lutherville, Maryland.

Mary Frances Keen, 1970, is a coauthor of *Our Shared Legacy.* A former president of the Johns Hopkins Nurses' Alumni Association, in 1996 she became the first nurse alumna and the first woman to serve as president of the Johns Hopkins University Alumni Association. She is director of the undergraduate program and an associate professor at Villanova University College of Nursing.

Bernard Keenan, 1986, was president of the historic first class of the Johns Hopkins University School of Nursing. He received an MSN degree from the school in 1993. A part-time member of the faculty, he is also a psychiatric nurse the Johns Hopkins Hospital. The first male president of the alumni association, Keenan was interviewed on June 23, 2004.

Kate Knott, 2002, pursued nursing as a second career. After graduation she joined the adolescent unit of the Children's Medical and Surgical Center at the Johns Hopkins Hospital. A member of the board of the alumni association, she was interviewed on August 3, 2004.

Elaine Larson was the first to hold the M. Adelaide Nutting Chair in Clinical Nursing at the Johns Hopkins University School of Nursing. She arrived in 1985 and by 1987 she had instituted a postdoctoral program. She became the first director of the Center for Nursing Research in 1990, before leaving to become the dean of nursing at Georgetown University. She was interviewed at Columbia University, where she is associate dean and professor of pharmaceutical and therapeutic nursing, on March 14, 2003.

Maureen Maguire joined the faculty in 1985 as coordinator of nursing for child health and to teach strategies in nursing. She was interviewed on July 29, 2003.

Medea Marella, doctor of education from Columbia University, was the vice president of nursing at Sinai Hospital in 1982, when she was invited to serve on the steering committee for the formation of the Consortium for Nursing Education at the Johns Hopkins University. She remained a member of the consortium board as long as Sinai Hospital continued its membership. Once students arrived in 1984, Dr. Marella was responsible for their education as they participated in clinical rotations at Sinai. She was interviewed on August 5, 2004.

Stephen McClain was vice provost for academic planning and budget at the Johns Hopkins University when the School of Nursing was established, and he worked closely with the deans until he left that position in 2000. He was interviewed on January 15, 2005.

Betsy Mumaw McGeady, 1955, earned an associate's degree at Mount St. Agnes College before entering the hospital school, so she was awarded a BSN degree from the Johns Hopkins University's McCoy College at the time of her graduation. After raising her children, she returned to nursing at the Johns Hopkins Hospital, retiring in 1996 from the Children's Medical and Surgical Center. A former president of the alumni association, she was interviewed on June 21, 2004.

Steven Muller served as president of the Johns Hopkins University from 1972 to 1990 and of the Johns Hopkins Hospital from 1972 to 1983. He is on the faculty of the School of Advanced International Studies in Washington, D.C., where he was interviewed on March 15, 2001.

Cathy Novak, 1973, president of the last class of the hospital School of Nursing, received the Anna D. Wolf Award, for which the former director sent Novak the alumna pin she had received upon her own graduation in 1915. Today Novak is a manager for the National Center for Health Statistics, which sponsors the National Health and Nutrition Examination Survey. She was interviewed in Rockville, Maryland, on June 28, 2004.

Kay Partridge received a PhD degree from the Johns Hopkins School of Public Health in 1971. She assumed the directorship of the Nursing Education Program in the School of Health Services in 1974 and resigned in 1977. Subsequently, Partridge practiced law in Columbia, Maryland, until retiring to Rockport, Massachusetts, where she was interviewed on July 16, 2004.

William C. Richardson served as president of the Johns Hopkins University from 1990 to 1995. He is the president of the W. K. Kellogg Foundation in Battle Creek, Michigan, where he was interviewed on February 23, 2004.

Linda Emerson Sabin, 1967, is a coauthor of *Our Shared Legacy,* editor of the *Bulletin,* a publication of the American Association for the History of Nursing, and author of *Struggles and Triumphs: The Story of Mississippi Nurses, 1800–1950.* She is a professor in the Department of Concepts in the School of Nursing at the University of Louisiana at Monroe.

Betty Borenstein Scher, 1950, graduated from the College of William and Mary before attending the School of Nursing. As a result, she received a BSN degree from Johns Hopkins at the time she received her diploma, as did everyone else in her college-educated class at the School of Nursing. She pursued much of her nursing career at Sinai Hospital and has been active in the alumni association for more than fifty years, including serving as its president. She was interviewed on June 26, 2004.

Frances Schlosser Scherer, 1944, was born in China, where her parents were missionaries, and she returned there to work as a nurse educator after graduation from the School of Nursing. Her memoir, "To Be a Pilgrim," was published privately by her family. She was interviewed in Oak Park, Illinois, on May 14, 2002.

Stella Shiber was on the faculty of the hospital school and of the Nursing Education Program in the School of Health Services, and she was the first associate dean for undergraduate education at the Johns Hopkins University School of Nursing, where she was responsible for developing the curriculum. She retired in 2002 and was interviewed on September 16, 2003.

Marni Sommer, 1999, is a returned Peace Corps volunteer who completed the thirteen-month accelerated program. After completing a dual MSN/MPH degree in 2001, she worked for the Bureau of Global Health for three years. Sommer then began a doctoral program in social and behavioral medicine at Columbia University and became managing editor of the new journal *Global Public Health.* On June 3, 1999, Sommer addressed the Isabel Hampton Robb Society's annual dinner.

Benita Walton-Moss, 1978, was in the second class of the Nursing Education Program in the School of Health Services. She returned to Johns Hopkins to join the faculty of the master's program of the university school and to conduct research in the Center on Health Disparities Research. She was interviewed on June 29, 2004.

Ethel Rainey Ward, 1947, was a member of the U.S. Cadet Nurse Corps while a student during World War II. After graduation she was a psychiatric nurse in the Phipps Clinic for ten years. Ward was a director on the alumni board and chaired the M. Adelaide Nutting Endowment Fund Committee for many years. She was interviewed in Columbia, Maryland, on June 24, 2004.

Mame Warren is a coauthor and the editor of *Our Shared Legacy* and *Johns Hopkins: Knowledge for the World.* She is the director of Hopkins History Enterprises, based in the Sheridan Libraries. Before coming to Johns Hopkins, she produced a book for Washington and Lee University and was the author of six photographic books relating to Maryland history. A prominent oral historian, Warren is the former curator of photographs at the Maryland State Archives.

Constance Cole Heard Waxter, 1944, worked at Johns Hopkins Hospital after graduation. A past president of the alumni association, she was interviewed on July 14, 2004.

Herb Zinder, 1971, completed nurse anesthetist school at Johns Hopkins Hospital after becoming one of only two male graduates from the Johns Hopkins Hospital School of Nursing. He heads a private practice of nurse anesthetists. His son, Matt, graduated in the class of 1999, making them the first father/son nursing graduates of Johns Hopkins. Herb Zinder was interviewed on March 10, 2004, in Westminster, Maryland.

The Johns Hopkins Nursing Historical Collection, which is housed in the Alan Mason Chesney Medical Archives, now located on the Mount Washington campus, is a treasure trove of source materials pertaining to the history of nursing at Johns Hopkins and elsewhere. I encourage readers interested in pursuing further studies on the subject to explore its riches. The Chesney Medical Archives and the Ferdinand Hamburger Jr. Archives, on the Homewood campus, include vast amounts of useful information. The staffs at both facilities are extremely knowledgeable and helpful.

The endnotes of this book indicate precise citations for materials referenced. In general, all three authors consulted original documents, personal and official collections, biographical files, and newspaper clippings at the Chesney Medical Archives. I discovered records pertaining to early decisions regarding the hospital and its training school for nurses among the Gilman Papers in the Hamburger Archives, which is also the repository for the Records of the Office of the Provost. The latter include many details regarding the short-lived Nursing Education Program in the School of Health Services and decisions relating to the creation of the Johns Hopkins University School of Nursing. The university website, www.jhu.edu, is a readily available and invaluable source of information on a myriad of topics and people.

Publications concerning nursing and nursing education at Johns Hopkins were particularly helpful. I reviewed every issue of the *Johns Hopkins Nurses' Alumnae Magazine*, as well as copies of its later iterations, the *Vigilando* and *Johns Hopkins Nursing*. Information gleaned there and in Ethel Johns and Blanche Pfefferkorn's *Johns Hopkins Hospital School of Nursing, 1889–1949*—the essential reference work for the early years of nursing education at Johns Hopkins—and complete runs of the *Routine* and the *Dome*, the two yearbooks published by students, provided the basis for information included in the chronology and illustration captions.

A number of books and manuscripts were particularly helpful reference works:

Alumnae Association of the Johns Hopkins Hospital School of Nursing. *Alumnae Directory*. Baltimore: Alumnae Association of the Johns Hopkins Hospital School of Nursing, 1951.

Alumnae Association of the Johns Hopkins Hospital School of Nursing. *Within the Gates of the Johns Hopkins Hospital*. Baltimore: Alumnae Association of the Johns Hopkins Hospital School of Nursing, 1939.

Baldick, Jacqueline, and Paula Einaudi. *Hopkins Nursing, 1889–1989*. Baltimore: Johns Hopkins University, School of Nursing, [1989].

Cavagnaro, Louise. "Buildings of the Johns Hopkins Medical Institutions." 1989. Typescript. Rev. 1993 by Michael Iati; rev. 1994 by L. Cavagnaro and W. R. Day Jr.

French, John C. *A History of the University Founded by Johns Hopkins*. Baltimore: Johns Hopkins Press, 1946.

Gray, Carol J. "The Legacy and the Vision: The Johns Hopkins School of Nursing, 1982–1994." Johns Hopkins University, School of Nursing, 1998. Typescript.

Harvey, A. McGehee, Gert H. Brieger, Susan L. Abrams, and Victor A. McKusick. *A Centennial History of Medicine at Johns Hopkins*. Vol. 1 of *A Model of Its Kind*. Baltimore: Johns Hopkins University Press, 1989.

Harvey, A. McGehee, Gert H. Brieger, Susan L. Abrams, Jonathan M. Fishbein, and Victor A. McKusick. *A Pictorial History of Medicine at John Hopkins*. Vol. 2 of *A Model of Its Kind*. Baltimore: Johns Hopkins University Press, 1989.

Johns, Ethel, and Blanch Pfefferkorn. *The Johns Hopkins Hospital School of Nursing, 1889–1949*. Baltimore: Johns Hopkins Press, 1954.

Scherer, Frances E. "To Be a Pilgrim." Privately published, 1988.

Turner, Thomas B., MD. *Heritage of Excellence: The Johns Hopkins Medical Institutions, 1914–1947*. Baltimore: Johns Hopkins University Press, 1974.

Warren, Mame. *Knowledge for the World*. Baltimore: Johns Hopkins University, 2001.

Credits and Sources

a=above
al=above left
ar=above right
b=below
bl=below left
br=below right
c=center
l=left
r=right

Index

accommodations, 266–68
    See also Hampton House; Main Residence
Allen, Jerilyn, 212, *213*
Allison, Sarah, 97, *98*, *140*, 141–42, 152, 155, 168, 278–80
alumni association, 4–5, 30, 152, 251
    archives project, 284, 286–87
    clubhouse, 40, *40–41*, 263, *263*
    code of ethics, 112, *112*, 263, 274, 276, 293n61
    cookbook, 280
    Endowed Bed Fund, 41, 153, 284
    endowment fund, 42–45, *81*, 265–67
    History Committee, 276, 282–83
    history of school, 112–13, *113*, 276
    history research, 271, 274–75
    and JHU SON building, 246, *246*, *249*, *255*
    library, 272–73
    magazines, 284, 287
    membership changes, 283, 285
    motto, 42, *44*, 262
    name changes, 114, 270, 277, 279, 281–82, 294n3
    newsletter, 283
    100th anniversary, 284
    origins, 42, *43*, 262
    recommendations for future nursing education, 133, 155, 169–70
    75th Anniversary, 152–53, *154–55*
    Sick Benefit Fund, 262, 277–78, 284
    symposium on university nursing education, 152–53, *154–55*
    See also Gate House Shop; *Johns Hopkins Nurses' Alumni Magazine*; M. Adelaide Nutting Endowment Fund for the School of Nursing
Amberson, Katherine Good, *116*
American Association of Superintendents of Training Schools for Nurses, 11, 263
    See also National League for Nursing
American Journal of Nursing, 10, 37
American Nurses Association (ANA), 10–12, 87–88, 133, 230, 278
American Red Cross, *31*, *32–33*
    Nursing Service, 32, 34, *267*, 271–72, *273*
    alumni serving in, 32, 34, *266*, 266, *272*
Ames, Joseph Sweetman, 269
Ames, Miriam, *21*, 95, 272–73
Andrews, Margaret, 278
Angell, Sandra Stine, xvi, *221*, 244, 248, *254*, 259, 285
    and alumni, 193, 203, 205, 242, 282
    director of admissions, 212, 214, 219–20, 234
    student, 118, 130, 133, 136, *144*, 146, 155, 278
Anna D. Wolf Chair, 283–84
Appling, Sue, 120, 145, *170*, *183*, 185, 187, 192, 194, 197, *199*, 238, 246
    faculty member, 212, *215*, 215, 218–20, 222
Arenth, Linda, *283*, 283
Armstrong, Doris, 168–69, *169*, 171–72, 175–76, 279–81
Army Nurse Corps, 15
Aronson, Jeanne Regan, *152*
Aschenbrenner, Diane, *240*
Associated Alumnae of Trained Nurses of the United States and Canada, 11, 263
    See also American Nurses Association
Association of Collegiate Schools of Nursing, 87
Athey, Helen Wilmer, 23–25, 56, *82–83*, *89*, 150
    donations, *264*, 264, 271, 275, 277
    Gate House shopkeeper, *114*, 114
Aydelotte, Jeannie, *185*

Babcock, Charity, *30–31*, 31–32, *156*
Backscheider, Joan, 142, 278, 280
Backwash of War (LaMotte), *39*, 39–40,
Bagwell, Maude Magill, 20, 268–69
Bahne, Emily, *287*
Baker, Bessie, *15*, *34–35*, 34–35, 265
Baldick, Jackie, 249
Baretto, Pam, *iv*, *1*
Barnard, Helena, 42, 262–63
Barnard, Mildred E., 114, 275
Bartlett, Vashti, 32, *32–33*, *116*, *156*
Barwick, Ethel, 41, 263
Base Hospital No. 18, 34–35, *35–37*, 37, 266
basketball league, *145*, 146, 277
Baxter, Grace, 35, *36*, 37
Beach, Janet, 277
Beaux, Cecilia, 264
Becker, Kathleen, *258*
Bellevue Hospital, 9–10
Benson, Linda, 189–90
Berger, Olive, *66–67*
Berk, Ronald, *238*, 285
Bernhard, Barbara, 185–86, 279
Betzold, K. Virginia, 27, 59–60, 127, 153, *154–55*, 167, 280, 283, 293n4
    associate director of JHH SON, 63–64, *97*, 100–101, 138–39, 143
    instructor, *21*, *61*, 270
    retirement, 139, 277
Big Sister–Little Sister program, 118, 120, *144*, 144, 147–48, *185*
Billings, John Shaw, xiv, 6
Billman, Linda, *178*
Blalock, Alfred, 66, *66–67*, 90, 104
Bledsoe, Turner, 175, 280
Block, James A., 242, *243*, 284
Bloomberg, Michael, *244*, 246, 285
Boise, Margaret G., *269*
Boland, Mary, *43*
Boley, Elizabeth, *9*
Bolton Act of 1943, 80
Bonovich, Leah, 212
Booker, Sophie, *48–49*
Borowicz, Jeanne, *189*
Bowling, Gertrude H., 32
Bowman, Isaiah, 274
Boykin, Nancy, 195
Boyle, Katherine, *190*
Brack, Annabelle Gleason, 283
Brady, James Buchanan ("Diamond Jim"), 265
Brager, Rosemarie, 247
Bridgeman, Margaret, 91–94
Bridgeman Report, 91–94, 96, 100, 103
Brinkley, Jean, *143*
Brix, Adele Sparks, 106
Brizendine, Elizabeth, 283
Brody, William R., 253, 286–87
Brooks, Ethel A., 150
Brown, Esther Lucille, 65, 292n32
Brown Report, 65, 100, 110, 292n32
Bryn Mawr College, 59
Bullough, Bonnie, xiv
Bullough, Vern, xiv

Numerals in **bold italics** refer to illustration and photo caption pages. Page numbers preceding an "n" refer to endnotes pages, followed by the specific note number. JHU refers to the Johns Hopkins University. JHH refers to the Johns Hopkins Hospital. SON refers to the Johns Hopkins Schools of Nursing.

Bushel, Arthur, 175, 280
Butz, Arlene, 226, 283
Buzzard, Jim, 121
Byrnes, Geri, 170

Cabot, Richard, 110, 133, 292n55
Campbell, Jacquelyn, 212, 234–35, 259, 284
candlelight ceremony, 108, 118, 185–86, 272, 275, 279
caps
    See uniforms, caps
Carlson, Dennis, 169, 171, 278–79, Carr, Ada, 264–65
Carpenter Foundation
    See E. Rhodes and Leona B. Carpenter Foundation
Cater, George, 266
Caulfield, Kathleen, 48–49
Cavell, Edith, 291n64
Center for Allied Health Careers, 169–74, 279
Center for Experimentation and Development in Nursing, 140, 142, 278–80
Center for Health Disparities Research, 247, 287
Center for Nursing Research, 213, 226, 251, 259, 284
Cerniglia, Laurie, 213
Chadwick, Debbie, 186
Chapman, Emma, 46–47
Chesney, Alan M., 64
Child Life Program, 60, 60, 273
Children's Medical and Surgical Center, 119, 123, 125, 126–27, 253, 278
Christus Consolator, 72
Church Home and Hospital, 203–5, 207, 209–11, 216, 218–19
Cohen, Hal, 203
Collegiate Education for Nursing
    See Bridgeman Report
Collins, Mary B., 142, 278, 280
Committee for the Study of Nursing Education. See Goldmark Report
Committee for the 21st Century at Hopkins, 253
Committee on Allied Medical Professions, 134
Committee to Secure by Act of Congress the Employment of Women Nurses in the Hospital Service of the United States Army Nurse Corps, 12–13, 15
community outreach, 130, 196–99, 196–99, 241
Connors, Peter, 232–33
Conover, Alice B., 263
Consortium for Nursing Education, 201, 207, 243, 282
Cook, Susan Dieterle, 152
Cooley, Denton, 90
Courtney, Margaret, 100–101, 128, 135, 138, 146, 155, 286, 293n4
    assistant director of JHH SON, 139, 275, 277
    associate director of JHH SON, 139, 140–41, 277
    director of JHH SON, 168, 172, 180, 279
    director of Nursing Education Program, 180–81, 184–85, 281
    faculty member, Evening College, 180, 204–5, 281
Coverdell, Paul, D., 248, 283

Cox, Mary Claire, 78
Coyne, Karin, 286
Craig, Margaretta, 150–51
Crosby, Edwin L., 63, 90–91, 91, 273–74, 276
Cushman, Peg, 146
Cuthbert, Betty L., xvi, 152–53, 168, 193, 195, 195, 246, 280, 282, 284
    faculty member, 131, 140, 141, 184–85
    and Nutting Fund, 202, 208–9, 281–82
    student, 22, 68

Daniels, Worth, 213
Davis, Ada, xii, xvi, 4–5, 207–9, 212, 238, 239, 241, 246, 247, 250
    on Hill, 253, 255
Davis, Carolyne, 179–80, 206
Dear, Margaret, 212
Delano, Jane, 32, 34
DeLong, Katherine, 263
DeYoung, Joan Verlee, 60
Diabetic Nurse Management Clinic, 142, 278
Dias, Dana Cohen, 189
Dick, Christine, 21, 81, 81, 105, 158, 266, 273
Diehl, Isabelle C., 271
Dienemann, Jacqueline, 285
Diggs, Angela, 165
Diller, Doris, 66
Dines, Alta Elizabeth, 114, 114
Dispensary Visiting Nurse Service, 95–96, 196–98, 276
Dittberner, Donna, 133, 139–40, 202
    faculty member, 149, 170, 207
    student, 118–19, 125, 129, 137, 143–44, 147, 151
Dixon, Mary Bartlett, 263
D'Lugoff, Marion Isaacs, 199, 234–35, 241, 284
Dobratz, Marjorie Clowry, 282
Dock, Lavinia, 10, 12, 22, 22, 109, 262, 265, 277
Dodge Commission, 13, 15
Doetsch, Agnes J., 102, 277
Donaho, Barbara Russell, I, III, 241, 244
Donaldson, Sue, xv, 194
    compared to Gray, 234, 236–39
    dean of JHU SON, 234, 234–35, 238–41, 253, 259, 284, 286
    faculty member, 251, 287
    and Pinkard Building, 242–44, 243–45, 246, 248, 285
Donough, Mary Jane, 92, 141, 185
Donovan, Ann Poorman, 142, 278
Dougherty, Jeanne, 122–23
Dunbar, Virginia, 80, 109–10, 114

Earnest, Mary, 273
East Baltimore campus, 252
Eastern Health District, 196–97, 198, 258, 269–70, 272, 276
"Education and Professional Position of Nurses, The" (Nutting), 12
Einaudi, Paula
    and alumni, 42, 166, 192, 255
    JHH SON background, 4, 25, 53, 66, 92
    and JHU SON, 207, 226, 230, 236, 249–50, 253
    and Pinkard Building, 241–42, 244, 245, 246, 248

Eisenhower, Milton, 103, 127–28, 130–31, 134, 171, 277–78, 294n11
Elsie M. Lawler Professorship, 216, 283
E. Rhodes and Leona B. Carpenter Foundation, 285
Evans-Agnew, Robin, 258
Evans, G. Heberton, 128
Evening College, Division of Nursing, 168, 180, 204–6, 277–79, 281, 285
    See also McCoy College
Everhart, David, 278
Ewell, Charlotte, 40, 263

Fall-Dickson, Jane, 237
Fallon, Helen Grose, 113
Filler, Dorothy D., 44
Finkelstein, Harold, 28
Finney, Helen Peters, 204
Finney, John M. T., 34, 125
Fischer, Charlotte, 77, 272
Fitzgerald, Alice, 35, 36–37, 37–38, 39, 150, 271
Fitzpatrick, Louise, 278
Flatley, Anna Buchko, 204
Flexner, Abraham, 293n55
Flexner Report, xiii, 110
Fliedner, Pastor, xi
Florence Nightingale Medal, 109, 110, 150, 150
Foard, Virginia McMaster, 266
Foreman, Spencer ("Spike"), 200–201, 203–5, 210
Fox, Elizabeth, 267
Fralic, Maryann, 240–41, 284
France-Merrick Foundation, 243, 243, 248, 284–85
Freadkin, Esther Weber, 21
Frederick, Hester, 21, 21–22, 68, 81, 269
Freeman, Ruth, 134, 196
Frei, Colleen, iv, I
French, Helen, 89
Frisby, Ben, 28, 269
Fry, Elizabeth, xi
Furgess, Lois Ann, 172–73, 279
"Future of the School of Nursing," 166

Gaintner, Richard, 208
Gaston-Johansson, Fannie, 234–35, 247, 259, 286
Gate House Shop, 114–15, 202, 267–68, 271, 274
    closure, 125, 277
    committee, 69, 70, 114, 276
Gautier, Mary Agnes, 72, 75–76, 78, 80
Geiser, Dara Lawrence, 257, 286
General Hospital No. 18, 58, 75, 75–78, 272–73
General Hospital No. 118, 47, 58, 72, 72, 75–79, 160, 272–73
George, Mary Flynn, iv, I
Gerhart, Mabel, 275
Gilman, Daniel Coit, 9, 153
Glaser, Erika, 146
Goldmark, Josephine, xiii, 293n55
Goldmark Report of 1923, xiii, 44, 110, 266
Goldthwaite, Mary, 69
Gonsalves, Stephen, 287

Good, Jan, *131*

Goodnow, Frank, 44

Goodrich, Annie, 109

Gordon, Dorothy, *216*, 283

Gordon, Lincoln, 134–35, 167–68, 171, 278–79, 294n11

Goucher College, 59, 131, 135, 272–73

graduations, *28*, 28, *64*, 277–78

Graffin, George W., 40, 263

Graffin, William, 263

Grainger, Margaret, 56, 68, *68–69*

Gray, Carol, *iv*, 44, 211, *249*, **283**
  characteristics, 206–7
  compared to Donaldson, 234, 236–39
  dean of JHU SON, *201*, 203, *203*, **209**, 212, *215*, 230, *231*, *248*, 253, 259, *261*
  director of Evening College's Division of Nursing, 206–7, *207*, 281
  and Pinkard, 231, *243*, 243, 248, 286
  and Heyssel, 227
  resignation, 230–31, 284

Great Depression, 16–18, 48, 84, *158*, 269

Greenfield, Lucy, *160*

Griggs, Carolyn, *134*, *279*

Gross, Mary, 290n35

Guerrero, Christiani, *121*

Guthrie, Mary, 275–76

Hahn, Anne, *21*, 64

Hall, Sue, *198*

Haller, Karen, *234–35*, 257

Halsted, William, *15*

Hamburger, Maravene Deveney, 16–18, 20, 23

Hampton, Isabel
  See Robb, Isabel Hampton

Hampton House, 27, 59, *61*, *74*, *105*, 144, *159*, 267–69, 271
  opening of, *26*, 26, 268, *270*

Hanson, Rebecca, *iv*, *1*

Harlan, Henry D., 269

Harms, Mary T., 114

Harriet Lane Home for Invalid Children, *17*, *19*, *55*, *101*, 125, *253*, 265, *268*, 273, *278*
  integration of patients, 27, 87

Harriman, E. Roland, 150

Harris, Julia, 275

Harrison, Valerie Simmons, *202*

Hawkins, Margaret, 71

Hay, Mabel, *21*, 28

Health Services Cost Review Commission (HSCRC) of Maryland, 209–10

Heeg, Mary Farr, *96*, 116, 127, *141*, 141, *198*, 277, 284
  with General Hospital No.118, *46–47*, 79, 79, *160*
  instructor, 80, *92*, 101
  student, 27–28

Heeg, Tom, 141

Hemler, Cathy, *191*

Henderson, Alice E., 32

Heriot, Mary, 263

Heyman, Amy Berman, *218*

Heyssel, Robert M., xii, 173–74, *200–201*, 202, 204–5, 208, 210, **227**, 227, 280–81
  JHU SON creation, 203, 206–7, 209, 257, 284

Hickey, Shelagh, *143*

Higgins Mill Pond meeting, 128–31, 277, 293n12

Hill, Martha Norton, 20, 175, 196, 198, 211–12
  dean of JHU SON, 248, *251*, 251–53, 255, 257, 259–61, 287
  director of Center for Nursing Research, *213*, 251, 284
  faculty member, *184–85*, 185, 204–6, 220, *234–35*, *237*, *251*
  on Pinkard Building, 241, 243
  president of American Heart Association, 252–53, 259, 285
  student, 129, *132–33*, 133, 137, *139*, 144, *145*, 151

History of Nursing (Dock & Nutting), 22

Hodges, Trudy Jones, 93, 96, 99, 104, 106, 119, 277

Hoffer, Lois Grayshan, xvi, 205, 239
  student, 86, 95, 108, 117, 130, *131*, 142, 156
  on faculty, 140, 143, 147

Hollowell, Mabel Gerhart, *70*, 101, 107

Holmes, Deborah Chadwick, *170*

Hopkins, Johns, xii, 6, **27**, 262

Hopkins, Kathy, 95

Hoptown, *159–60*

Horn, Francis, 64, 87, 274

Hospital for Consumptives of Maryland, 125

Hurd, Henry, xii, 9, 40, 42, **262**, 262

Hurlock, Paul, *90*

Hutchins, Marie, *21*

Immelt, Susan Carroll, 177, *188*, 189, 194, 202, 206, 251–52
  on Donaldson, 234, 239
  on PhD program, 236–37, *237*, 286

infirmary, 270–71

influenza pandemic of 1918, 266

Institute for Johns Hopkins Nursing, 240–41, 285, 287

Instructive Visiting Nurse Association, 41, 265

Irvine, Agnes Ysobel, 13

Jacoby, Esther, *80*, 80, 100, 141

Jarrett, Mary, *185*

James, Janet, xii

James, Lucy Wortham, 267

Jammé, Anna, 267

Jenkins, Nancy, *183*

Johns, Ethel, xiv, 112–13, 274–76, 282

Johns Hopkins Hospital, 6, 262, 268, 270, 277
  budget, *9*
  expansion, 17, 125
  integration, 27, 87

Johns Hopkins Hospital School of Nursing
  accelerated program, 58–59
  accreditation, 94, 103
  admission requirements, 60–61, 84–86, 136–37, 273
  Advisory Board, 17–18, 45, 57, 60, 86, 131, 135, 271, 279–80
  alumnae, *127*, 150–51, *151*
  baccalaureate program, 64–65, 125–29, 134, 271, 277
  Christmas at, *28–29*, *107*, 107
  closing of diploma school, 166, 175, 183, 185–88, 192
  commencement, *165*, *186*, 187–88
  curriculum changes, 18, 56–58, 103, 144, 273, 275–76
  diploma model, 84–87, 93, 130
  dual track, 91, 92–93, 96
  enrollments, 143–44, 266, 272
  faculty, 18, *21*, 66, 68, 94–95, *99*, 101, *138–139*, *167*, 185, 271
  founding of, xii, 6, 9
  grading system, *99*, 99
  history of school, 112–13
  integration of, *87*, 99, 106, *111*, 148
  international students, *96*
  library, 22, 22, *61*, *104*, 270
  recruitment, 59–60, *95*, 96, 103
  relationship to JHU, xiii–xiv, 60–61, 64–66, *66*, 127–31, 267, 271, 273
  relationship to Teachers College, 18, 20, 54–55, 271
  scholarships, 96, 276
  Student Association, 56, 69

Johns Hopkins Hospital School of Nursing, 1889–1954 (Johns and Pfefferkorn), xiv, 112–13, *113*, 276

Johns Hopkins Hospital Training School for Nurses of Baltimore City, 6, 9, *42*, 262–63, 269–70
  applicants, 263–64

Johns Hopkins Medical Institutions. *See* East Baltimore campus

Johns Hopkins Nurses Alumnae Magazine, 42, 264–65, 280

Johns Hopkins Nurses' Registry, 40, 263, 273–74

Johns Hopkins University School of Health Services, 173–76, 207–8
  academic council, 176
  baccalaureate program, 177, 190
  closing of, 181, 190, 192, 281
  feasibility study, 134–35, 278
  See also Nursing Education Program

Johns Hopkins University School of Hygiene and Public Health, 236

Johns Hopkins University School of Nursing, *201*, 202, 261, 282, 287
  accelerated program, 222–24, 250, 283, 286–87
  accreditation, 219–21, 239, 285, 287
  Anne M. Pinkard Building, iv, 241–44, *243–45*, 246, *247*, 248, *249*, *260–61*, 285, 285–86
  classroom space, *209*, *215*, *220–21*, 241, *242*, 250, 257
  clinical rotations, 253, 255–57, *256*
  consortium with Church Home and Sinai Hospitals, 203–5, 207, 209, 210–11, *216*, 217–19, 283
  curriculum, *215*, 217, 225, 283
  DNSc program, 286
  enrollment, 214, 287
  Johnson & Johnson funding, 224–25, 283
  library, *252*
  master's program, *226*, 282–83
  MSN/MBA program, 236, 251, 257, 285
  MSN/MPH program, 198, 236, 251, 257, 285
  partnership with Peking Union Medical College, 287
  PhD program, 230, 234, 236–37, 285
  rankings, 239, *254*, 261, 285–87

Johns Hopkins University School of Professional Studies in Business and Education, 236

Johnson, Jean, 180

Johnson & Johnson, 224–25, 283

Jones, H. Alvan, 76, 78, 273

Jones, Margaret Porter, *iv*, *1*
Jones, Ross, 281
Jordan, Betty, *287*
Jordan, Gerry, *92*

Kaschel, Eleanor Summers, 70
Kazamek, Marlene, *165*
Keeler, Mary, *160*
Keen, Mary Frances, *191*, 251, 285
Keenan, Bernard, 121, 246, 251
    on Appling, 217–18, 220
    on JHU SON, 205–6, 208, 218–21, 230,
       236, 259
    on Shiber, *213*, 214–15, 220
Kelly, Edmund S., 28
Kelly, Howard, *267*, 267
Kennedy, John F., 124
Kennedy, Katie, *105*
Kennedy, Loula E., *21*, *61*, 63, *89*, 275
    library, *22*, 22, *61*, *104*
Kidd, Langford, *222*
Kiger, Alice, 147
Kim, Miyong T., *239*
King, Francis, xi
King, Martin Luther Jr., *146*, 146, 278
Kinlein, M. Lucille, 142, 278
Kinney, Dita H., 15
Kirby, Carolyn, *170*, *185*
Kirby, Nell, 172, 279
Knight, Harold, 268
Knott, Kate, 121, 197, 224, 238, 251, 253, 256–57
Koch, Moses S., 169
Kolb, Louisa, *21*
Komoroski, Chris, *170*
Korniewicz, Denise, *226*, 283
Kuntz, Mary, 57–58
Kurtz, Ethna, *21*
Kushto-Reese, Kathy, *236*
Kuzmikis, Dennis, *248*

Lambert, Claire, *120*
LaMotte, Ellen, *15*, *39*, 39–40
Larson, Elaine, 4, 12, 15, 212, 217–18, 224–26,
    236, 259
    director of Center for Nursing Research,
      226
    Nutting Chair, *225*, 282–83
Lashinsky, Jean, *120*
Lawler, Elsie, *ii*, *iv*, 2, *14–15*, 26–27, 44, 76, *82–83*,
    89, 101–2, 114, 150, *158*, 270–71, 277
    achievements, 20–21
    discipline, 20, 25
    retirement, 21, 51, *52*, 68, *102*, 114
    superintendent of nurses and principal of
      JHH SON, 3, *16*, 16–18, *21*, 27–29, 196, *265*,
      266–68, 275
League of Red Cross Societies, *39*, 39
Leahy, Eileen Gallagher, 190
Lee, Peggie-Louise, *105*
Legters, Elva McMahon, *151*
LeHew, Bonnie, *167*, *170*, *182–83*
Lemkau, Paul, 127
Lent, Mary, 41, 267

Leone, Lucile Petry, 26, 109, 150, 152, 175, 280,
    285
    assistant surgeon general of U.S. Public
      Health Service, 80, 275, 277
    director of U.S. Cadet Nurse Corps, *59*, 80,
      275
Letocha, Phoebe Evans, 287
Levya, Jim, *149*, 149, 152, 278–79
Liechty, Jacqueline, *151*
Lillian D. Wald Community Nursing Center,
    199, *241*, 284–85
Lochow, Mafalda, 172, *173*, 279
Loeffler, Catherine M., 21
Long, Laurel Gene, *151*
Long, Loretta, *198*
Longaker, Richard P., 179, 180–81, 204, 207, 212,
    281
Lowder, Marlene, *85*
Lowe, Marie, 27, 271
Lucy, Joan, *90*

M. Adelaide Nutting Chair of Nursing, 15,
    194–95, *225*, 280, 282
M. Adelaide Nutting Endowment Fund for
    the School of Nursing, 63, 81, 192–95,
    269–71, 285, *286*
    committee, 42–45, 192–93, 265, 268
    contributions to School of Health Services,
      193, 208, 281
    and SON's advisory board, 193–94, 217,
      279–81
    and university-based nursing, 152, 155
MacSherry, Mary, *97*
Maguire, Maureen, 12, 174, 181
    faculty member, 212, *214*, 218–19, 221, 223–24,
      234–36, 249
    on clinical rotations, 255–56, 257
Main Residence, *12–13*, *24*, 26, 59, 192, *264*, 265,
    280
    library, *22*, 22, *61*, *104*, 112, 280
    Mary Adelaide Nutting Educational Unit,
      83, *89*, *93*, *275*, 275
male nurses, 8–9, 149, 211, 214, *223*, 275, 278
Mallory, Cynthia, *68–69*
Maltese cross pin, *44*, 64, 120, 190, *261*, 262,
    276, 282, 285, 291n73
Marburg, Charles L., 265
Marchum, Melinda, *216*
Marella, Medea, 45, 203, 205, 207, 209–12, *216*,
    217, 224, 257–60
Martineau, Harriet, xi
Maryland State Association of Graduate
    Nurses, 264, 268
Maryland State Board of Examiners of
    Nurses, 281–82
Mason, Phyllis, *232–33*
McClain, Stephen, 204, 210–11, 218–19, 224–25,
    282
    on Donaldson, 237–38, 240
    on Heyssel, 206–9, 227
    on Hill, 248, 252, 255, 260
McCoy College, 64–65, 87, 127–29, 274–75,
    277, 285
    See also Teachers College; Evening College
McDonnell Foundation, 283
McGaw, George K., 266

McGeady, Betsy Mumaw, 160, 192, 211–12, 250,
    252–53
    alumni activity, 41, 112, 155, 193, *202*, 246
    nurse, 110, 120
    student, 84, 88, 92, 97, 99, 103–5, 118
McLaughlin, Elizabeth, 76, 272
McVicar, Jessie Black, 63, 113, *131*, *139*, 152, 272,
    274, 277
Medicaid, 136, 150
Medicare, 136, 150
Meerholz, Ed, 211
Meloche, John, 277
Melosh, Barbara, xiii
Mercy Ship, 32
Miller, Amy P., 44, 275
Miller, Dawn, *183*
Miller, Edward, *249*
Miller, Hilda, *21*
Morgan, Russell, 133–34, 153, 278
Morris, Ira, 185
Moser, Elizabeth, 70, 277
Muldrew, Gertrude, 32
Muller, Steven, 172, 175, 280–82
    president of JHH and JHU, 174, *175*, 178–81
    and JHU SON, 203–5, 207, 224
Mullin, Bernadette, *21*
Mumma, Richard, 64, 127–29, 168, 293n4
Murphy, Marion, 175, 280
Musco, Pauline, 281

Nathans, Dan, 242
National Association of Colored Graduate
    Nurses, 87
National Association of Student Nurses, 230
National Center for Medical Rehabilitation
    Research, *216*
National Council Licensure Examination for
    Registered Nurses (NCLEX), 219, 287
National League for Nursing, 12, 87–88, 94,
    103, 149, 230, 239, 276, 285
    exams, 220–21
    and Nursing Education Program, 177–78,
      204, 281
National League for Nursing Education, 11,
    66, 87, 266, 276
National Nursing Council, 65
National Nursing Council for War Service, 58
National Organization of Public Health
    Nurses, 87
Nelson, Karen, *186*
Nelson, Russell, xii, 16, 103, *107*, 174, 279–80
    director of Johns Hopkins Hospital, 90–91,
      91, 277
    and nursing education, 127–31, *131*, *138–39*,
      142, 152, *153*, 166–68, 175, 278–79
Nelson, Ruth Jeffcoat, 16, 91, 139, *153*
Nevins, Georgia, 12, 42, *43*
Newpher, Sue, *170*
Nightingala, 284
Nightingale, Florence, xi–xii, 6, *31*, 266–67, 275
Nikel, Edith D., 281
Nix, Kathy, *186*
Norris, Linda, 195
Northam, A. Ethel, *89*
Notes on Nursing (Nightingale), xi

Novak, Cathy, xv, 10, 15, 65, 117, 141, 162, 168, 171–72, 176, 227
  Anna D. Wolf Award, 188, 280
  on closing of JHH SON, 183–88
Noyes, Clara Dutton, 32, 34, 34–35, 267
Nunn, Edith A., 78
nurse anesthetists, 66–67, 269
nurses in the military, 13, 15, 30, 31–32, 34, 72, 74–80, 272
  See also Base Hospital No. 18; General Hospital No. 18; General Hospital No. 118
Nurses' Club, 40–41, 40–41, 263, 263, 271
Nurses' Home
  See Main Residence
Nurses' Journal Club, 262
Nursing
  history of, xii–xiii, 12
  philosophy of, viii, 87–88
  as a profession, xii, 10, 15, 20, 89–90, 133, 252, 258, 262, 278
  shortages, 61, 63, 72, 84–86, 95, 202–4, 272, 274, 287
Nursing Council on National Defense, 48
nursing education, general, 133, 267, 278
  PhD programs, 234
  two-year programs, 103
Nursing Education Program in the School of Health Services, 163, 169, 172, 177, 281
  acting director, 180–81
  accreditation issues, 177–80, 204, 281
  alumni, 190–91
  director search, 175–76, 280
  nursing subcommittee, 172–73, 279
  students, 183, 188–90, 188–91, 280, 281
  See also JHU School of Health Services
Nursing for the Future
  See Brown Report
Nursing News, 283
nursing students, 265
  activities, 27–28, 69–71, 70, 144–46, 156–63
  caroling, 27–28, 28, 106
  classes, 19, 56–57, 88, 94, 103
  and Harriet Lane Home, 55, 101, 253, 265, 268, 273
  in 1950s, 104–9
  in 1960s, 124, 144–4
  preclinical, 71, 108
  probationers, 23, 24, 26, 54, 71, 264, 271
  schedules (1930s), 17, 19, 23–27, 74, 103
  service v. education, 10, 60, 96, 274
  volunteers, 71
  and World War II, 72, 74–76, 78
  yearbooks, 26, 137, 267–69
Nutting, Mary Adelaide, xiii, 62–63, 63, 266, 281
  and alumnae, 30, 42–45, 62–63
  death of, 63, 81, 275
  instructor, 14–15, 16, 22
  and military, 12–13, 15
  student, 22, 45, 262
  superintendent of nurses and principal of JHH Training School, 12, 12–13, 25, 25, 263–64, 268
  at Teachers College, Columbia University, 15, 45, 264–65, 275
  and university-based nursing education, 15, 155

Olmstead, Katherine, 38–39, 38–39, 41
ophthalmia neonatorum, 41
Ordered to Care (Reverby), xiii

Orem, Dorothea D., 142, 278
O'Shea, Joyce, 207
Osler, William, xii, 6, 9, 9, 40–41, 188, 262, 280
Osler Medical Clinic, 85

Packer, Liz, 216
Packer, Sophie, 16, 21
Parran, Thomas, 80
Parsons, Louisa, 262
Partridge, Kay, 166, 169, 172, 174–76, 177, 189–190, 195, 279, 280
  resignation from Nursing Education Program, 177–81, 191, 281
Peace Corps program, 248, 249–51, 283
Peck, Steve, 244
Pennington, Caroline, 283
Peterson, Malcolm L., 280–81
  dean of School of Health Services, 173–74, 188, 195
  nonsupporter of nursing, 175, 177, 180–81
  and Partridge, 176–78, 191
Pfefferkorn, Blanche, xiv, 89, 112–14, 113, 275–76, 282
  "On Nursing Education," 267
Phipps, Henry, 265
Phipps Building, 3, 209, 215, 220–21, 231, 241, 242, 266, 282
Phipps Psychiatric Clinic, 17, 25, 125, 220, 265
Physician's Hand (Melosh), xiii
Pierson, Jane, 75–76, 272
Pinkard, Anne Merrick (Nan), 206–7, 231, 243, 243, 248, 249, 286
Pinkard (Anne M.) Building, iv, 241–44, 243–45, 246, 247, 248, 249, 260–61, 285, 285–86
Pinkard family, 243, 249
Pinneo, Rose, 71
Piper, Mary Ann, 183
Pipkin, Kate, 254, 287
Pithotomy Club, 105–6
Play Activities Program
  See Child Life Program
Poe, Andre, 178
poisonous gas, 35, 36
Price, Harry, 78, 78, 100, 139, 147, 277
Price, Mary Sanders, 154–55, 283
  bachelor's program in nursing committee, 128–29, 133–35
  commencement address, 101–2
  director of JHH SON, 100, 100–103, 114, 138, 138–39, 147, 168, 206, 277–79
  and General Hospital No. 118, 75–76, 75–76, 78, 78, 272
Professional Nurse Traineeship Program, 149
public-health nursing, 95–96, 196–98, 258, 269–70, 276, 279
Pugh, Linda, 287
Purcell, Mary, 21, 48–49

Raboy, Judith, 218
Reed, Lowell J., 275
Reed Hall, 190
Reikenis, Gale, 189–90
Reiter, Frances, 110, 133, 150, 150

Rennoe, Robin, 183
Reverby, Susan, xi, xiii
Rice, Gertrude, 218
Richards, Esther, 28
Richardson, William C., 234, 243, 284
Roary, Mary, 198
Robb, Hunter, 11, 263
Robb, Isabel Hampton, 6–7, 12, 23, 26, 42, 112, 230
  biography of, 271, 274
  death of, 11, 265
  superintendent of nurses and principal of JHH Training School, 6, 9, 9–10, 103, 262–63
  and university-based nursing education, 15, 155
Robert Garrett Fund for the Surgical Treatment of Children, 125
Robert Wood Johnson Foundation, 280, 294n28
Roberts, Doris, 179–81
Roberts, Jean Stauffer, 186, 188, 192
Robertson, Dorothea, 204, 205, 277
Rockefeller Foundation, 44–45, 50, 264, 266
Rodgers, Karen, iv
Rogers, Mildred, 146
Rohde, Charles, 237
Roosevelt, Eleanor, 60, 60, 76, 273
Rose, Melinda, 205, 251, 254, 283
Ross, Georgina Caird, 14–15, 15, 264–65
Ross, Richard S., 203, 282
Rowe, Ella, 141, 167
Russell Sage Foundation, 91

Sabatier, Kathy, 234–35
Sabin, Florence, 11, 265
Sacci, Martha, 207, 208, 281, 283
Sam, Ann, 257
Sanborn, Allie, 98
Sanford, Katherine K., 55
Santmeyer, Karen Shank, 189, 280
Sarbanes, Paul, 226
Saunderlin, Shelia, 247
Scher, Betty Borenstein, viii, 20, 114, 167, 173, 195, 246
  and alumni association, 114, 279
  student, 56, 68, 69, 70, 86, 90, 104, 117, 119, 161
  on Wolf, 58, 70, 86, 91, 113, 159
Scherer, Frances Schlosser, 54, 64, 69–71
Schlotfeldt, Rozella M., 153
Schnider, Janet, iv
Scholl, Anna, 172, 196, 279
School of Allied Health Sciences, 153, 155
  See also Johns Hopkins University School of Health Services
Schuler, Ann, 112
Seidel, Henry, 175, 280
Selway, Janet, 257
Shaffer, Wilson, 128
Shallenberger, Clyde, 137–38, 139
Sheets, Buelah Mae, 160
Sheetz, Dena, 284
Sherman, Ruth Brewster, 266

Sherwood, Elizabeth, *21*

Sherwood Forest (Dick) Cottage, **69-70**, 69-70, *161*, 266, 274
   named for Christine Dick, *81*, 105, 273
   sold, 148-49, 277

Shiber, Stella, xvi, 87, 100, 135, 138, 176, 181, 191, 202, 215
   associate dean of JHU SON, 205-6, 208, 214, 217-19, 221-22, 224-26, 249, 252, 259, 282
   faculty member, 173, 179, *183*, 191, 212, *213*
   and Pinkard Building, 242-43, *245*, 246, *247, 261*
   and professional organizations, 230

Sigma Theta Tau, 283

Sinai Hospital, 203-5, 207, 209-11, *216*, 217-19

Skinner, Leila, 103, 138, 143

Sloand, Beth, *248*

Smellie, Elizabeth Lawrie, 80

Smith, Florence, *46-47*

Smith, Winford, xii, xiii, 3-4, 20, 44-45, 63, 266, 268, 273
   and Wolf, 51, *52*, 54, *91*

Snelling, Matilda, *105*

societal changes, 84, 124, 146-47

Society of Teresians, 264

Sommer, Marni, 199, 286

Spanish-American War, 13, 30-31, *31*

Special Committee for the Consideration of a University School of Nursing, 64-66

Spence, William Wallace, *72*

Spencer, Tillie, 23

Spring, Faye, 167

Stafford, Edward, 128-29, 293n4

State Pool Licensing examinations, 88

Stehly, Betty, *65*

Stevens, Mary Betty, 133, 175, 280

Stewart, Isabel, 114

Stewart, Mary Agnes Hull, *74*, 86

Stone, Harvey B., 266

Straub, Jean, 175, 280

Street, Wendell, *190*

Strickland, Ann, 273

Struve, Mildred, *21*, 56, 64, 75, *154-55*

St. Thomas's Hospital, xi

Student Teams Using Research (STUR), 225

Stulman Charitable Foundation, 287

Sturm, Patrice, *183, 185*

suffrage movement, 265

Sullivan, Pat, *178*

Sutton, Bertha, *48-49*

Sutton, Joan, 185, 193-95, *195*, 281-82, 284
   and Nutting Fund, 202, 208

swimming pool, 147-48, *148*, 277

Swort, Arlowayne, *221*, 236, 282-83

Taylor, Casper, 285

Taylor, Effie J., 17, 25, 44, *109*, 109, *113*, 114, 150

Taylor, Harriet, *142*

Teachers College at JHU, 18, 20, 54-55, 271
   See also McCoy College

Telinde, Richard, 64, 89-90

Thayer, Susan Read, 23, 42, *43*, 264, 290n35

Thayer, William, 125, 264

Thomas, Louise, 90

Thompson, Doris Higgins, 106

Thompson, Sharon, *232-33*

Thompson, Virginia, 78

Thorswaldsen, Bertel, *72*

Trimble, I. Ridgeway, 171, 175, *213*, 279, 283

Tumulty, Philip, 128, 173

Turner, Thomas B. (Tommy), 128, 131, 269

turtle derby, 27-28, 71, *105*, 105, 147, *183*, 269

uniforms, 81, *116-21, 167, 184-85*, 187, 227, 266, 277, 280
   caps, 23, 26, 64, 70, *99, 120, 152*, 190, 267, 271, 277, 282, 290n35
   community nursing, *130, 196-98*
   early, *23*, 23
   exhibit of, 280, *282*
   1950s, *108*, 276
   1970s, *178, 188*, 279
   after World War I, 26, 267
   during World War II, *57*, 64, 70-71, *104*, 271, 275
   See also Maltese cross pin

University of Maryland, 87, 260

U.S. Cadet Nurse Corps, 59, *59-60*, 63, 80, 84, 273

Van Blarcom, Carolyn, *40-41*

VandeGrift, Emma, 278

VandeGrift, W. B., *79*, 160

Van Horn, Lena, 138

Ventura, Emma, 278

Ventura, Michael, 193

Verhaalen, Roman, 205, 281

Villepique, Holly, *244*

Vincent, George E., 44

Wagley, Philip, 173

Waid, Helen, 271

Waites, Rosemary, *186*

Wald, Lillian, 30

Wald Clinics, *199, 241*, 284-85

Waldhauser, Josephine ("Teeny"), 263, 290n14

Walton-Moss, Benita, 178, 199, 239-40, 259

Ward, Ethel Rainey, 55, 60, 72, 80-81, 103, 148, 161, 180

Ware, Edith, 271

Wasserberg, Chelly, *21*

Waters, Yssabella, 30-31, 44

Waxter, Constance Cole Heard, 5, 58-59, 74, 130, 151, 195, 244, 281

Waybright, Geraldine, *105*

Weber, Helen J., 78

Weiland, Karen, *218*

Weinberg Foundation, 285

Weissman, Wendy, *170*

Welch, William H., xiii, 9, 15, 44-45, 265, 268

Welch Medical Library, 22, 57, 269, 280

Wessel, Genevieve Lipa, 175, *186, 188*, 280

Weymouth, Clarice, *21*

Whedbee, Thomas Gillam (Gil) Jr., *200-201*, 204-5, 210

Wheeler, Margaret, *46-47*

White, Kathy, *183*

White, Richard, 266

Whiteside, Faye, *48-49*, 63

Wickson, Judy Jacoby, *183, 185*

Wiedenbach, Ernestine, 270

Wiener, Joan, *178*

Wilcox, Mabel, 41

Wilcox, Patti, *244*

William, Vivian Weinhardt, 26

Williams, Joyce, *183*

Wilmer, William Holland, 268

Wilmer Ophthalmological Institute, *23*, 268

Winslow, Becky, 180

Within the Gates, 271

Witmer, Kathryn, *21*

Wolf, Anna Dryden, 41, 44, *59, 65, 82-83*, 112, *113*, 271, 276, 280, 282
   accomplishments at JHH SON, 98-99
   admissions changes, 60-61, 64-66, *66*, 84-87, 91
   background, 48, 50
   challenges, 84-86, 97-98
   conditions for employment, 51-53
   dean of nursing at Peking Union Medical College (China), 48-49, 50, 266, 287
   director of JHH SON and nursing service, 51, *51-52*, 55-58, 63, 89, 97, *102*, 131, 271, *277*
   director of nursing at New York-Cornell Medical Center, 51, 54
   and Lawler, 17, 21, 54
   and Nutting, *25*, 25, 50, 54, 65
   relationship with faculty and staff, 66, 68, 89
   response to Bridgeman Report, 92-94
   retirement, 97-98
   and students, 74, 159
   superintendent of nurses at Billings Hospital, University of Chicago, 50-51
   and World War II, 56-58, 72

Wolf, Karen, *183*

Wolman, M. Gordon ("Reds"), *248*, 283

Woman's Clinic, 176, *198*, 267

Wood, Barry, 128

Wood, Ellen M., 12

Woolf, Harry, 280

World War I, 16-17, 30, *31*, 32, 34-35, 38-41, 72, *266*

World War II, 48, 56-58, 271-72, *272*

Wright, Christine, *iv, 1*

Wright, Sue, ix

Wu, Lillian, *48-49*

Yale University School of Nursing, xiii, 44

Yen, F. C., 271

Young, Hugh, 161, 266

Young, John P., 54, 134

Zafman, Nelli Bogdanovskaia, *232-33*

Zdanis, Richard, 177

Zinder, Herb, *149*, 149, 152-53, 211, 223, 236, 278-79, *287*

Zinder, Matt, 287

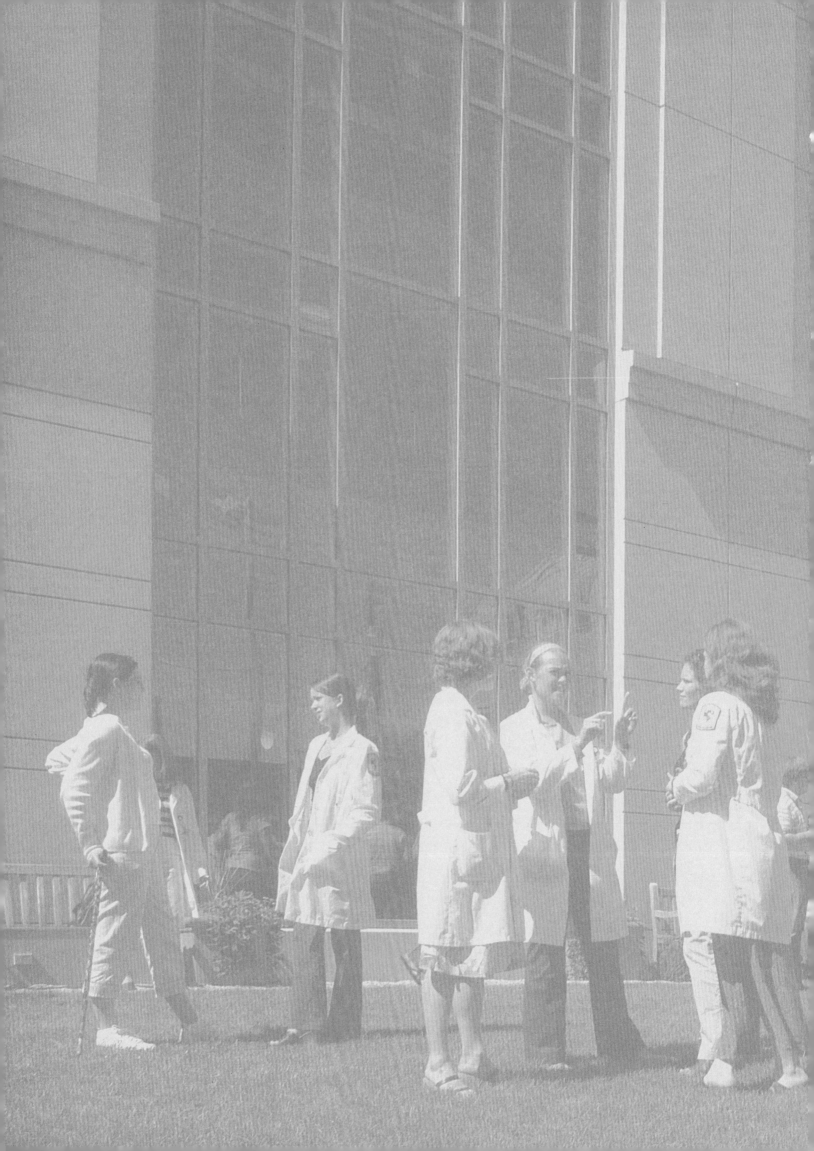